OPHTHALMOLOGY SECRETS

OPHTHALMOLOGY SECRETS

JAMES F. VANDER, MD
Associate Surgeon, Retina Service
Wills Eye Hospital
Jefferson Medical College of Thomas Jefferson University
Philadelphia, Pennsylvania

JANICE A. GAULT, MD
Instructor, Cataract and Primary Eye Care Service
Wills Eye Hospital
Philadelphia, Pennsylvania

HANLEY & BELFUS, INC./ Philadelphia

Publisher: HANLEY & BELFUS, INC.
                  Medical Publishers
                  210 South 13th Street
                  Philadelphia, PA 19107
                  (215) 546-7293; 800-962-1892
                  FAX (215) 790-9330
                  Web site: http://www.hanleyandbelfus.com

Note to the reader: Although the information in this book has been carefully reviewed for correctness of dosage and indications, neither the authors nor the editors nor the publisher can accept any legal responsibility for any errors or omissions that may be made. Neither the publisher nor the editors make any warranty, expressed or implied, with respect to the material contained herein. Before prescribing any drug, the reader must review the manufacturer's current product information (package inserts) for accepted indications, absolute dosage recommendations, and other information pertinent to the safe and effective use of the product described. This is especially important when drugs are given in combination or as an adjunct to other forms of therapy.

Library of Congress Cataloging-in-Publication Data

Ophthalmology secrets : questions you will be asked—on rounds, in the clinic,
   on oral exams / [edited by] James F. Vander.
      p.   cm. — (The Secrets Series)
   Includes bibliographical references and index.
   ISBN 1-56053-165-7 (alk. paper)
      1. Ophthalmology—Miscellanea.   2. Eye—Diseases—Miscellanea.
   I. Vander, James F., 1960–   . II. Series.
      [DNLM: 1. Eye Diseases examination questions.   WW 18.2 0612 1998]
   RE48.0666 1998
   617.7'0076—dc21
   DNLM/DLC
   for Library of Congress   97-52287
                                                                  CIP

OPHTHALMOLOGY SECRETS   ISBN 1-56053-165-7

Last digit is the print number: 9   8   7   6   5   4   3   2   1

CONTENTS

I. GENERAL

1. Clinical Anatomy of the Eye. 1
   Kenneth B. Gum, M.D.

2. Anatomy of the Orbit and Eyelid 7
   Edward H. Bedrossian, Jr., M.D.

3. Optics and Refraction 11
   Janice A. Gault, M.D.

4. Color Vision 24
   William E. Benson, M.D.

5. The Electroretinogram, the Electro-oculogram, and Dark Adaptation. 30
   Caroline R. Baumal, M.D., and Elizabeth L. Affel, M.S.

6. Ophthalmic Ultrasonography 38
   Caroline R. Baumal, M.D., FRCSC

7. Visual Fields 45
   David S. Friedman, M.D., M.P.H.

II. CORNEA AND EXTERNAL DISEASES

8. The Red Eye 48
   Janice A. Gault, M.D.

9. Corneal Infections. 61
   Terry Kim, M.D., Richard C. Rodman, M.D., and Elisabeth J. Cohen, M.D.

10. Ophthalmia Neonatorum 72
    Janine G. Tabas, M.D.

11. Topical Antibiotics and Steroids. 76
    Stephen Y. Lee, M.D.

12. Dry Eyes 84
    Peter R. Laibson, M.D.

13. Corneal Dystrophies 89
    Sadeer B. Hannush, M.D., and Lorena Riveroll, M.D.

14. Keratoconus 95
    Irving Raber, M.D.

15. Refractive Surgery 102
    *Richard C. Rodman, M.D., Terry Kim, M.D., René Dinh, M.D.,
    and Christopher J. Rapuano, M.D.*

III. GLAUCOMA

16. Glaucoma 111
    George L. Spaeth, M.D.

17. Angle Closure Glaucoma 117
    Anup K. Khatana, M.D., and George L. Spaeth, M.D.

18. Secondary Open-angle Glaucoma 130
    Janice A. Gault, M.D.

19. The Medical Treatment of Glaucoma 136
    Richard P. Wilson, M.D.

20. Trabeculectomy Surgery 142
    Marlene R. Moster, M.D.

21. Traumatic Glaucoma and Hyphema 151
    Annette K. Terebuh, M.D., and Martha Motuz Leen, M.D.

IV. CATARACTS

22. Cataracts 162
    Richard Tipperman, M.D.

23. Techniques of Cataract Surgery 165
    Sydney Tyson, M.D., M.P.H.

24. Complications of Cataract Surgery 171
    Robert S. Bailey, Jr., M.D.

V. OCULAR DEVIATIONS

25. Amblyopia 176
    Steven E. Brooks, M.D.

26. Esodeviations 183
    Scott E. Olitsky, M.D., and Leonard B. Nelson, M.D.

27. Miscellaneous Ocular Deviations 190
    Janice A. Gault, M.D.

28. Strabismus Surgery 198
    Bruce M. Schnall, M.D.

29. Nystagmus 202
    Robert D. Reinecke, M.D.

VI. NEURO-OPHTHALMOLOGY

30. The Pupil 206
    Barry Schanzer, M.D., and Peter Savino, M.D.

31. Diplopia 212
    Julian D. Perry, M.D.

32. Optic Neuritis 218
    Barry Schanzer, M.D., and Peter Savino, M.D.

33. Miscellaneous Optic Neuropathies and Neurologic Disturbances 221
    Janice A. Gault, M.D.

VII. OCULOPLASTICS

34. Tearing and the Lacrimal System 226
    Nancy G. Swartz, M.D., and Marc S. Cohen, M.D.

35. Orbital Imaging. 231
   Patrick De Potter, M.D.

36. Proptosis 234
   David G. Buerger, M.D.

37. Thyroid-related Ophthalmopathy 239
   Robert B. Penne, M.D.

38. Orbital Inflammations. 244
   Marlon Maus, M.D., F.A.C.S.

39. Ptosis. 248
   Carolyn S. Repke, M.D.

40. Eyelid Tumors. 252
   Janice A. Gault, M.D.

VIII. UVEITIS

41. Granulomatous Uveitis 257
   Caroline R. Baumal, M.D., F.R.C.S.C.

42. Masquerade Syndromes 263
   Vinay N. Desai, M.D., and Jay S. Duker, M.D.

43. Ocular Manifestations of AIDS 267
   Tamara R. Vrabec, M.D., and Vincent F. Baldassano, M.D.

IX. RETINA

44. Toxic Retinopathies 274
   Philip G. Hykin, FRCS, FRCOphth

45. Coats' Disease. 279
   William Tasman, M.D.

46. Fundus Trauma 283
   Jeffrey P. Blice, M.D.

47. Age-related Macular Degeneration. 288
   Joseph I. Maguire, M.D., F.A.C.S.

48. Retinopathy of Prematurity. 294
   J. Arch McNamara, M.D.

49. Diabetic Retinopathy 300
   James F. Vander, M.D.

50. Retinal Arterial Obstruction 306
   Jay S. Duker, M.D.

51. Retinal Venous Occlusive Disease 312
   Vernon K. W. Wong, M.D.

52. Retinal Detachment 315
   Michael J. Borne, M.D.

53. Retinoblastoma. 322
   Carol L. Shields, M.D.

54. Pigmented Lesions of the Ocular Fundus.................................327
     Jerry A. Shields, M.D.

X. NEOPLASMS

55. Ocular Neoplasms..332
     Ralph C. Eagle, Jr. M.D.

56. Orbital Tumors 340
     Jurij R. Bilyk, M.D.

INDEX 349

CONTRIBUTORS

Elizabeth L. Affel, M.S., RDMS
Department of Visual Physiology and Ultrasound, Wills Eye Hospital, Philadelphia, Pennsylvania

Robert S. Bailey, Jr., M.D.
Instructor, Department of Ophthalmology, Jefferson Medical College of Thomas Jefferson University; Associate Surgeon, Wills Eye Hospital, Philadelphia, Pennsylvania

Vincent F. Baldassano, M.D.
Clinical Assistant Professor, Department of Ophthalmology, Temple University, Philadelphia, Pennsylvania

Caroline R. Baumal, M.D., FRCSC
Assistant Professor, Department of Ophthalmology, Tufts University School of Medicine and Vitreoretinal Service, New England Eye Center, Boston, Massachusetts

Edward H. Bedrossian, Jr., M.D., FACS
Associate Clinical Professor, Department of Ophthalmology, Jefferson Medical College of Thomas Jefferson University; Chief, Oculoplastic and Reconstructive Surgery Division, Temple University Hospital; Associate Surgeon, Oculoplastic Surgery Department; Founding Director, Fascia Lata Bank, Wills Eye Hospital, Philadelphia, Pennsylvania

William E. Benson, M.D.
Professor, Department of Ophthalmology, Jefferson Medical College of Thomas Jefferson University; Attending Surgeon and Director of the Retina Service, Wills Eye Hospital, Philadelphia, Pennsylvania

Jurij R. Bilyk, M.D.
Instructor, Oculoplastics and Orbital Surgery, Wills Eye Hospital, Philadelphia, Pennsylvania

Jeffrey P. Blice, M.D.
Department of Ophthalmology, National Naval Medical Center, Bethesda, Maryland

Michael J. Borne, M.D.
Assistant Clinical Professor, Department of Ophthalmology, University of Mississippi School of Medicine, Jackson, Mississippi

Steven E. Brooks, M.D.
Assistant Professor, Departments of Ophthalmology and Pediatrics, Director of Pediatric Ophthalmology and Adult Strabismus, Medical College of Georgia, Augusta, Georgia

David G. Buerger, M.D.
Clinical Instructor, Department of Ophthalmology, University of Pittsburgh Medical Center, Eye & Ear Institute of Pittsburgh, Pittsburgh, Pennsylvania

Elisabeth J. Cohen, M.D.
Professor, Department of Ophthalmology, Jefferson Medical College of Thomas Jefferson University; Co-Director, Cornea Service, Wills Eye Hospital, Philadelphia, Pennsylvania

Marc S. Cohen, M.D., FACS
Associate Surgeon, Department of Oculoplastic Surgery, Wills Eye Hospital, Philadelphia, Pennsylvania

Patrick De Potter, M.D.
Professor, Department of Ophthalmology, Cliniques Universitaires St-Luc, Université Catholique
de Louvain, Brussels, Belgium

Vinay N. Desai, M.D.
New England Eye Center, Tufts University School of Medicine, Boston, Massachusetts

René Dinh, M.D., FRCS(C)
Cornea Fellow, Jefferson Medical College of Thomas Jefferson University; Cornea Service, Wills
Eye Hospital, Philadelphia, Pennsylvania

Jay S. Duker, M.D.
Associate Professor, Department of Ophthalmology, Tufts University School of Medicine;
Director, Retina Service, New England Eye Center, Boston, Massachusetts

Ralph C. Eagle, Jr., M.D.
Professor, Departments of Ophthalmology and Pathology, Jefferson Medical College of Thomas
Jefferson University; Director, Department of Pathology, Wills Eye Hospital, Philadelphia,
Pennsylvania

David S. Friedman, M.D., M.P.H.
Assistant Professor, Department of Ophthalmology, Johns Hopkins University School of
Medicine and Wilmer Eye Institute, Baltimore, Maryland

Janice A. Gault, M.D.
Instructor, Cataract and Primary Eye Care Service, Wills Eye Hospital, Philadelphia, Pennsylvania

Kenneth B. Gum, M.D.
Section Chief, Department of Ophthalmology, Munson Medical Center, Transverse City,
Michigan

Sadeer B. Hannush, M.D.
Assistant Professor, Department of Ophthalmology, Jefferson Medical College of Thomas
Jefferson University; Associate Surgeon, Cornea Service, Wills Eye Hospital, Philadelphia,
Pennsylvania

Philip G. Hykin, FRCS, FRCOphth
Consultant Ophthalmic Surgeon, Medical Retina Service, Moorfields Eye Hospital, London,
United Kingdom

Anup K. Khatana, M.D.
Assistant Clinical Professor, Department of Ophthalmology, University of Missouri–Kansas City
School of Medicine; Director, Glaucoma Service, Eye Foundation of Kansas City, Kansas City,
Missouri

Terry Kim, M.D.
Assistant Professor, Department of Ophthalmology, Cornea and External Disease Division, Duke
University School of Medicine, Durham, North Carolina

Peter R. Laibson, M.D.
Professor, Department of Ophthalmology, Jefferson Medical College of Thomas Jefferson
University; Director, Cornea Service, Wills Eye Hospital, Philadelphia, Pennsylvania

Stephen Y. Lee, M.D.
Instructor, Cornea Service, Wills Eye Hospital, Jefferson Medical College of Thomas Jefferson
University, Philadelphia, Pennsylvania

Martha Motuz Leen, M.D.
Clinical Assistant Professor, Department of Ophthalmology, University of Washington School of Medicine, Seattle, Washington; Harrison Memorial Hospital, Bremerton, Washington

Joseph I. Maguire, M.D., FACS
Associate Professor, Department of Ophthalmology, Jefferson Medical College of Thomas Jefferson University; Assistant Surgeon, Wills Eye Hospital, Philadelphia, Pennsylvania

Marlon Maus, M.D., FACS
Assistant Professor, Department of Ophthalmology, Jefferson Medical College of Thomas Jefferson University; Associate Surgeon, Department of Oculoplastic Surgery, Wills Eye Hospital, Philadelphia, Pennsylvania

J. Arch McNamara, M.D.
Associate Surgeon, Retina Service, Wills Eye Hospital; Assistant Professor, Department of Ophthalmology, Jefferson Medical College of Thomas Jefferson University, Philadelphia, Pennsylvania

Marlene R. Moster, M.D.
Associate Professor, Department of Ophthalmology, Jefferson Medical College of Thomas Jefferson University; Attending Surgeon, Glaucoma Service, Wills Eye Hospital, Philadelphia, Pennsylvania

Leonard B. Nelson, M.D.
Associate Professor, Departments of Ophthalmology and Pediatrics, Jefferson Medical College of Thomas Jefferson University; Co-Director, Pediatric Ophthalmology, Wills Eye Hospital, Philadelphia, Pennsylvania

Scott E. Olitsky, M.D.
Assistant Professor, Department of Ophthalmology, State University of New York at Buffalo and Children's Hospital of Buffalo, Buffalo, New York

Robert B. Penne, M.D.
Assistant Professor, Department of Ophthalmology, Jefferson Medical College of Thomas Jefferson University; Active Staff, Lankenau Hospital, Wills Eye Hospital, West Jersey Health System, Pennsylvania Hospital, Philadelphia, Pennsylvania

Julian D. Perry, M.D.
Assistant in Ophthalmology, Wilmer Eye Institute, Johns Hopkins University Hospitals, Baltimore, Maryland

Irving M. Raber, M.D.
Clinical Associate Professor of Ophthalmology, Department of Surgery, Allegheny University of the Health Sciences; Clinical Assistant Professor of Surgery, Jefferson Medical College of Thomas Jefferson University; Associate Surgeon, Cornea Service, Wills Eye Hospital, Philadelphia, Pennsylvania

Christopher J. Rapuano, M.D.
Associate Professor, Department of Ophthalmology, Jefferson Medical College of Thomas Jefferson University; Cornea Service Co-Director, Refractive Surgery Unit, Wills Eye Hospital, Philadelphia, Pennsylvania

Robert D. Reinecke, M.D.
Professor, Department of Ophthalmology, Jefferson Medical College of Thomas Jefferson University; Attending Surgeon, Wills Eye Hospital, Philadelphia, Pennsylvania

Carolyn S. Repke, M.D.
Instructor, Cataract and Primary Eye Care Service, Wills Eye Hospital, Philadelphia, Pennsylvania

Lorena Riveroll, M.D.
Assistant Professor, Department of Ophthalmology, Cornea Service, Hospital Associatión Para Evitar la Ceguera en Mexico, Mexico City, Mexico

Richard C. Rodman, M.D.
Assistant Clinical Professor, Department of Surgery (Ophthalmology), Brown University School of Medicine and Rhode Island Hospital, Providence, Rhode Island

Peter Savino, M.D.
Chief, Neuro-Ophthalmology Service, Wills Eye Hospital, Philadelphia, Pennsylvania

Barry Schanzer, M.D.
Assistant Attending Physician, John F. Kennedy Medical Center, Edison, New Jersey

Bruce M. Schnall, M.D.
Assistant Surgeon, Department of Ophthalmology, Wills Eye Hospital, Philadelphia, Pennsylvania

Carol L. Shields, M.D.
Associate Professor, Department of Ophthalmology, Jefferson Medical College of Thomas Jefferson University; Associate Surgeon, Ocular Oncology Service, Wills Eye Hospital; Consultant, Children's Hospital of Philadelphia, Philadelphia, Pennsylvania

Jerry A. Shields, M.D.
Professor of Ophthalmology, Jefferson Medical College of Thomas Jefferson University; Director, Ocular Oncology Service, Wills Eye Hospital; Consultant, Children's Hospital of Philadelphia, Philadelphia, Pennsylvania

George L. Spaeth, M.D.
Professor, Department of Ophthalmology, Jefferson Medical College of Thomas Jefferson University; Director and Attending Surgeon, William and Anna Goldberg Glaucoma Service, Wills Eye Hospital, Philadelphia, Pennsylvania

Nancy G. Swartz, M.D.
Clinical Associate, University of Pennsylvania School of Medicine; Instructor, Neuro-Ophthalmology Service, Wills Eye Hospital; Instructor, Jefferson Medical College of Thomas Jefferson University, Philadelphia, Pennsylvania

Janine G. Tabas, M.D.
Instructor, Cataract and Primary Eye Care Service, Wills Eye Hospital, Philadelphia, Pennsylvania

William Tasman, M.D.
Professor and Chairman, Department of Ophthalmology, Jefferson Medical College of Thomas Jefferson University; Ophthalmologist-in-Chief, Wills Eye Hospital, Philadelphia, Pennsylvania

Annette K. Terebuh, M.D.
Instructor, William and Anna Goldberg Glaucoma Service and Research Laboratories, Wills Eye Hospital, Jefferson Medical College of Thomas Jefferson University, Philadelphia, Pennsylvania

Richard Tipperman, M.D.
Assistant Professor, Cataract and Primary Eye Care Service, Wills Eye Hospital, Philadelphia, Pennsylvania

Sydney Tyson, M.D., M.P.H.
Associate Surgeon, Cataract and Primary Eye Care Service, Wills Eye Hospital, Philadelphia, Pennsylvania

James F. Vander, M.D.
Associate Surgeon, Retina Service, Wills Eye Hospital, Jefferson Medical College of Thomas Jefferson University, Philadelphia, Pennsylvania

Tamara Vrabec, M.D.
Retina Service, Wills Eye Hospital; Clinical Assistant Professor, Center for Preservation of Vision, Allegheny University of the Health Sciences; Adjunct Assistant Professor, Department of Ophthalmology, Temple University School of Medicine; Instructor, Department of Ophthalmology, Jefferson Medical College of Thomas Jefferson University, Philadelphia, Pennsylvania

Richard P. Wilson, M.D.
Associate Professor, Department of Ophthalmology, Jefferson Medical College of Thomas Jefferson University; Attending Surgeon, Glaucoma Service, Wills Eye Hospital, Philadelphia, Pennsylvania

Vernon K. W. Wong, M.D.
Assistant Clinical Professor, Division of Ophthalmology, Department of Surgery, University of Hawaii School of Medicine, Honolulu, Hawaii

PREFACE

Much of the information in this book can be found in a number of other ophthalmology text-books. The table of contents is similar to that of many other books already in print. So why bother to write a new ophthalmology text? The value of this book is in the unique manner in which the material is presented, continuing the tradition of the Secrets Series® established in numerous other specialties. The question-and-answer format reflects the process by which a large portion of clinical medical education actually takes place. Our purpose is not to displace the comprehensive textbooks of ophthalmology from the shelves of clinicians and students. Instead we hope that we have filled a useful spot beside them. We greatly appreciate the efforts of the talented contributors who have shared their wisdom and experience to help fill this void. In addition, thanks must go to Mary Rafferty and Kathy Martin for their substantial help in the production of this book. We have enjoyed preparing it, and we hope that clinicians and students will enjoy this book and find it valuable.

James F. Vander, MD
Janice A. Gault, MD

COLOR PLATES

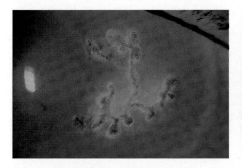

FIGURE 1. Herpes simplex. (See p. 49.)

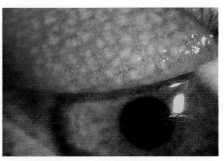

FIGURE 2. Giant papillary conjunctivitis. (See p. 51.)

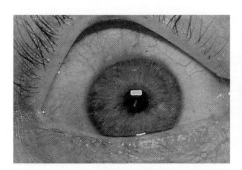

FIGURE 3. Superior limbic kerato-conjunctivitis. (See p.56.)

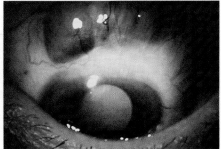

FIGURE 4. Scleromalacia perforans. (See p. 58.)

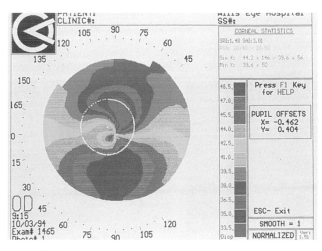

FIGURE 5. Map showing symmetric inferior steepening. (See p. 97.)

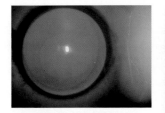

FIGURE 6. Fleischer ring.
(See p. 98.)

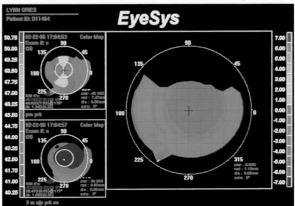

FIGURE 7. Corneal topography.
(See p. 103.)

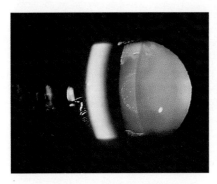

FIGURE 8. Pseudoexfoliation with
deposits in a bull's eye pattern.
(See p. 130.)

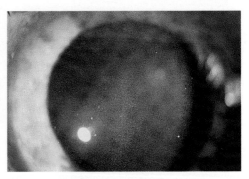

FIGURE 9. Krukenberg spindle.
(See p. 131.)

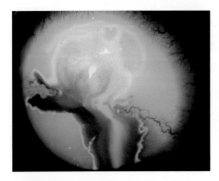

FIGURE 10. Buttonhole at dome of
bleb. (See p. 146.)

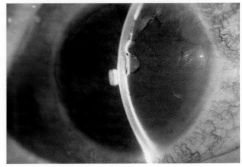

FIGURE 11. Flat anterior chamber.
(See p. 149.)

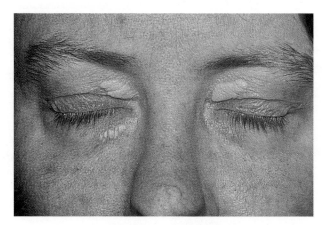

FIGURE 12. Xanthelasma.
(See p. 253.)

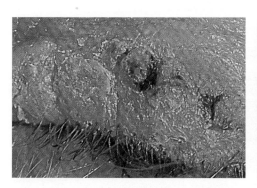

FIGURE 13. Squamous cell carcinoma.
(See p. 255.)

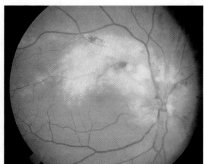

FIGURE 14. CMV retinitis.
(See p. 268.)

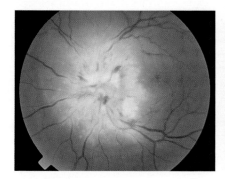

FIGURE 15. Papilledema in AIDS.
(See p. 271.)

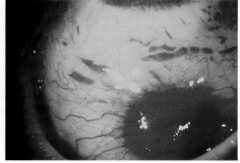

FIGURE 16. Kaposi's sarcoma.
(See p. 272.)

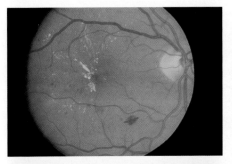

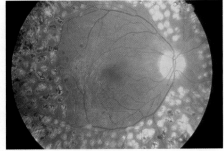

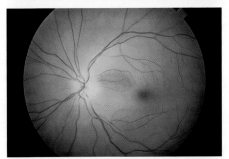

FIGURE 17 *(Above left).* Background diabetic retinopathy. (See p. 300.)

FIGURE 18 *(Above right).* Panretinal photocoagulation. (See p. 303.)

FIGURE 19 *(Left).* Central retinal artery obstruction. (See p. 308.)

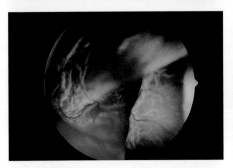

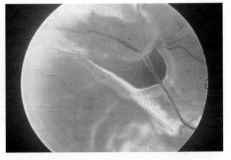

FIGURE 20. Rhegmatogenous bullous detachment. (See p. 315.)

FIGURE 21. Horseshoe retinal tear. (See p. 317.)

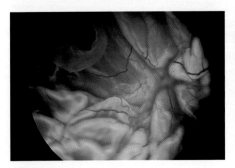

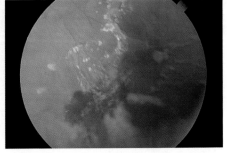

FIGURE 22. Severe proliferative vitreo-retinopathy. (See p. 320.)

FIGURE 23. Proliferative traction retinal detachment. (See p. 320.)

I. General

1. CLINICAL ANATOMY OF THE EYE

Kenneth B. Gum, M.D.

1. Name the seven bones that make up the bony orbit and describe which location is most prone to damage in an orbital blowout fracture.

The seven orbital bones are the frontal, zygoma, maxillary, sphenoid, ethmoid, palatine, and lacrimal. A true blowout fracture most commonly affects the orbital floor posteriorly and medially to the infraorbital nerve. The ethmoid bone of the medial wall often is broken.

2. Which nerves and vessels pass through the superior orbital fissure? Which motor nerve to the eye lies outside the anulus of Zinn, leaving it unaffected by retrobulbar injection of anesthetic?

The superior orbital fissure transmits the third, fourth, and sixth cranial nerves as well as the first division of the fifth cranial nerve, which has already divided into frontal and lacrimal branches. The superior ophthalmic vein and sympathetic nerves also pass through this fissure. The fourth cranial nerve supplying the superior oblique muscle lies outside the anulus. This position accounts for residual intortion of the eye sometimes seen during retrobulbar anesthesia.

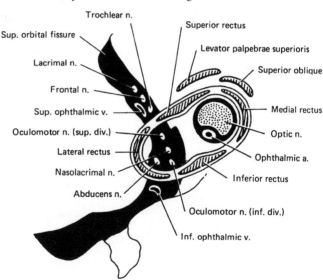

Relationships of the superior orbital fissure, inferior orbital fissure, anulus of Zinn, and optic foramen and their contents. (From McCord, Tannenbaum, and Nunery: Oculoplastic Surgery, 3rd ed. Philadelphia, Lippincott-Raven, 1995, with permission.)

3. A 3-year-old is referred for evaluation of consecutive exotropia after initial bimedial rectus recessions for esotropia performed elsewhere. Review of the operative notes discloses that each muscle was recessed 4.5 mm for a 30-prism diopter deviation. Unfortunately, the child had mild developmental delay and presents with a 25-prism diopter exotropia. You decide to advance the recessed medial rectus of each eye back to its original insertion site. Where is this site in relation to the limbus? Identify the location of each of the rectus muscle insertion sites relative to the limbus.

Reattach each medial rectus muscle 5.5 mm from the limbus. Insertion of the inferior rectus is 6.5 mm from the limbus; the lateral rectus is 6.9 mm from the limbus; and the superior rectus, 7.7 mm. The differing distances of rectus muscle insertions from the limbus make up the spiral of Tillaux. An important caveat in developmentally delayed children is to postpone muscle surgery until much later, treating any amblyopia in the interim. Early surgery frequently leads to overcorrection.

4. You have just begun a ptosis procedure. A lid crease incision was made, and the orbital septum has been isolated and opened horizontally. What important landmark should be readily apparent? Describe its relation to other important structures.

The orbital fat lies directly behind the orbital septum and directly on the muscular portion of the levator (see figure). A separate medial fat pad often herniates through the septum in later years.

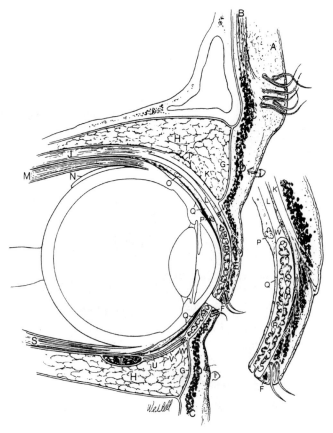

Schematic cross-section of eyelids and anterior orbit. *A*, skin; *B*, frontalis muscle; *C,* orbicularis muscle (orbital portion); *D*, orbicularis muscle (preseptal portion); *E*, orbicularis muscle (pretarsal portion); *F*, orbicularis muscle (muscle of Riolan); *G*, orbital septum; *H*, orbital fat; *I*, superior transverse (check) ligament; *J*, levator muscle; *K*, levator aponeurosis; *L*, Müller's muscle; *M*, superior rectus muscle; *N*, superior oblique tendon; *O*, gland of Krause; *P*, gland of Wolfring; *Q*, conjunctiva; *R*, tarsus; *S*, inferior rectus muscle; *T*, inferior oblique muscle; *U*, inferior tarsal muscle; *V*, capsulopalpebral fascia; *W*, peripheral arterial arcade. (From Beard C: Ptosis, 3rd ed. St. Louis, Mosby, 1981, with permission.)

5. To what glands do the lymphatics of the orbit drain?

There are no lymphatic vessels or nodes within the orbit. Lymphatics from the conjunctivae and lids drain medially to the submandibular glands and laterally to the superficial preauricular nodes.

6. What is the orbital septum?

The septum is a thin sheet of connective tissue that defines the anterior limit of the orbit. In the upper lid it extends from the periosteum of the superior orbital rim to insert at the levator aponeurosis, slightly above the superior tarsal border (see figure, previous page). The lower lid septum extends from the periosteum of the inferior orbital rim to insert directly on the inferior tarsal border.

7. A 70-year-old patient presents with herpes zoster lesions in the trigeminal nerve distribution. Classic lesions on the side and tip of the nose increase your concern about ocular involvement. Why?

This sign, called Hutchinson's sign, results from involvement of the infratrochlear nerve. The infratrochlear nerve is the terminal branch of the nasociliary nerve, which gives off the long ciliary nerves (usually two) that supply the globe.

8. Where is the sclera the thinnest? Where are globe ruptures after blunt trauma most likely to occur?

The sclera is thinnest just behind the insertion of the rectus muscles (0.3 mm). Scleral rupture usually occurs opposite the site of impact and in an arc parallel to the limbus at the insertion of the rectus muscles or at the equator. The most common site of rupture is near the superonasal limbus.

9. Describe the surgical limbus and Schwalbe's line.

The surgical limbus can be differentiated into an anterior bluish zone that extends from the termination of Bowman's layer to Schwalbe's line, which is the termination of Descemet's membrane. The posterior white zone overlies the trabecular meshwork and extends from Schwalbe's line to the scleral spur.

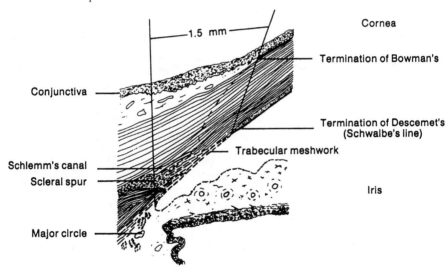

Anterior chamber angle and limbus, depicting concept of limbus. Solid lines represent the limbus as seen by pathologists; the dotted line represents the limbus as seen by anatomists. (From American Academy of Ophthalmology: Basic and Clinical Science Course, Section 2. San Francisco, American Academy of Ophthalmology, 1993–1994, with permission.)

10. You are preparing to do an argon laser trabeculoplasty. Describe the gonioscopic appearance of the anterior chamber angle.

The ciliary body is a visible concavity anterior to the iris root. The scleral spur appears as a white line anterior to the ciliary body. Above this are the trabecular meshwork and canal of Schlemm. Treatment is applied to the anterior trabecular meshwork.

11. After a filtering procedure, your patient develops choroidal effusions. Explain the distribution of these fluid accumulations based on uveal attachments to the sclera.

The uveal tract is attached to the sclera at the scleral spur, the optic nerve, and the exit sites of the vortex veins. The fluid dissects the choroid from the underlying sclera but retains these connections.

12. Describe the structure of Bruch's membrane. Name two conditions in which defects develop in this structure spontaneously.

Bruch's membrane consists of five layers: internally, the basement membrane of the pigment epithelium, the inner collagenous zone, a central band of elastic fibers, and the outer collagenous zone; externally, the basement membrane of the choriocapillaris. Pseudoxanthoma elasticum and myopia may cause spontaneous defects in this membrane, making the patient prone to development of choroidal neovascularization.

13. Less laser power is required for photocoagulation in darkly pigmented fundi. What determines this pigmentation?

The pigmentation of the fundus seen ophthalmoscopically is largely determined by the number of melanosomes in the choroid. The darker macular area results from taller pigment epithelial cells that contain more and larger melanosomes than the periphery.

14. What is the blood-retinal barrier?

The inner blood-retinal barrier consists of the retinal vascular endothelium, which is nonfenestrated and contains tight junctions. The outer blood-retinal barrier is the retinal pigment epithelium. Bruch's membrane is permeable to small molecules.

15. Which retinal layer is referred to as the fiber layer of Henle in the macular region?

The outer plexiform layer, which is made up of connections between photoreceptor synaptic bodies and horizontal and bipolar cells, becomes thicker and more oblique in orientation as it deviates away from the fovea. At the fovea this layer becomes nearly parallel to the retinal surface and accounts for the radial or star-shaped patterns of exudate in the extracellular spaces under pathologic conditions causing vascular compromise.

16. What are three clinically recognized remnants of the fetal hyaloid vasculature?

Mittendorf dot, Bergmeister's papilla, and vascular loops (which are 95% arterial).

17. A patient presents with a central retinal artery occlusion and 20/20 visual acuity. How do you explain this finding?

Fifteen percent of people have a cilioretinal artery that supplies the macular region. Thirty percent of eyes have a cilioretinal artery supplying some portion of the retina. These are perfused by the choroidal vessels, which are fed by the ophthalmic artery.

18. Where do branch retinal vein occlusions occur? Which quadrant of the retina is most commonly affected?

Branch retinal vein occlusions occur at arteriovenous crossings, most commonly where the vein lies posterior to the artery. The superotemporal quadrant is most often affected because of a higher number of arteriovenous crossings on average.

19. Discuss the organization of crossed and uncrossed fibers in the optic chiasm.

Inferonasal extramacular fibers cross in the anterior chiasm and bulge into the contralateral optic nerve (Willebrand's knee). Superonasal extramacular fibers cross directly to the opposite optic tract. Macular fibers are located in the center of the optic nerve. Temporal macular fibers pass uncrossed through the chiasm, whereas nasal macular fibers cross posteriorly. However, in albinism, many temporal fibers also cross.

20. A patient presents with a chief complaint of tearing and ocular irritation. As she dumps the plethora of eye drops from her purse, she explains that she has seen seven different doctors and none has been able to help her. The exam shows mild inferior punctate keratopathy, but a normal tear lake and normal Schirmer's testing. Of interest, she had blepharoplasty surgery 6 months previously. What is the diagnosis?

You are already patting yourself on the back as you ask if the irritation is worse in the morning or evening. She replies emphatically that it is much more severe upon awakening. You ask her to close her eyes gently and see two millimeters of lagophthalmos in each eye. This is a frequently overlooked cause of tearing in otherwise normal eyes.

21. During orbital surgery, a patient's lacrimal gland is removed. Afterward, there is no evidence of tear deficiency. Why not?

Basal tear production is provided by the accessory lacrimal glands of Krause and Wolfring. The glands of Krause are located in the superior fornix, and the glands of Wolfring are located above the superior tarsal border. They are cytologically identical to the main lacrimal gland.

22. Describe anatomically the macula and fovea.

The macula is defined as the area of the posterior retina that contains xanthophyllic pigment and two or more layers of ganglion cells. It is centered approximately 4 mm temporal and 0.8 mm inferior to the center of the optic disc. The fovea is a central depression of the inner retinal surface and is approximately 1.5 mm in diameter.

23. Fluorescein angiography typically shows perfusion of the choroid and any cilioretinal arteries prior to visualization of the dye in the retinal circulation. Why?

Fluorescein enters the choroid via the short posterior ciliary arteries, which are branches of the ophthalmic artery. The central retinal artery, also a branch of the ophthalmic artery, provides a more circuitous route for the dye to travel, resulting in dye appearance in the retinal circulation 1–2 seconds later.

24. Explain why visual acuity in infants does not reach adult levels until approximately 6 months of age based on retinal differentiation.

The differentiation of the macula is not complete until 4–6 months after birth. Ganglion cell nuclei initially are found directly over the foveola and gradually are displaced peripherally, leaving this area devoid of accessory neural elements and blood vessels as neural organization develops to adult levels by age 6 months. This delay in macular development is one factor in the inability of newborns to fixate, and improvement in visual activity parallels macular development.

25. A neonate presents with an opacification in her left cornea. What is the differential diagnosis?

Neonatal cloudy cornea usually falls into one of the following categories (which can easily be recalled by using the mnemonic **STUMPED**): **s**clerocornea, **t**rauma, **u**lcers, **m**etabolic disorder, **P**eter's anomaly, **e**ndothelial dystrophy, and **d**ermoid.

26. Describe the innervation of the lens.

The lens is anatomically unique because it lacks innervation and vascularization. It depends entirely on the aqueous and vitreous for nourishment.

27. Describe the innervation of the cornea.

The long posterior ciliary nerves branch from the ophthalmic division of the trigeminal nerve and penetrate the cornea. Peripherally, 70–80 branches enter the cornea in conjunctival, episcleral, and scleral planes. They lose their myelin sheath 1–2 mm from the limbus. The network just posterior to Bowman's layer sends branches anteriorly into the epithelium.

28. What are the three layers of the tear film? Where do they originate?

1. The **mucoid layer** coats the superficial corneal epithelial cells and creates a hydrophilic layer that allows for spontaneous, even distribution of the aqueous layer of the tear film. Mucin is secreted principally by the conjunctival goblet cells but also from the lacrimal gland.

2. The **aqueous layer** is secreted by the glands of Kraus and Wolfring (basal secretion) and the lacrimal gland (reflex secretion). The aqueous layer contains electrolytes, immunoglobulins, and other solutes, including glucose, buffers, and amino acids.

3. The **lipid layer** is secreted primarily by the Meibomian glands and maintains a hydrophobic barrier that prevents tear overflow, retards evaporation, and provides lubrication for the lid/ocular interface.

29. What are the differences in the structure of the central retinal artery and retinal arterioles?

The central retinal artery contains a fenestrated internal elastic lamina and an outer layer of smooth muscle cells surrounded by a basement membrane. The retinal arterioles have no internal elastic lamina and lose the smooth muscle cells near their entrance into the retina. Hence, the retinal vasculature has no autoregulation.

30. Where is the macula represented in the visual cortex?

Macular function is represented in the most posterior portion at the tip of the occipital lobe. However, there may be a wide distribution of some macular fibers along the calcarine fissure.

BIBLIOGRAPHY

1. American Academy of Ophthalmology: Basic and Clinical Science Course, Section 2. San Francisco, American Academy of Ophthalmology, 1993-1994.
2. Gass JDM: Stereoscopic Atlas of Macular Diseases, 4th ed. St. Louis, Mosby, 1997.
3. Fine BS, Yanoff M: Ocular Histology, 2nd ed. Hagerstown, MD, Harper & Row, 1979.
4. Jaffe NS: Cataract Surgery and its Complications, 5th ed. St. Louis, Mosby, 1990.
5. Justice J, Lehman RP: Cilioretinal arteries: A study based on review of stereofundus photographs and fluorescein angiographic findings. Arch Ophthalmol 94:1355–1358, 1976.
6. Miller NR: Walsh and Hoyt's Clinical Neuro-Ophthalmology, vol 1, 4th ed. Baltimore, Williams & Wilkins, 1982.
7. Stewart WB: Surgery of the Eyelid, Orbit, and Lacrimal System. Ophthalmology Monographs, vol 1. San Francisco, American Academy of Ophthalmology, 1993.
8. Weinberg DV, Egan KM, Seddon JM: The asymmetric distribution of arteriovenous crossing in the normal retina. Ophthalmology 100:31–36, 1993.

2. ANATOMY OF THE ORBIT AND EYELID

Edward H. Bedrossian, Jr., M.D.

ORBIT

1. Name the bones of the orbit.
1. Medial wall: sphenoid, ethmoid, lacrimal, maxillary
2. Lateral wall: zygomatic, greater wing of sphenoid
3. Roof: frontal, lesser wing of sphenoid
4. Floor: maxillary, zygomatic, palatine

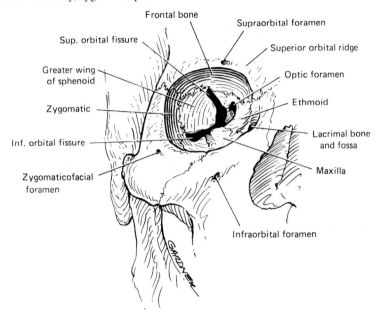

Frontal view of the orbit. (From McCord, Tannenbaum, and Nunery: Oculoplastic Surgery, 3rd ed. Philadelphia, Lippincott-Raven, 1995, with permission.)

2. What are the weak spots of the orbital rim?
1. Frontozygomatic suture
2. Zygomaticomaxillary suture
3. Frontomaxillary suture

3. Describe the most common location of blowout fractures.
The posteromedial aspect of the orbital floor.

4. What is the weakest bone within the orbit?
The lamina papyracea portion of the ethmoid bone.

5. Name the divisions of cranial nerve V that pass through the cavernous sinus.
1. Ophthalmic division (V1)
2. Maxillary division (V2)

7

6. What is the anulus of Zinn?
The circle defined by the superior rectus muscle, inferior rectus muscle, lateral rectus muscle, and medial rectus muscle (see figure on p. 1).

7. What nerves pass through the superior orbital fissure but outside the anulus of Zinn?
Frontal, lacrimal, and trochlear nerves.

EYELID

8. List the factors responsible for involutional entropion.
1. Lower lid laxity
2. Override of the preseptal orbicularis oculi muscle onto the pretarsal orbicularis oculi muscle
3. Dehiscence/disinsertion of the lower lid retractors
4. Orbital fat atrophy

9. Describe the sensory nerve supply to the upper and lower eyelids.
1. The ophthalmic nerve (V1) provides sensation to the upper lid.
2. The maxillary nerve (V2) provides sensation to the lower lid.

10. What are the surgical landmarks in locating the superficial temporal artery during temporal artery biopsies?
The superficial temporal artery lies deep to the skin and subcutaneous tissue but superficial to the temporalis fascia.

11. What structures would you pass through during a transverse blepharotomy 3 mm above the upper eyelid margin?
1. Skin
2. Pretarsal orbicularis muscle
3. Tarsus
4. Palpebral conjunctiva

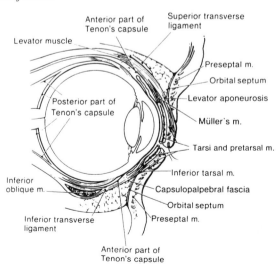

Sagittal view of the orbit and eyelid structures. (From McCord, Tannenbaum, and Nunery: Oculoplastic Surgery, 3rd ed. Philadelphia, Lippincott-Raven, 1995, with permission.)

12. What is meant by the term *lower lid retractors*?

The lower lid retractors consist of the capsulopalpebral fascia and the inferior tarsus muscle. The capsulopalpebral fascia of the lower lid is analogous to the levator complex in the upper lid The inferior tarsus muscle of the lower lid is analogous to Müller's muscle in the upper lid.

13. What structures would be cut in a full-thickness lower-lid laceration 2 mm below the lower tarsus (see figure, previous page)?
1. Skin
2. Preseptal orbicularis oculi muscle
3. Conjoint tendon (fused orbital septum and lower lid retractors)
4. Palpebral conjunctiva

14. What structures would be cut in a full-thickness lower-lid laceration 6 mm below the lower tarsus (see figure, previous page)?
1. Skin
2. Preseptal orbicularis oculi muscle
3. Orbital septum
4. Fat
5. Lower lid retractors (capsulopalpebral fascia and inferior tarsus muscle)
6. Conjunctiva

15. Discuss the bony attachments of Whitnall's superior suspensory ligament.

Medially it attaches to the periosteum of the trochlea. Laterally the major attachment is to the periosteum at the frontozygomatic suture. It also sends minor attachments to the lateral orbital tubercle.

16. What structure separates the medial fat pad from the central (also called the preaponeurotic) fat pad in the upper eyelid?

The superior oblique tendon.

17. Lester Jones divided the orbicularis oculi muscle into three portions. Name them.
1. Orbital portion
2. Preseptal portion
3. Pretarsal portion

18. What portions of the orbicularis oculi muscle are important in the lacrimal pump mechanism?

The preseptal and pretarsal portions.

BIBLIOGRAPHY

1. Anderson R, Dixon R: The role of Whitnall's ligament in ptosis surgery. Arch Ophthalmol 97:705–707, 1979.
2. Dutton J: Atlas of Clinical and Surgical Orbital Anatomy. Philadelphia, W.B. Saunders, 1994.
3. Gioia V, Linberg J, McCormick S: The anatomy of the lateral canthal tendon. Arch Ophthalmol 105:529–532, 1987.
4. Hawes M, Dortzbach R: The microscopic anatomy of the lower eyelid retractors. Arch Ophthalmol 100:1313–1318, 1982.
5. Jones LT: The Anatomy of the Lower Eyelid. Am J Ophthalmol 49:29–36, 1960.
6. Lemke B, Della Rocca R: Surgery of the Eyelids and Orbit: An Anatomical Approach. Norwalk, CT, Appleton & Lange, 1990, pp 173–182, 190–192.
7. Lemke B, Stasior O, Rosen P: The surgical relations of the levator palpebrae superioris muscle. Ophthal Plast Reconstr Surg 4:25–30, 1988.
8. Lockwood CB: The anatomy of the muscles, ligaments and fascia of the orbit, including an account of the capsule of tenon, the check ligaments of the recti, and of the suspensory ligament of the eye. J Anat Physiol 20:1–26, 1886.

9. Meyer D, Linberg J, Wobig J, McCormick S: Anatomy of the orbital septum and associated eyelid connective tissues: Implications for ptosis surgery. Ophthal Plast Reconstr Surg 7:104–113, 1991.
10. Sullivan J, Beard C: Anatomy of the eyelids, orbit and lacrimal system. In Stewart W (ed): Surgery of the
Eyelids, Orbit and Lacrimal System. American Academy of Ophthalmology Monograph no. 8, 1993,
pp 84–96.
11. Whitnall SE: The levator palpebrae superioris muscle: The attachments and relations of its aponeurosis.
Ophthalmoscope 12:258–263, 1914.
12. Whitnall SE: The Anatomy of the Human Orbit and Accessory Organs. London, Oxford Medical
Publishers, 1985, pp 122, 131–135, 136–140.

3. OPTICS AND REFRACTION

Janice A. Gault, M.D.

1. What is the primary focal point (f)?

The point along the optical axis at which an object must be placed for parallel rays to emerge from the lens. Thus, the image is at infinity.

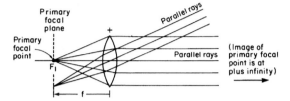

The primary focal point has an image at infinity. (From American Academy of Ophthalmology: Basic and Clinical Science Course. Section 3, Optics, Refraction, and Contact Lenses. San Francisco, American Academy of Ophthalmology, 1992, with permission.)

2. What is the secondary focal point (f')?

The point along the optical axis at which parallel incoming rays are brought into focus. It is equal to 1/lens power in diopters (D). The object is now at infinity.

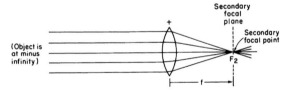

The secondary focal point has an object at infinity. (From American Academy of Ophthalmology: Basic and Clinical Science Course. Section 3, Optics, Refraction, and Contact Lenses. San Francisco, American Academy of Ophthalmology, 1992, with permission.)

3. Where is the secondary focal point for a myopic eye? A hyperopic eye? An emmetropic eye?

The secondary focal point for a myopic eye is anterior to the retina in the vitreous. The object must be moved forward from infinity to allow the light rays to focus on the retina. A hyperopic eye has its secondary focal point posterior to the retina. An emmetropic eye focuses light rays from infinity onto the retina.

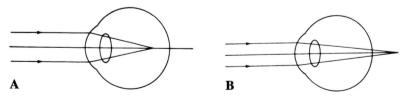

A, In myopia, the focus is in the vitreous. B, In hyperopia, the focus is behind the retina. (From American Academy of Ophthalmology: Basic and Clinical Science Course. Section 3, Optics, Refraction, and Contact Lenses. San Francisco, American Academy of Ophthalmology, 1992, with permission.)

4. What is the far point of an eye?

The term *far point* is used only for the optical system of an eye. It is the point at which an object must be placed along the optical axis for the light rays to be focused on the retina when the eye is not accommodating.

5. Where is the far point for a myopic eye? A hyperopic eye? An emmetropic eye?

The far point for a myopic eye is between the cornea and infinity. A hyperopic eye has its far point beyond infinity or behind the eye. An emmetropic eye has light rays focused on the retina when the object is at infinity.

6. How do you determine which lens will correct the refractive error of the eye?

A lens with its focal point coincident with the far point of the eye allows the light rays from infinity to be focused on the retina. The image at the far point of the eye now becomes the object for the eye.

7. What is the near point of an eye?

The point at which an object will be in focus on the retina when the eye is fully accommodating. Moving the object closer will cause it to blur.

8. Myopia can be caused in two ways. What are they?

Refractive myopia is caused by too much refractive power due to steep corneal curvature or high lens power. Axial myopia is due to an elongated globe. Every millimeter of axial elongation causes about three diopters of myopia.

9. The power of a proper corrective lens is altered by switching from a contact lens to a spectacle lens or vice versa. Why?

Moving a minus lens closer to the eye increases effective minus power. Thus, myopes have a weaker minus prescription in their contact lenses than in their glasses. Patients near presbyopia may need reading glasses when using their contacts but can read without a bifocal lens in their glasses (see question 45). Moving a plus lens closer to the eye decreases effective plus power. Thus, hyperopes need a stronger plus prescription for their contact lenses than for their glasses. They may defer bifocals for a while. The same principle applies to patients who slide their glasses down their nose and find that they can read more easily. They are adding plus power. This principle works for both hyperopes and myopes.

10. What is the amplitude of accommodation?

The total number of diopters that an eye can accommodate.

11. What is the range of accommodation?

The range of clear vision obtainable with accommodation only. For an emmetrope with 10 D of accommodative amplitude, the range of accommodation is infinity to 10 cm.

12. What is the near point of a 4-D hyperope with an amplitude of accommodation of 8?

The far point is 25 cm behind the cornea. The patient must use 4 D of accommodation to overcome hyperopia and focus the image at infinity on the retina. Thus, he has 4 D to accommodate to the near point, which is 25 cm anterior to the cornea. However, when wearing a 4.00 lens, he has the full amplitude of accommodation available. His near point is now 12.5 cm.

13. What is the near point of a 4-D myope with an amplitude of accommodation of 8?

The far point is 25 cm in front of the eye. The patient can accommodate 8 D beyond this point. The near point is 12 D, which is 8.3 cm in front of the cornea.

14. When a light ray passes from a medium with a lower refractive index (n) to a medium with a higher refractive index (n′), is it bent toward or away from the normal?

It is bent toward the normal.

When light passes from a medium with lower refractive index (n_i) to a medium of higher refractive index (n_r), it slows down and is bent toward the normal to the surface. Snell's law determines the amount of bending. i = angle of incidence, r = angle of refraction. (From American Academy of Ophthalmology: Basic and Clinical Science Course. Section 3, Optics, Refraction, and Contact Lenses. San Francisco, American Academy of Ophthalmology, 1992, with permission.)

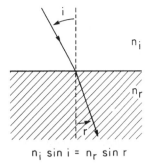

$$n_i \sin i = n_r \sin r$$

15. What is the critical angle?

The incident angle at which the angle of refraction is 90° to normal. The critical angle occurs only when light passes from a more dense to a less dense medium.

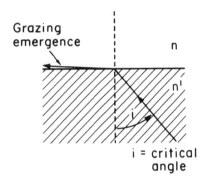

The critical angle. (From American Academy of Ophthalmology: Basic and Clinical Science Course. Section 3, Optics, Refraction, and Contact Lenses. San Francisco, American Academy of Ophthalmology, 1992, with permission.)

16. What happens if the critical angle is exceeded?

Total internal reflection. The angle of incidence equals the angle of reflection.

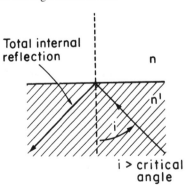

Total internal reflection occurs when the critical angle is exceeded. (From American Academy of Ophthalmology: Basic and Clinical Science Course. Section 3, Optics, Refraction, and Contact Lenses. San Francisco, American Academy of Ophthalmology, 1992, with permission.)

17. Give examples of total internal reflection.

Total internal reflection at the tear-air interface prevents a direct view of the anterior chamber. To overcome this limitation, the critical angle must be increased for the tear-air interface by applying a plastic or glass goniolens to the surface. Total internal reflection also occurs in fiberoptic tubes and indirect ophthalmoscopes.

18. What is the formula for vergence?

$$U + P = V$$

where U is the vergence of light entering the lens, P is the power of the lens (the amount of vergence added to the light by the lens), and V is the vergence of light leaving the lens. All are expressed in diopters. By convention, light rays travel left to right. Plus signs indicate anything to the right of the lens, and minus signs indicate points to the left of the lens.

19. What is the vergence of parallel light rays?

Zero. Parallel light rays do not converge (which would be positive) or diverge (which would be negative). Light rays from an object at infinity or going to an image at infinity have zero vergence.

20. How does a diopter relate to meters?

A diopter is the reciprocal of the distance in meters.

21. What is the image point if an object lies 25 cm to the left of a + 5.00 lens?

Everything must be expressed in diopters: 25 cm is 4 D (1/0.25 m). Because the image is to the left of the lens,

$$U = -4\,D$$
$$P = +5\,D$$
$$-4 + 5 = 1$$

The vergence of the object is + 1 D. Converted to centimeters, the object lies 1 meter to the right of the lens (1/1 D = 1 m = 100 cm).

22. Draw the schematic eye with power (P), nodal point (np), principal plane, primary (f) and secondary (f′) focal points, refractive indices (n, n′), and respective distances labeled.

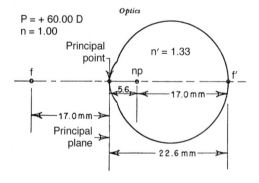

The reduced schematic eye. (From American Academy of Ophthalmology: Basic and Clinical Science Course. Section 3, Optics, Refraction, and Contact Lenses. San Francisco, American Academy of Ophthalmology, 1992, with permission.)

23. How is the power of a prism calculated?

The power of a prism is calculated in prism diopters (Δ) and is equal to the displacement in centimeters of a light ray passing through the prism measured 100 cm from the prism. Light is always bent toward the base of the prism. Thus, a prism of 15 Δ displaces light from infinity 15 cm toward its base at 100 cm.

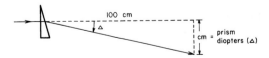

A prism diopter is the displacement of light passing through the prism at 100 cm. (From American Academy of Ophthalmology: Basic and Clinical Science Course. Section 3, Optics, Refraction, and Contact Lenses. San Francisco, American Academy of Ophthalmology, 1992, with permission.)

24. What is Prentice's rule?

$$\Delta = hD$$

The prismatic power of a lens (Δ) at any point on the lens is equal to the distance of that point from the optical axis in centimeters (h) multiplied by the power of the lens in diopters (D). It follows that a lens has no prismatic effect at its optical center; a light ray will pass through the center undeviated.

25. How is Prentice's rule used in real life?

In a patient who has anisometropia, the reading position may cause hyperdeviation of one eye due to the prismatic effect.

26. How can the prismatic effect be alleviated?

1. Contact lenses move with the eye and allow patients to see through their optical center, preventing the prismatic effect.
2. Lowering the optical centers decreases the h of Prentice's rule.
3. Slab off (removing the prism inferiorly from the more minus lens) helps to counteract the prismatic effect.

27. How does Prentice's rule affect the measurement of strabismic deviations when the patient is wearing glasses?

Plus lenses decrease the measured deviation, whereas minus lenses increase the measured deviation. The true deviation is changed by approximately 2.5 D% where D is the spectacle power. The plus lenses have the base of the prism peripherally, whereas the minus lenses have the base of the prism centrally.

28. Bifocals can cause significant problems induced by prismatic effect. What is the difference between image jump and image displacement?

Image jump is produced by the sudden introduction of the prismatic power at the top of the bifocal segment. The object that the patient sees in the inferior field suddenly jumps upward when the eye turns down to look at it. If the optical center of the segment is at the top of the segment, there is no image jump. Image jump is worst in glasses with a round-top bifocal because the optical center is far from the distance lens optical center. A flat-top bifocal is better because the optical center is close to the distance optical center.

Image displacement is the prismatic effect induced by the addition of the bifocal and the distance lenses in the reading position. Image displacement is more bothersome than image jump for most people. A flat-top lens is essentially a base-up lens whereas a round-top lens is a base-down lens. A myopic distance lens has base-up prismatic power in the reading position; thus, image displacement is worsened with a flat-top lens. The prism effects are additive. Similarly, a hyperopic correction is a base-down lens in the reading position; thus, a round-top lens makes image displacement an issue.

29. Should a hyperope use a round-top or flat-top reading lens?

A plus lens will have significant image displacement with a flat-top lens. Image displacement is lessened with a round-top lens. Although image jump will be present, it is the less disturbing of the two.

30. Should a myope use a flat-top or round-top reading lens?

A round-top lens has significant image displacement with a minus lens. A flat-top lens minimizes image displacement and image jump.

31. What is the circle of least confusion?

Patients with astigmatism have two focal lines formed by the convergence of light rays. The first focal line is nearer the cornea and created by the more powerful corneal meridian. The second focal line is further away, created by the less powerful meridian. The circle of least confusion is the circular cross-section of the conoid of Sturm, dioptrically midway between the two focal lines. The goal of refractive correction is to choose a lens that places the circle of least confusion on the retina.

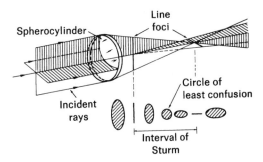

The circle of least confusion. (From American Academy of Ophthalmology: Basic and Clinical Science Course. Section 3, Optics, Refraction, and Contact Lenses. San Francisco, American Academy of Ophthalmology, 1992, with permission.)

32. What is the spherical equivalent of $-3.00 + 2.00 \times 125$?
Take half the cylinder and add it to the sphere. The spherical equivalent is -2.00 sphere.

33. Change the following plus cylinder refraction to minus cylinder form: $-5.00 + 3.00 \times 90$.
First, add the sphere and cylinder to each other. Then change the sign of the cylinder, and add 90° to the axis. Thus, the minus cylinder form is $-2.00 - 3.00 \times 180$.

34. After cataract surgery, a patient has the following refraction: $+1.00 + 3.00 \times 100$. Does the patient have with-the-rule or against-the-rule astigmatism?
With-the-rule astigmatism is corrected with a plus cylinder at 90° (± 15–20°). Against-the-rule astigmatism is corrected with a plus cylinder at 180° (± 15–20°). The patient has with-the-rule astigmatism.

35. How should you proceed with the patient's care?
Check the remaining sutures. Cutting the 11:00 suture will relax the wound and decrease the amount of astigmatism.

36. What if a postoperative patient has a refraction of $+2.00 - 2.00 \times 90$? Where should you cut the suture?
Changing the refraction to plus cylinder form, you see that the patient is plano $+2.00 \times 180$ and has against-the-rule astigmatism. You cannot cut any sutures to relax the astigmatism. The only option is to do a relaxing incision of the cornea, but it is likely that the patient will tolerate glasses, especially if the refraction is close to the preoperative correction. Also, check the preoperative keratometry. The patient may have had against-the-rule astigmatism before surgery.

37. Thick lenses have aberrations. List them.
1. **Spherical aberration.** The rays at the peripheral edges of the lens are refracted more than the rays at the center, thus causing night myopia. The larger pupil at night allows more spherical aberration than the smaller pupil during daylight.
2. **Coma.** A comet-shaped blur is seen when the object and image are off the optical axis. Coma is similar to spherical aberration but occurs in the nonaxial rays.
3. **Astigmatism of oblique incidence.** When the spherical lens is tilted, the lens gains a small astigmatic effect that causes curvature of the field (i.e., spherical images produce

curved images of flat objects). This effect is helpful in the eye because the retina has a similar curvature.

4. **Chromatic aberration.** Each wavelength has its own refractive index; the shorter wavelengths are bent the most.

5. **Distortion.** The higher the spherical power, the more significantly the periphery is magnified or minified in relation to the rest of the image. A high plus lens produces pincushion distortion; a high minus lens produces barrel distortion.

The aberration caused by the astigmatism of oblique incidence is helpful in the eye because the curvature of the field that it induces is almost identical to the retinal curvature.

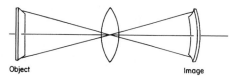

Object   Image

Because each wavelength has a different refractive index, light passing through a prism will reveal the characteristic visible spectrum. (From American Academy of Ophthalmology: Basic and Clinical Science Course. Section 3, Optics, Refraction, and Contact Lenses. San Francisco, American Academy of Ophthalmology, 1992, with permission.)

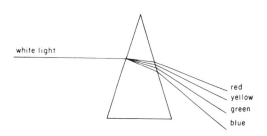

38. Are red or green light rays refracted more by a plus lens?

The shorter green rays are bent more than the longer red rays. This distinction causes chromatic aberration and is the basis for the red-green duochrome test. Green rays are focused 0.50 D closer to the lens than red rays. When a corrected myopic patient is fogged to prevent accommodation, the red letters should be clearer than the green. Slowly add more minus in 0.25 increments until the green and red letters are equal in clarity. This technique prevents overcorrection of myopia.

39. A myopic patient tilts his glasses to see in the distance. What does this tell you?

The patient is using the principle of astigmatism of oblique incidence to strengthen the power of his glasses. He needs a refraction. Tilting a minus lens induces a minus cylinder with axis in the axis of tilt. Tilting a plus lens induces a plus cylinder with axis in the axis of tilt. A small amount of additional sphere of the same sign is induced as well.

40. What measurements are necessary in determining the intraocular lens implant calculation?

Axial length in millimeters and keratometry readings in diopters. The desired postoperative refraction is also necessary. The SRK formula is commonly used. For emmetropia, the formula is $P = A - 2.5$ (axial length) $- 0.9$ (K_{avg}), where P equals the implant power, A is the implant constant as determined by the manufacturer, and K_{avg} is the average of the keratometry readings. The A constant also can be individualized by analysis of previous cases. For each diopter of desired ametropia, add 1.25 to 1.50 D. For example, if the SRK formula reveals a calculation of + 18.0 D for emmetropia, implant a + 19.50 D lens for − 1.00 D.

41. How does an axial error that is incorrect by 0.1 mm affect the intraocular lens calculation?

For every 0.1-mm error, the calculation is impacted by 0.25 D. Recheck the A scan if the axial length is less than 22 mm or more than 25 mm or if there is more than a 0.3-mm difference in the measurement between the two eyes.

42. How does an error in keratometry readings affect the intraocular lens calculation?

For every error of 0.25 D, the calculation is in error by 0.25 D. Recheck the keratometer measurements if the average corneal power is less than 40 D or more than 47 D. Also check if there is a difference of more than 1 D in the average keratometer readings between eyes.

43. What is the formula for transverse magnification?

Also known as linear or lateral magnification, transverse magnification equals I/O = v/u, where I is the size of the image, O is the size of the object, v is the distance from the lens to the image, and u is the distance of the object from the lens. All are measured in millimeters.

44. What is the formula for axial magnification?

The square of the transverse magnification. Magnification along the visual axis causes distortion in three-dimensional images.

45. What is the effect of axial magnification on accommodative requirements for a given near-viewing distance?

Hyperopes must accommodate more through glasses than through contact lenses, and myopes must accommodate less through glasses than through contact lenses. This effect can be clinically significant in early presbyopic years. The effect is greatest with high refractive errors. For example, a – 5.00 myope may be able to read without bifocal glasses but require reading glasses with contact lenses. Conversely, a hyperope may be able to forego reading glasses with contact lenses but need bifocal glasses.

46. What is angular magnification?

The magnification of a simple magnifier, such as viewing something with an eye or a single lens. Magnification is D/4, where D is the power of the lens used.

47. What is the magnification of a direct ophthalmoscope?

The examiner uses the optics of the patient's eye as a simple magnifier. Estimating the power of the eye as + 60 D, the magnification is 15 ×. Thus, the retina appears 15 times larger than it is.

48. Does an astronomic telescope form an upright or an inverted image?

An inverted image, which has few uses in ophthalmic optics.

49. Does a Galilean telescope form an upright or an inverted image?

An upright image, which is used often in ophthalmic optics. An aphakic eye corrected with spectacles or contact lens is an example. The eyepiece is the aphakic eye estimated to be – 12.50 D, and the objective is the corrective lens.

50. What is the magnification formula for a telescope?

$$\text{Magnification} = D \text{ eyepiece}/D \text{ objective}$$

This formula applies to both astronomic and Galilean telescopes. For the aphakic eye with a spectacle correction of + 10.00 D, the magnification is 1.25 or 25%. For a contact lens, this translates to + 11.75 D, accounting for the vertex distance of 10 mm. Magnification now is 1.06 or 6%. Thus, aniseikonia with a contact lens is better tolerated than aniseikonia with glasses if the patient needs less powerful correction in the other eye.

51. When using the direct ophthalmoscope, which patient provides the larger image of the retina—the hyperope or the myope?

The myope functions as a Galilean telescope and provides extra magnification. The eyepiece (spectacle lens) is a minus lens, and the objective (the patient's own lens) is a plus lens. The hyperope functions as a reverse Galilean telescope and provides minification in comparison. In this situation, the eyepiece is a plus lens, and the objective is a minus lens.

52. What do you need to determine the best low vision aid for a patient?

Best refraction, visual acuity, visual field, and practical needs of the patient.

53. What are the advantages and disadvantages of using a high add in a bifocal for a low vision aid?

The advantages include a large field of view. Disadvantages include a short reading distance as well as significant cost.

54. What are the advantages and disadvantages of using a high-power single-vision lens as a low vision aid?

High-power single-vision lenses come in monocular and binocular forms. They also afford a large field of view but have a short reading distance.

55. How do you estimate the strength of plus lens needed to read newspaper print without accommodation?

The reciprocal of the best Snellen acuity is equal to the plus power of the lens required. For example, if a patient can read 20/60, a + 3.00 D will suffice. The reciprocal of the diopter power gives the reading distance (i.e., 33 cm).

56. What adjustment is necessary when a binocular high-power single-vision lens is used?

Base in prisms to augment the natural ability to converge. Otherwise, patients develop exotropia at near when looking through high plus lenses.

57. What are the advantages and disadvantages of hand-held magnifiers for low vision aids?

Hand-held magnifiers have a variable eye-to-lens distance and are easily portable. They enjoy a high rate of acceptability. However, they have a small field of view when the lens is held far from the eye and are difficult to manipulate by patients with tremors and arthritis. A stand magnifier may be more useful for such patients.

58. What are the advantages and disadvantages of using loupes as a low vision aid?

Loupes are basically prefocused telescopes. They allow a long working distance and keep the hands free. But they have a small field of view, limited depth of field, and are expensive.

59. The devices mentioned thus far are for magnifying at near. What is available for distance aids?

The only magnifying device for distance is a telescope. Telescopes are monocular or binocular and can be hand-held or mounted on glasses. They also have an adjustable focus. Unfortunately, they have a restricted field of view (approximately 8°). Thus, the object of regard may be difficult to find.

60. Do convex mirrors add plus or minus vergence?

Convex mirrors add minus vergence like minus lenses. Concave mirrors add plus vergence like plus lenses. Plane mirrors add no vergence.

61. What is the reflecting power in diopters of a mirror?

$D = 2/r$, where r is the radius of curvature. The focal length is one-half the radius.

62. What instrument uses the reflecting power of the cornea to determine its readings?

The keratometer uses the reflecting power of the cornea to determine the corneal curvature. The formula is $D = (n - 1)/r$, where D is the reflecting power of the cornea and n is the standardized refractive index for the cornea (1.3375).

63. How much of the cornea is measured with a keratometer?

Only the central 3 mm. A peripheral corneal scar or defect may be missed by using a keratometer instead of a corneal map.

64. Why does a keratometer use doubling of its images?

To avoid the problems of eye movement in determining an accurate measurement. Doubling is done with prisms.

65. What is a Geneva lens clock?

A device to determine the base curve of the back surface of a spectacle. It is often used clinically to detect plus cylinder spectacle lenses in a patient used to minus cylinder lenses. It is specifically calibrated for the refractive index of crown glass. A special lens clock is available for plastic lenses.

66. Do you measure the power of spectacles in a lensmeter with the temples toward you or away from you?

The distance is measured with the temples facing away from you (back vertex power). The add is measured with the temples pointing toward you (front vertex power). You must measure the difference between the top and bottom segments, especially if the patient has a highly hyperopic prescription.

67. If you obtain "with" movement during retinoscopy, is the far point of the patient in front of the peephole, at the peephole, or beyond the peephole?

Beyond the peephole. The goal is neutralization of the light reflex so that the patient's far point is at the peephole. The light at the patient's pupil fills the entire space at once. More plus must be added to the prescription to move the far point to neutralization. "Against" movement means that the far point is in front of the peephole; more minus must be added to move the far point to neutralization.

68. What does a pachymeter measure?

The corneal thickness or anterior chamber depth.

69. How does the Hruby lens give an upright or inverted image?

A Hruby lens is – 55 D and gives an upright image. The Goldman lens is – 64 D and also provides an upright image. The Volk 90-D lens provides an inverted image.

70. Why does the indirect ophthalmoscope provide a larger field of view than the direct ophthalmoscope?

The condensing lens used with the indirect ophthalmoscope captures the peripheral rays to give a field of view of 25° or more depending on the lens power used. The direct ophthalmoscope does not use the condensing lens and thus provides only a 7° field of view.

71. What are the wavelengths of the spectrum of visible light?

The range is from 400 nm for violet light to 700 nm for red light. Anything shorter than 400 nm is considered ultraviolet, and anything longer than 700 nm is in the infrared spectrum.

72. Antireflective coatings on spectacle lenses are based on what principle?

Interference. Antireflective coatings use destructive interference. The crest of one wavelength cancels the trough of another.

73. What is the most effective pinhole diameter?

A pinhole diameter of 1.2 mm neutralizes up to 3 D of refractive error. A 2-mm pinhole neutralizes only 1 D. An aphakic patient may need a + 10-D lens in addition to the pinhole to obtain useful visual acuity.

74. When is a cylcoplegic refraction indicated?

1. Patients younger than 15 years, especially if they have strabismus. Make sure to measure the deviation before cycloplegia.

2. Hyperopes younger than 35 years, especially if they experience asthenopia.

3. Patients with asthenopia suggestive of accommodative problems.

Note: Check accommodative amplitudes and reading adds before cycloplegia.

75. Which cycloplegic agent lasts the longest? The shortest?

Atropine lasts for 1–2 weeks. Watch for toxic effects in small children and elderly patients. Tropicamide (Mydriacyl) lasts 4–8 hours and is not strong enough for cylcoplegia in children. One or two diopters of hyperopia may remain. Cyclogyl lasts 8–24 hours; homatropine, 1–3 days; and scopolamine, 5–7 days.

76. What are the signs and symptoms of systemic intoxication from cylcoplegic medications? How are they treated?

Dry mouth, fever, flushing, tachycardia, nausea, and delirium. Treatment includes counteraction with physostigmine.

77. When is it important to measure the vertex distance in prescribing glasses?

When the patient has a strong prescription of more than ± 5.00 D.

78. What is the threshold for prescribing glasses in a child with astigmatism?

When visual acuity is not developing properly, as noted by amblyopia or strabismus. Give the full correction. Children tolerate full correction better than adults. Most often, amblyopia or strabismus occurs with at least 1.50 D of astigmatism. Anisometropia that presents with 1.00 D or more of hyperopic asymmetry also requires full correction.

79. What may cause monocular diplopia?

- Corneal or lenticular irregularity
- Decentered contact lens
- Inappropriate placement of reading add
- Transient sensory adaptations after strabismus surgery
- Distortion from retinal lesions (rare)

80. What conditions may give a false-positive reading with a potential acuity meter?

Macular scotomas in a patient with amblyopia or retinal disease, such as age-related macular degeneration. Acute macular edema also may elevate the reading, but the elevation disappears with chronic edema. An irregular corneal surface can falsely improve the potential acuity; however, wearing a contact lens may help.

81. What do you check when patients complain that their new glasses are not as good as their previous pair?

1. Ask specifically what the complaint is: distance reading? near problems? asthenopia? diplopia? pain behind the ears or at the nose bridge from ill-fitting glassses?

2. Read the new and old glasses on the lensmeter and compare. Make sure that the old glasses did not have any prism. Check the patient for undetected strabismus with cover testing.

3. Refract the patient again, possibly with a cycloplegic agent if the symptoms warrant.

4. Check the optical centers in comparison with the pupillary centers.

5. Check whether the reading segments are in the correct position—level with the lower lid.

6. Make sure that the new glasses fit the patient correctly.

7. Check whether the old glasses were made with plus cylinder by using the Geneva lens clock.

8. Check whether the base curve has changed with the Geneva lens clock.

9. Evaluate the patient for dry eye.

10. If the patient has a high prescription, check the vertex distance. Often it is easier to refract such patients over their old pair of glasses to keep the same vertx distance.

11. Check the pantoscopic tilt. Normally the tilt is 10–15° so that when the patient reads, the eye is perpendicular to the lens. If the tilt is off, especially in relation to the old glasses, the patient may notice.

12. With postoperative glasses, evaluate for diplopia in downgaze due to anisometropia.

13. Perhaps the add is too strong or too weak. Check the patient using trial lenses and reading material.

14. Sometimes if the diameter of the lens is much larger in the newer frames, the patient notices significant distortion in the peripheral lens. Encourage a small frame.

15. Above all, try to test the new prescription in trial frames with a walk around the office. You do not want to go through this process again.

82. If after repeat refraction the patient suddenly develops more hyperopia than you previously noted, what do you look for?

A cause of acquired hyperopia, such as a retrobulbar tumor, central serous retinopathy, posterior lens dislocation, or a flattened cornea from a contact lens.

83. What if the patient has more myopia than previously noted?

Check the cycloplegic refraction to make sure that it is true. Acquired myopia may be caused by diabetes mellitus, sulfonamides, nuclear sclerosis, pilocarpine, keratoconus, a scleral buckle for retinal detachment, and anterior lens dislocation.

84. What about acquired astigmatism?

Lid lesions such as hemangiomas, chalazions, and ptosis may cause acquired astigmatism. A pterygium or keratoconus may reveal a previously undetected astigmatism. And, of course, healing cataract wounds may change the previous astigmatism.

85. If the astigmatism has changed and the patient has difficulty with tolerating the new prescription, what are the options?

If the astigmatism is oblique, try rotating the axis toward 90 or toward the old axis. The astimgatic power may be reduced, but keep the spherical power the same. Sometimes a gradual change in prescription over time may allow the patient to adapt. For example, if a patient's prescription is $-3.00 + 2.00 \times 110$, a possibility is $-2.50 + 1.00 \times 90$. The spherical equivalent of -2.00 D has been maintained.

86. What does laser stand for?

Light amplification by stimulated emission of radiation.

87. To steepen a contact lens fit, do you increase the diameter of the lens or the radius of curvature?

Increasing the diameter of the lens or decreasing the radius of curvature will steepen the lens. This information is useful for lenses that fit too tightly.

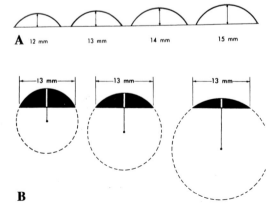

A 12 mm 13 mm 14 mm 15 mm

B

A, When the radius of curvature is kept constant while the diameter of the contact lens is increased, the fit steepens. *B,* Conversely, increasing the radius of curvature while maintaing the same diameter of the contact lens allows a flatter fit. (From American Academy of Ophthalmology: Basic and Clinical Science Course. Section 3, Optics, Refraction, and Contact Lenses. San Francisco, American Academy of Ophthalmology, 1992, with permission.)

88. How many seconds of arc does the "E" on the 20/20 line of the Snellen eye chart subtend?
Five seconds. The Snellen eye chart measures the minimal separable acuity.

89. When the Jackson cross is used to define the astigmatic axis, is the handle of the lens parallel to the axis or 45° from it?
Parallel. To define the astigmatic power, the handle is 45° to the axis. Define the axis before the power.

90. A 25-year-old patient has a manifest refraction of + 0.50 OU and complains of asthenopia. What do you do?
Check the patient's accommodative amplitude and look for an exophoria at near to evaluate for convergence insufficiency. Then do a cycloplegic refraction to check for undercorrection. On exam, the amplitude of accommodation is 3 D OU. Because this value is low for a young person, suspect undercorrection of hyperopia. Indeed, the cycloplegic refraction is + 2.50 OU. The patient has accommodative spasm. Try giving one-half of the cycloplegic findings. Sometimes atropine is needed to break the spasm.

91. What instrument is useful to measure the accommodative amplitude?
Prince rule.

92. Define absolute hyperopia, facultative hyperopia, manifest hyperopia, and latent hyperopia.
A 35-year-old man has 20/40 uncorrected vision. With + 0.50 glasses, he is 20/20. He will remain 20/20 with a + 1.50 manifest refraction. With cycloplegia, he has a refraction of + 4.00.

Total hyperopia—found by cycloplegia	+ 4.00
Manifest hyperopia—found without cycloplegia; more plus will blur vision	+ 1.50
Latent hyperopia—total minus manifest hyperopia	+ 2.50
Absolute hyperopia—the minimal correction that the patient needs to see distances	+ 0.50
Facultative hyperopia—manifest minus absolute hyperopia; compensation accomplished by accommodation	+ 1.00

BIBLIOGRAPHY

1. American Academy of Ophthalmology: Basic and Clinical Science Course. San Francisco, American Academy of Ophthalmology, 1992.
2. Milder B, Rubin ML: The Fine Art of Prescribing Glasses without Making a Spectacle of Yourself, 2nd ed. Gainesville, FL, Triad Publishing, 1991.
3. Rubin ML: Optics for Clinicians, 2nd ed. Gainesville, FL, Triad Publishing, 1974.

4. COLOR VISION

William E. Benson, M.D.

1. What are photons?

Atoms consist of a nucleus (composed of protons and neutrons) and electrons, which revolve around the nucleus of orbits of more or less fixed diameter. An electron can move to a higher orbit if it receives energy from an external source (e.g., heating). However, it remains in the higher orbit for only a one-hundred-millionth of a second. As it falls back to its original lower orbit, it releases its excess energy by emitting a small "packet" of energy called a quantum or a photon.

2. Describe the physical properties of photons.

In a vacuum, all photons move at the speed of light. As they travel, they vibrate, causing measurable electric and magnetic effects (wave properties). The further an electron falls to reach its original lower orbit, the greater its frequency of vibration, and the shorter its wavelength (λ), which is the straight-line distance a photon moves during one complete vibration. Frequency and wavelength are related by the formula $f = c/\lambda$, where f = frequency of vibration, λ = wavelength, and c = speed of light. Thus, f and λ are inversely proportional (i.e., as frequency increases, wavelength decreases). For example, gamma rays have a very high frequency and a very short wavelength, and radio waves have a very low frequency and a rather long wavelength.

3. What is the electromagnetic spectrum?

Light, x-rays, gamma rays, and radio waves are all forms of electromagnetic energy. When photons (quanta) are classified according to their wavelength, the result is the electromagnetic spectrum. The photons with the longest wavelengths are radio and television waves; those with the shortest are gamma rays. The photons we see (visible light) are near the middle of the spectrum.

4. Why can we "see" light, but not other types of electromagnetic energy?

The rods and cones of the retina (photoreceptors) contain pigments that preferentially absorb photons with wavelengths between 400 and 700 nm (a nanometer is a billionth of a meter) and convert their energy into a neuronal impulse that is carried to the brain. Wavelengths longer than 700 nm and shorter than 400 nm tend to pass through the sensory retina without being absorbed.

5. What is the light spectrum?

Photons can be classified not only by their wavelength but also by the sensation they cause when they strike the retina. Photons of the shortest wavelengths that we can see are perceived as blue and green; those of longer wavelengths are perceived as yellow, orange, and red.

6. How does a prism break white light into the colors of the rainbow?

Photons travel at the speed of light in a vacuum, but if they enter a denser medium, such as glass, their wavelength and speed decrease. The frequency of vibration remains the same. The shorter the wavelength, the more the speed is decreased. For example, imagine two photons traveling through a vacuum, one of wavelength 650 nm and the other of wavelength 450 nm. As long as they remain in a vacuum, they keep pace with one another. When they strike the glass perpendicularly, the 450 nm photon is slowed down more than the 650 nm photon. If they enter the glass obliquely, their paths are bent in proportion to how much their speed is slowed. In other words, the shorter the wavelength, the greater the bending. The blue is bent more and is separated from the red.

7. How do rods differ from cones?

Both rods and cones are photoreceptors, which are defined as retinal cells that initiate the process of vision. Rods function best when the eye is dark-adapted (i.e., for night vision). They cannot distinguish one color from another. Cones, on the other hand, function when the retina is light-adapted (i.e., for day vision).

8. What are the visual pigments?

There are four visual pigments: rhodopsin, which is present in rods, and the three cone pigments. All visual pigments are made up of 11-cis retinal (vitamin A aldehyde) and a protein called an opsin. When a photon is absorbed, the 11-cis retinal is converted to the all-trans form and is released from the opsin, initiating an electrical impulse in the photoreceptor that travels toward the brain. The eye then resynthesizes the rhodopsin.

9. Describe the three cone pigments.

Our ability to distinguish different colors depends on the fact that there are three different kinds of cone pigment. All visual pigments use retinal, but each has a different opsin. The function of the different opsins is to rearrange the electron cloud of retinal, thereby changing its ability to capture photons of different wavelength. Red-catching cones (R cones) contain erythrolabe, which preferentially absorbs photons of long wavelengths. It is best stimulated by 570 nm photons, but also absorbs adjoining wavelengths. Blue-catching cones (B cones) contain cyanolabe, which absorbs the shortest wavelengths best. Its maximal sensitivity is at 440 nm. Green-catching cones (G cones) contain chlorolabe, which is most sensitive to the intermediate wavelengths. Its maximal sensitivity is at 540 nm.

10. How does the sensation of light get to the brain?

The electrical signals initiated by absorption of photons by the photoreceptors are transmitted to bipolar cells and then to ganglion cells. Horizontal and amacrine cells modify these messages. For example, if a cone is strongly stimulated, it sends inhibitory messages by way of a horizontal cell to neighboring cones, thereby reducing "noise" and sharpening up the message the brain receives. Bipolar cells send similar inhibitory messages by way of amacrine cells. The axons of ganglion cells form the optic nerve, which carries information to the brain. In the brain is the "hue center," which adds up the information from the different color channels and determines which color we see. In general, the hue we see depends on the relative number of photons of different wavelength that strike the cones.

11. What three attributes are necessary to describe any color?

To accurately describe any color, one must specify three attributes: hue, saturation, and brightness.

12. What is hue?

Hue is synonymous with "color" and is the attribute of color perception denoted by blue, red, purple, and so forth. Hue depends largely on what the eye and brain perceive to be the predominant wavelength present in the incoming light. In simplest terms, this means that if light of several wavelengths strikes the eye and if more light of 540 nm is present than is light of other wavelengths, we will see green.

13. What is saturation?

Saturation (chroma) corresponds to the purity or richness of a color. When all the light seen by the eye is the same wavelength, we say that a color is fully saturated. Vivid colors are saturated. If we add white to a saturated color, the hue does not change, but the color is paler (desaturated). For example, pink is a desaturated red.

14. What is brightness?

Brightness (luminance, value) refers to the quantity of light coming from an object (the number of photons striking the eye). If we place a filter over a projector or gradually (with a rheostat) lower its intensity, the brightness decreases.

15. What are complementary colors?

When equal quantities of complements are added, the result is white. Blue-green and red are complements as are green and magenta. (We are talking of colored lights, not paints.)

16. What is the color wheel?

The color wheel is made up of all hues arranged in a circle so that each hue lies between those hues it most closely resembles and complementary hues lie opposite each other. Using the color wheel, we can predict the color that will result when two different lights are mixed. When noncomplements are mixed, the resultant color lies between the two original colors. The exact color seen depends on the quantity of each color used. For example, equal quantities of red and green result in yellow, whereas a large quantity of red and a relatively small quantity of green result in orange.

17. How does the eye differ from the ear?

Unlike the ear, which can distinguish several musical instruments playing at once, our eye and brain cannot determine the composition of a color we see. For example, if we present the eye with a light composed purely of 589 nm photons, the eye sees yellow. However, if we mix green and red lights in the proper proportions, the eye also sees yellow and cannot differentiate this from the other. Similarly, when two complements are mixed, we see white and cannot distinguish this white from the white seen when equal quantities of all wavelengths are present. Further, if we add white light to our original 589 nm yellow, the eye still sees yellow. Similarly, a light composed only of 490 nm photons is seen as blue-green and cannot be distinguished from an appropriate mixture of blue and green.

18. What are the primary colors?

When speaking of colored lights, the primary hues (also called the additive primaries) are red, green, and blue. Any color, including white, can be produced by overlapping red, green, and blue lights on a screen in the proper proportions. The reflecting screen can be regarded as a composite of an infinite number of tiny projectors. The eye, bombarded by all these photons "adds up" their relative contribution. The color we see is determined by how many quanta of each wavelength reach the eye. Color television relies on this ability of the eye to add up tiny adjacent points of light. If one looks at a color television from six inches away, one sees tiny dots of only three colors: red, green, and blue. If one then backs away, the full range of colors becomes apparent and the eye can no longer distinguish the tiny dots. It synthesizes (adds up) the adjacent colors (e.g., tiny dots of red and blue = purple, red and green = yellow, red and green and blue = white, and so forth).

19. Where is the final determination of color made?

The hue center, localized in the cortex, synthesizes information it receives from two "intermediate centers"; the R-G center and the B-Y center. The information sent to the hue center from the R-G center depends on the relative stimulation of the R and G cones. For example, when light of 540 nm strikes the retina, it will stimulate both R and G cones. However, because the G cones are stimulated much more than the R cones, the message received by the hue center is predominantly "green." On the other hand, if light of 590 nm strikes the retina, the R cones are stimulated more than the G cones and we see yellow. When light of 630 nm strikes the retina, the G cones are not stimulated at all and we see red. The B cones send information to the B-Y center. The Y information does not come from Y cones because there are no Y cones. Information from R and G cones has the effect of of yellow in the B-Y center.

20. Why is brown, which is definitely a color, not on the color wheel?

This is because brown is a yellow or orange of low luminance.

21. Describe the Bezold-Brucke phenomenon.

As brightness increases, most hues appear to change. At low intensities, blue-green, green, and yellow-green appear greener than they do at high intensities, when they appear bluer. At low intensities, reds and oranges appear redder and at high intensities, yellower. The exceptions are a blue of about 478 nm, a green of about 503 nm, and a yellow of about 578 nm. These are the wavelengths of invariant hue.

22. What is the Abney effect?

As white is added to any hue (desaturating it), the hue appears to change slightly in color. All colors except a yellow of 570 nm appear yellower.

23. What are the relative luminosity curves?

The relative luminosity curves illustrate the eye's sensitivity to different wavelengths of light. They are constructed by asking an observer to increase the luminance of lights of various wavelength until they appear to be equal in apparent brightness to a yellow light whose luminance is fixed. When the eye is light-adapted, yellow, yellow-green, and orange appear brighter than do blues, greens, and reds. The cones' peak sensitivity is to light of 555 nm. A relative luminosity curve can also be constructed for the rods in a dark-adapted eye, even though the observer cannot name the various wavelengths used. The rods' peak sensitivity is to light of 505 nm (blue).

24. Define lateral inhibition.

As mentioned above, as cones of one kind (e.g., R cones) are stimulated, they may send an inhibitory message by way of horizontal and amacrine cells to adjacent cones of the same kind (e.g., other R cones). Therefore, when a purple circle is surrounded by a red background, the R cones in the purple area are inhibited, making the purple (a combination of red and blue) appear bluer than it really is. If the purple is surrounded by blue, it appears redder.

25. What are afterimages?

If one stares at a color for 20 seconds, it begins to fade (desaturate). Then, if one gazes at a white background, the complement of the original color (afterimage) appears. These two phenomena depend on the fact that even when cones are not being stimulated, they spontaneously send a few signals toward the brain. For example, when red light is projected onto the retina, the eye sees red because the R cones are stimulated much more than the G cones and B cones. The G and B contribution to the hue center is far outweighed by the R. After several seconds, the red color fades (becomes desaturated) because the red cones, being more strongly stimulated, cannot regenerate their pigment fast enough to continue to send such a large number of signals (fatigue). Now the G and B cone contribution to the hue center increases relative to that of the R cones and the brain "sees" a desaturated or paler red. It is as if we added blue-green light to the red. (Recall that blue-green is the complement of red and that mixing complements yields white). When the red light is turned off, the frequency of the spontaneous messages sent to the brain by the fatigued R cones is far less than that sent by the G and B cones, so the brain sees blue-green, or cyan, the complement of red.

26. Why are white flowers white?

The color of any object that is not white or black depends on the relative number of photons of each wavelength that it absorbs and reflects. Our ambient light, derived from the sun, contains approximately equal numbers of all the photons that make up the light spectrum. White paint reflects all photons equally well, so white flowers appear white.

27. Why is charcoal black?

Charcoal absorbs most of the light that strikes it. Because very few photons are reflected toward the eye, the photoreceptors are not stimulated and no color is seen.

28. Why are blue flowers blue?

The pigments in blue flowers absorb red and yellow photons best, green next best, and blue least of all; therefore, more blue photons are reflected than others, and the eye sees blue. A green leaf is green because chlorophyll strongly absorbs blue and red and reflects green.

29. Why does mixing red and blue-green lights result in white, but mixing red and green paint results in brown?

Oil paints are made by mixing (suspending) tiny clumps of pigment in an opaque medium (the binder). Pigments reflect and absorb some wavelengths of light better than others. The dominant wavelength reflected is the color of the paint. When two lights are mixed, we speak of an "additive" mixture. But when two paints are mixed, each pigment subtracts some of the light the other would reflect. The resultant mixture is darker than either of the two originals. Red paint mixed with green paint results in brown because enough light is subtracted that the eye sees a yellow of low luminance.

30. Why does mixing paints yield unpredictable results?

An artist or home decorator never knows the exact absorption spectrum of the originals. Two greens may appear to be the same but, because their pigments are not identical, do not yield the same color when mixed with the same yellow.

31. Why do colors appear different under fluorescent light as opposed to incandescent lights?

Tungsten (incandescent) light bulbs emit relatively more photons of the longer (red) wavelengths than of the shorter (blue) wavelengths, whereas fluorescent light bulbs emit relatively more light in the blue and green wavelengths. A shopper who picks out material for drapes in a store that has fluorescent lighting may be surprised to find out that the material looks quite different at home. A purple dress appears redder under incandescent light than it does under fluorescent light.

32. Why is the sky blue?

The sun emits light of all of the spectral colors. If an astronaut in space looks at the sun, it appears white. If the astronaut looks away from the sun, he sees that the outer space is black, because the photons not coming directly at him pass through space unhindered and are not reflected toward him. On earth, the atmosphere, which contains ozone, dust, water droplets, and many other reflecting molecules and substances, is interposed between the sun and our eyes. The atmosphere scatters blue light more than it does green, yellow, or red. Therefore, if during the daytime we look away from the sun, we see the blue photons that are being bent toward us and the sky appears to be blue.

33. Why is the sunset red?

At dusk, in order to reach us, the light from the sun has to pass through much more of the earth's atmosphere than it does during the daytime. Therefore, even more of the blue and green photons are bent away from the atmosphere. The red and yellow photons penetrate better. If some of these are eventually reflected toward us by clouds or dust, we see a red sky. Similarly, the sun appears red.

34. Define trichromats.

Trichromats are the 92% of the population who have "normal" color vision. They have all three different kinds of cones, normal concentration of the cone pigments, and normal retinal wiring.

35. What is congenital dichromatism?

In dichromats, the cones themselves are normal, but one of the three contains the wrong pigment. For example, in deuteranopes, the "G" cones are normal in every way except that they contain erythrolabe (red pigment) instead of chlorolabe (green pigment). In protanopes, the "R" cones are normal in every way except that they contain chlorolabe (green pigment) instead of erythrolabe (red pigment). Tritanopia is a defect of "B" cones.

36. Why do deuteranopes have difficulty in distinguishing red from green?

In deuteranopia, because both R and G cones contain the same pigment, when red light strikes the retina, the R and G cones are stimulated equally and send an equal number of messages to the R-G center. Similarly, there is an increased R input to the B-Y center, where the R input now equals the G input. In other words, the hue center thinks that equal quantities of red and green light are striking the retina. When green or blue-green light strikes the retina, the R and G cones are again stimulated equally. An accurate analysis of the mechanics of color vision abnormalities would require a computer, but it should be apparent that because both red and green light stimulate the R and G cones equally, the information the hue center receives from the R-G center is not useful and the deuteranope would have difficulty distinguishing red from green. Similarly, protanopes also have difficulty seeing red from green.

37. What is anomalous trichromatism?

In anomalous trichromatism, two of the three cone pigments are normal, but the third functions suboptimally. Depending on which pigment is abnormal, the affected persons are termed **protanomalous, deuteranomalous,** or **tritanomalous.** Anomalous trichromats can distinguish between fully saturated colors but have difficulty distinguishing colors of low saturation (pastels) or low luminance (dark colors), or both. Deuteranomaly is present in approximately 5% of the population; deuteranopia, protanopia, and protanomaly in 1% each; and tritanopia or tritanomaly in only 0.002%.

38. How is abnormal color vision inherited?

All red-green disorders are inherited in a sex-linked recessive pattern. This means that men almost exclusively manifest the disorder. Women are carriers. In other words, the women have perfectly normal color vision, but approximately 50% of their sons are abnormal. Both men and women can have the tritan disorders, which are inherited as autosomal dominant traits.

39. What is Kollner's rule?

As a very general rule, the errors made by persons with optic nerve disease tend to resemble those made by protans and deutans, whereas those made by persons with retinal disease resemble those made by tritans.

BIBLIOGRAPHY

1. Boynton RM: Color, hue and wavelength. In Carterette EC, Friedman MP: Handbook of Perception, vol V. New York, Academic Press, 1975, pp 301–350.
2. Gerritsen F: Theory and Practice of Color. New York, Van Nostrand, 1974.
3. Krill AE: Hereditary retinal and choroidal diseases. In Krill AE (ed): Evaluation of Color Vision. Hagerstown, MD, Harper & Row, 1972, pp 309–340.
4. Linksz A: Reflections, old and new, concerning acquired defects of color vision. Surv Ophthalmol 17:229, 1973.
5. Rubin ML, Walls GL: Fundamentals of Visual Science. Springfield, IL, Charles C Thomas, 1969.
6. Smith VC: Color vision of normal observers. In Potts AM: The Assessment of Visual Function. St. Louis, C.V. Mosby, 1972, pp 105–135.

5. THE ELECTRORETINOGRAM, THE ELECTRO-OCULOGRAM, AND DARK ADAPTATION

Caroline R. Baumal, M.D., and Elizabeth L. Affel, M.S.

1. What is the electroretinogram?

The electroretinogram (ERG) is a recording of the electrical discharges from the retina elicited by a flash of light. This response occurs as a result of transretinal movement of ions induced by the light stimulus.

2. How is an ERG performed?

Light is delivered uniformly throughout the entire retina. This is called Ganzfeld or full-field stimulation and is typically achieved with a bowl perimeter. The electrical discharges induced by the light stimulus are recorded directly from the eye with a corneal contact lens electrode. The signal is then amplified and displayed on an oscilloscope or directly written out on an x–y plotter. International standardization of the technique for the full-field ERG has been established to permit comparison between clinical centers.

3. What are the three major components of the ERG?

The ERG is characterized by an initial negative waveform, the **a wave**, which arises from the photoreceptor cells (see figure). This is followed by a positive waveform, the **b wave**, which is generated by the Müller cells and bipolar cells in the outer retina. **Oscillatory potentials** are small wavelets that may be superimposed on the b wave. These oscillatory potentials arise from a number of cell types in the midretinal layers.

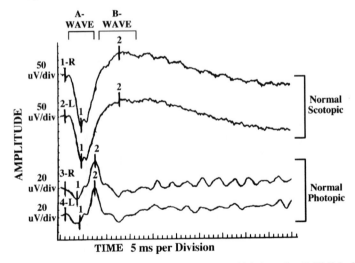

Normal scotopic (dark-adapted) and photopic ERG responses to a high-intensity (0 db) light flash demonstrating the a wave and b wave. Oscillatory potentials are present on the ascending limb of the b wave. The implicit time is measured from the stimulus onset to the peak of the a wave *(1)* or b wave *(2)*. The a wave amplitude is measured from the baseline to the trough of the a wave and b wave amplitude is measured from the trough of the a wave to the peak of the b wave.

4. Describe additional waveforms that may be recorded in the ERG.

Under certain recording conditions, additional waveforms may be noted. The **c wave** follows the b wave and reflects electrical activity at the level of the retinal pigment epithelium and is recorded in the dark-adapted eye. The **early receptor potential** is a rapid transient waveform that occurs immediately after a light stimulus, and this response originates from the bleaching of photopigments at the level of the photoreceptor outer segments.

5. What parameters are measured during evaluation of the ERG?

Two major parameters, the **amplitude** and the **implicit time**, are used to evaluate the ERG response (see figure in question 3). The amplitude is measured in microvolts (μV). The amplitude of the a wave is measured from baseline to the trough of the a wave, and the b wave amplitude is measured from the trough of the a wave to the peak of the b wave. The implicit time is measured in milliseconds (ms) and is defined as the time from the stimulus onset to the peak of the response.

6. How is ERG amplitude affected in retinal disorders?

The full-field light-evoked ERG is a mass response that reflects activity from the entire retina. The amplitude of the ERG is proportional to the area of functioning retina stimulated and is abnormal only when large areas of the retina are functionally impaired.

7. Describe different stimulus conditions and the associated photoreceptor response.

Certain light stimuli allow the isolation of either the cone or rod responses so that each photoreceptor can be studied independently. After sufficient dark adaptation (known as scotopic conditions), the rod responses are optimized. Under the light-adapted or photopic conditions, the rods are sufficiently dampened so that the response is primarily from the cones.

State of Adaptation	Light Stimulus	Photoreceptor Response
Scotopic	Dim white (24 db)	Rod
Scotopic	Dim blue (10 db)	Rod
Scotopic	Bright white (0 db)	Mixed response: maximal rod and cone
Scotopic	Red (0 db)	Mixed response: early cone, late rod
Scotopic	Bright white (0 db)	Cone oscillatory potentials
Photopic	Bright white (0 db)	Cone
Photopic	White flicker at 30 hertz	Pure cone (see figure)

db = decibels.

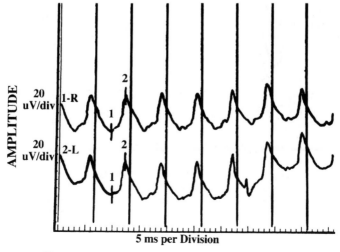

The normal cone response to a flicker light stimulus at 30 hertz.

8. What five responses are evaluated during a standard full-field ERG?
1. Rod response (dark-adapted)
2. Maximal combined rod–cone response (dark-adapted) (see table in question 7)
3. Oscillatory potentials
4. Single flash cone response (light-adapted)
5. 30 hertz flicker cone response (see table in question 7)

9. How is the ERG affected in age-related macular degeneration?
The entire retina is stimulated by a bright flash in the Ganzfeld; thus, the full-field ERG is not affected in either amplitude or implicit time if small areas of the retina are damaged. In eyes with small localized retinal lesions such as those of age-related macular degeneration, the full-field ERG is normal.

10. What does the ERG demonstrate in retinal ganglion cell disease?
The ganglion cells play no role in generation of the full-field ERG. Thus, disorders affecting the ganglion cells, such as glaucoma, do not alter the full-field ERG. On occasion, the b wave may be reduced in optic atrophy or central retinal artery occlusion. This is postulated to result from transsynaptic degeneration from the ganglion to the bipolar cell layer.

11. Describe a clinical application for the oscillatory potential.
A reduction in oscillatory potential amplitudes correlates with an increased risk of developing severe proliferative retinopathy in a diabetic patient.

12. Describe the clinical situations where the ERG is utilized.
• To diagnose a generalized degeneration of the retina
• To assess family members for a known hereditary retinal degeneration
• To assess decreased vision and nystagmus present at birth
• To assess retinal function in the presence of opaque ocular media or vascular occlusion
• To evaluate functional visual loss

13. List the retinal degenerations in which the ERG can be useful to clarify the diagnosis.
Retinitis pigmentosa and related hereditary retinal degenerations
Retinitis pigmentosa sine pigmento
Retinitis punctate albescens
Leber's congenital amaurosis
Choroideremia
Gyrate atrophy of the retina and choroid
Goldman-Favre syndrome
Congenital stationary night blindness
X-linked juvenile retinoschisis
Achromatopsia
Cone dystrophies
Disorders mimicking retinitis pigmentosa

14. What are the clinical features of retinitis pigmentosa?
Retinitis pigmentosa is an inherited retinal disorder characterized by progressive dysfunction of the photoreceptors and other cell layers in the retina. Inheritance may be autosomal dominant, autosomal recessive or X-linked. Both the rods and, to a lesser extent, the cones are abnormal in early retinitis pigmentosa. Clinical features include:
Decreased night vision (nyctalopia)
Positive or negative family history of retinitis pigmentosa
Visual field loss
Abnormal ERG

Ocular features, such as waxy pallor of the optic nerve head, attenuated retinal vessels, mottling of the retinal pigment epithelium with bone-spicule pigmentation, cellophane maculopathy, cystic macular edema, pigment cells in the vitreous, and posterior subcapsular cataract

15. Describe the ERG in retinitis pigmentosa.

Early in the course of retinitis pigmentosa, the ERG shows a reduced amplitude (usually of the b wave) and a prolonged photopic implicit time when compared with the normal ERG (see figure). Over time, the ERG becomes extinguished with no detectable rod or cone responses to a bright white light.

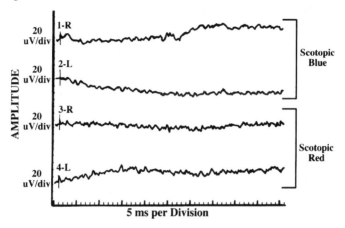

The ERG in retinitis pigmentosa reveals an extinguished response to scotopic blue and scotopic red light stimuli.

16. What does the ERG demonstrate in female carriers of X-linked retinitis pigmentosa?

Female carriers of X-linked retinitis pigmentosa may either have a normal retinal examination or demonstrate findings such as an unusual scintillating macular reflex or clumping of pigment in the periphery in the absence of subjective complaints. ERG abnormalities are noted in the majority of female carriers, even those without fundus abnormalities. These consist of a prolonged photopic b wave implicit time and/or a reduction in the amplitude of the scotopic b wave in the dark-adapted eye.

17. What does the ERG reveal in the congenital rubella syndrome?

Examination of the retina in the congenital rubella syndrome may reveal diffuse pigmentary changes that may be confused with retinitis pigmentosa. However, the ERG is normal in the congenital rubella syndrome. Additional signs associated with this syndrome may include deafness and congenital cataracts.

18. Describe the ERG in X-linked retinoschisis.

Clinical findings in X-linked retinoschisis may include peripheral retinoschisis cavities in 50% of cases and foveal cystic changes in almost all cases. The ERG reveals a reduced scotopic and photopic b wave amplitude, reflecting the widespread midretinal changes that result from the peripheral inner layer retinoschisis.

19. What does the ERG demonstrate in a progressive cone dystrophy?

The ERG reveals a markedly reduced photopic flicker response and a normal rod scotopic response. The ERG may establish this diagnosis prior to the development of symptoms. This disorder appears initially to affect peripheral cones with gradual progression to involve the central cones. When the central cones are intact, the visual acuity and color vision are good; however, the ultimate visual acuity is in the 20/200 range.

20. Why is the ERG useful in patients with congenitally decreased vision?

Three disorders characterized by nystagmus and a congenital decrease in vision may have a normal retinal examination and can be diagnosed with an ERG. These are achromatopsia (also known as rod monochromatism), Leber's congenital amaurosis, and congenital stationary nightblindness.

Achromatopsia is a nonprogressive congenital absence or near absence of cones and is inherited as autosomal recessive. Symptoms may include photophobia and poor color vision. The ERG reveals absent cone function and normal rod function. **Leber's congenital amaurosis** is a congenital form of retinitis pigmentosa and is inherited as autosomal recessive. The retina may appear normal in infancy but shows progressive changes during life. The ERG is extinguished or markedly reduced in amplitude, and vision is typically profoundly impaired. In **congenital stationary nightblindness**, the ERG indicates normal photoreceptors, as evidenced by the normal a wave, but an abnormality in the bipolar cell region as demonstrated by the absent b wave.

21. What does the ERG demonstrate in a central retinal vein occlusion?

Central retinal vein occlusions can be differentiated into nonischemic and ischemic types, with the latter having a poorer visual prognosis and a substantial risk of developing neovascular glaucoma. When large areas of retinal capillary nonperfusion are present, the ERG b wave will be affected. This occurs as the capillary plexus that is ischemic supplies the midretinal layers. In the ischemic variety of central retinal vein occlusion, the ERG may demonstrate a reduced b wave amplitude, a reduced b:a wave ratio and/or a prolonged b wave implicit time.

22. How can the ERG measure retinal function in the presence of opaque ocular media?

The full-field ERG can be used to assess the retinal function when the retina cannot be visualized, either because of a cataract or due to corneal or vitreous opacities. A normal ERG provides information regarding the overall retinal function, but does not indicate whether central vision is normal because macular degeneration and optic atrophy typically do not affect the ERG amplitude. A cataract or corneal opacities act as a diffuser of light, and, on occasion, a "supernormal" ERG may occur. Vitreous opacities hinder the amount of light stimulating the retina, so an intense "bright flash" ERG may be required to deliver light to the retina in order to assess overall retinal function.

23. What are variations on the standard ERG?

The **focal electroretinogram (FERG)** is induced by a focal directed flash of light, and the response is generated from the central cone photoreceptors and outer retina. The FERG can be used to evaluate or follow the progression of focal macular disorders such as early macular degeneration or to demonstrate normal central cone function in a subject with reduced vision.

The **pattern electroretinogram (PERG)** measures the electrical response to an alternating pattern stimulus that has a constant overall retinal luminance. It differs from the full-field and focal ERG as the response generated in the PERG appears to be localized to the ganglion cells. This was determined as the PERG was extinguished after transection of the optic nerve while the full-field was not altered. The PERG may be used to diagnose or monitor disorders such as glaucoma, ocular hypertension, optic neuritis, optic atrophy, and amblyopia. Although ganglion cells appear to generate the PERG, normal functioning retinal cells distal to the ganglion cells are required for a normal PERG. Thus, abnormal PERG responses can occur with retinal degenerations that affect the photoreceptor cells.

24. List the disorders that may demonstrate an extinguished ERG.

Retinitis pigmentosa and related disorders
Ophthalmic artery occlusion

Diffuse unilateral subacute neuroretinitis (DUSN)
Metallosis
Total retinal detachment
Drugs—phenothiazines, chloroquine
Cancer-associated retinopathy

25. List the disorders that may demonstrate a normal a wave and a reduced b wave amplitude.

Central stationary nightblindness
X-linked juvenile retinoschisis
Central retinal vein or artery occlusion
Myotonic dystrophy
Oguchi's disease
Quinine intoxication
Transsynaptic degeneration from the ganglion to the bipolar cell layer (for example, secondary to optic atrophy or central retinal artery occlusion)

26. List the disorders characterized by an abnormal photopic ERG and a normal scotopic ERG.

Achromatopsia (also known as rod monochromatism)
Cone dystrophy

27. What is an electro-oculogram?

The **electro-oculogram**, also known as the **EOG**, is an indirect measure of the standing potential of the eyes (see figure). This standing potential exists because of a voltage difference between the inner and outer retina. The EOG is measured by placing electrodes near the medial and lateral canthi of each eye and having a patient move the eyes back and forth over a specific distance.

The clinical measurement of the EOG relies on the fact that the amplitude of the response changes when the luminance conditions are varied. After dark adaptation, the response progressively decreases, reaching a trough in 8–12 minutes. With light adaptation, there is a progressive rise in amplitude, reaching a peak in 6–9 minutes. The greatest EOG amplitude achieved in light (light peak) is divided by the lowest amplitude in the dark (dark trough) and this calculated ratio is known as the **Arden ratio**. Normal subjects have a value of 1.80 or greater, while a ratio of less than 1.65 is distinctly abnormal.

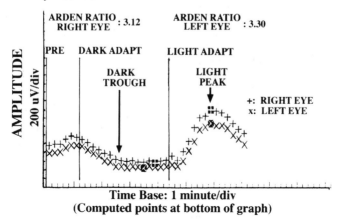

Normal EOG demonstrating the dark trough and light peak.

28. In what retinal location is the EOG response generated?

This electrical response in the EOG is generated by the retinal pigment epithelium with the light peak being produced by a depolarization of the basal portion of the retinal pigment epithelium. To generate the EOG potential, it is necessary to have intact photoreceptors in physical contact with the retinal pigment epithelium. Like the full-field ERG, the EOG reflects activity from the entire retina.

29. What are the clinical uses for the EOG?

The normalcy of the EOG is dependent on the total number of functioning photoreceptors. The EOG is often abnormal in any condition in which the ERG is abnormal. A patient with an extinguished ERG due to retinitis pigmentosa will show little or no EOG light rise, and this is similarly noted in any disorder with widespread generalized degeneration of the photoreceptor cells.

However, an abnormal ERG and a normal EOG may be noted in some disorders. In congenital stationary nightblindness and X-linked retinoschisis, there may be an abnormality in neural transmission in the bipolar cell region, and the EOG may be normal due to normal functioning rods. The EOG light rise is almost completely dependent on rod function, so it is normal in disorders of cone dysfunction.

30. In what disease is the EOG abnormal and the ERG normal?

An abnormal EOG and a normal ERG is the hallmark of dominantly inherited Best's disease (also known as vitelliform macular dystrophy). All patients with Best's disease have an abnormal EOG with an Arden ratio below 1.35. There is a wide range of expressivity in Best's disease such that an individual who has the gene may show no fundus abnormalities, but will have an abnormal EOG. The EOG helps to assess family members at risk, as well as individuals with atypical findings of Best's disease.

31. What are the characteristics of dark adaptation?

Dark adaptometry measures the absolute threshold of cone and rod sensitivity and is tested on an instrument known as the Goldmann-Weekers adaptometer. Initially, the subject is adapted to a bright background light, which is then extinguished. In the dark, the patient is presented with a series of dim lights. The threshold at which the light is just perceived is plotted against time. The normal dark adaptation curve is biphasic, where the first curve represents the cone threshold and is reached in 5–10 minutes, and the second curve represents the rod threshold and is reached after 30 minutes. The rod–cone break is a well-defined point between these 2 curves. Dark adaptometry is useful to evaluate retinal disorders with nightblindness and some conditions with cone dysfunction.

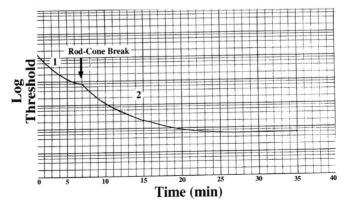

Normal dark adaptation curve demonstrates the rod–cone break at 7 minutes, separating the cone threshold *(1)* and the rod threshold *(2)*.

BIBLIOGRAPHY

1. Berson EL: Retinitis pigmentosa and allied diseases: Applications of electroretinographic testing. Int Ophthalmol 4:7–22, 1981.
2. Bresnick GH, Palta M: Predicting progression to severe proliferative diabetic retinopathy. Arch Ophthalmol 105:810–814, 1987.
3. Breton ME, Montzka DP, Brucker AJ, Quinn GE: Electroretinogram interpretation in central retinal vein occlusion. Ophthalmology 98:1837–1844, 1991.
4. Carr RE: Electroretinography. In Tasman W, Jaeger EA (eds): Duane's Clinical Ophthalmology, vol 2. Philadelphia, J.B. Lippincott, 1990.
5. Carr RE, Siegel IM: Electrodiagnostic Testing of the Visual System: A Clinical Guide. Philadelphia, F.A. Davis, 1990.
6. Deutman AF: Electro-oculography in families with vitelliform dystrophy of the fovea: Detection of the carrier state. Arch Ophthalmol 81:305–316, 1969.
7. Fish GE, Birch DG: The focal electroretinogram in the clinical assessment of macular disease. Ophthalmology 96:109–114, 1989.
8. Fishman GA, Sokol S: Electrophysiologic Testing in Disorders of the Retina, Optic Nerve, and Visual Pathways. American Academy of Ophthalmology, 1990.
9. Francois J, de Rouch A, Fernandez-Sasso D: Electro-oculography in vitelliform degeneration of the macula. Arch Ophthalmol 77:726–733, 1967.
10. Gass JDM: A clinicopathologic study of a peculiar foveomacular dystrophy. Trans Am Ophthalmol Soc 72:139, 1974.
11. Marmor MF, Arden GB, Nilsson SEG, Zrenner E (International Standardization Committee): Standard for clinical electroretinography. Arch Ophthalmol 107:816–819, 1989.

6. OPHTHALMIC ULTRASONOGRAPHY

Caroline R. Baumal, M.D., FRCSC

1. What are the indications for ophthalmic ultrasonography?
- Evaluation of the anterior or posterior segment in eyes with opaque ocular media
- Assessment of the dimensions of ocular tumors as well as their tissue characteristics such as calcium in retinoblastoma or choroidal osteoma
- Evaluation of orbital disorders
- Detection and localization of intraocular foreign bodies
- Measurement of distances within the eye and orbit (also known as biometry)

2. What frequency is used for standard ophthalmic ultrasonography?
Ultrasound is an acoustic wave that consists of an oscillation of particles within a medium. By definition, ultrasound waves have a frequency greater than 20 kHz. In standard ophthalmic ultrasound, frequencies are in the range of 8–10 MHz. This high frequency produces short wavelengths, which allow precise resolution of small ocular structures. In contrast, abdominal ultrasound typically uses a lower frequency in the range of 1–5 MHz, which produces longer wavelengths that permit deeper penetration into tissues. Resolution of structures is decreased, although resolution is less critical because the structures in the abdomen are much larger than those within the eye.

3. What are the principles of ultrasonography?
Ultrasound is based on physical principles of tissue-acoustic impedance mismatch and pulse-echo technology. As the acoustic wave is propagated through tissues, part of the wave may be reflected toward the source of the emitted wave (i.e., the probe). This reflected wave is referred to as an echo. Echoes are generated at adjoining tissue interfaces that have differential acoustic impedance. The greater the difference in acoustic impedance, the stronger the echo. For example, strong reflections occur at the interface between retinal tissue and vitreous, which is essentially water. When adjoining tissue interfaces have relatively small differences in acoustic impedance, (e.g, vitreous gel and mild vitreous hemorrhage or clumped intravitreal white blood cells), weak reflections are seen. Pulse-echo technology uses synthetic crystal transducers to produce ultrasonic wavefront pulses and to retrieve echoes for electronic display processing.

4. How is the clinical ophthalmic ultrasound displayed?
The reflected echoes are received, amplified, electronically processed, and displayed in visual format as an A-scan and/or a B-scan.

5. What is A-scan ultrasonography?
A-scan ultrasonography, or the A-mode, is a one-dimensional, time-amplitude display. The horizontal baseline represents the distance and depends on the time required for the sound beam to reach a given interface and for its echo to return to the probe. In the vertical dimension, the height of the displayed spike indicates the amplitude or strength of the echo. The A-scan may be accompanied by a simultaneous B-scan image with a vector line to demonstrate the position of the A-scan information.

6. What is B-scan ultrasonography?
B-scan ultrasonography, or the B-mode, produces a two-dimensional, cross-sectional display of the globe and orbit. The image is displayed in variable shades of gray, and the shade depends on the echo strength. Strong echoes appear white, and weaker reflections are seen as gray.

Examples of strong echoes include retinal tissue, sclera, and calcification. Weaker echoes are noted from clotted vitreous cells. B-scan images may be more easily interpreted than A-scan images, because the microscopic and gross cross-section evaluation of ocular abnormalities is often similar to the B-scan image.

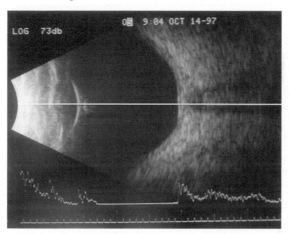

A-scan (bottom) and B-scan (top) of the normal globe. A cross-sectional anterior-posterior view is presented in the B-scan. The lens capsule is seen toward the left of the display, and the optic nerve is seen toward the right. A vector line through the B-scan demonstrates the position of the A-scan information.

7. What clinical information is provided by the A-scan and B-scan?

The A-scan is used predominantly for tissue characterization, whereas the B-scan is used to obtain architectural information. Information obtained from the A-scan and B-scan overlaps, and both scans may be required for ultrasound interpretation. Ultrasound results are most useful when combined with clinical and radiographic examination. A-scans are also helpful in determining intraocular lens calculations for cataract surgery (see question 10).

8. What lesion features are evaluated during the ultrasound examination?

1. The **topography** (location, configuration, and extension) of a lesion is evaluated most often by the two-dimensional B-scan.

2. The **quantitative features** include the reflectivity, internal structure, and sound attenuation of a lesion.

- The **reflectivity** of a lesion is evaluated by observing the height of the spike on the A-scan and the signal brightness on the B-scan. The internal reflectivity refers to the amplitude of echoes within a lesion and correlates with its histologic architecture.
- The **internal structure** refers to the degree of variation in the histologic architecture within a mass lesion. Regular internal structure indicates a homogeneous architecture and is noted by minimal or no variation in the height of spikes on the A-scan and a uniform appearance of echoes on the B-scan. In contrast, an irregular internal structure is noted in a lesion with a heterogeneous architecture and is characterized by variations in the echo appearance.
- **Sound attenuation** occurs when the acoustic wave is scattered, reflected, or absorbed by a tissue and is noted by a decrease in the strength of echoes either within or posterior to a lesion. It is indicated by a decrease in spike height on A-scan or a decrease in the brightness of echoes on B-scan. Sound attenuation may produce decreased signal strength and a void posterior to the lesion that is referred to as shadowing. Substances such as bone, calcium, and foreign bodies typically produce sound attenuation (see figure on next page).

3. The **dynamic features** of or within a lesion can be detected on B-scan.
   - **Aftermovement** is determined by observing the motion of lesion echoes after cessation of eye movements. The rapid movement of a vitreous hemorrhage is distinguished from the slower, undulating movement of the retina in an acute rhegmatogenous retinal detachment.
   - **Vascularity** is indicated by spontaneous motion of echoes within a lesion and represents blood flow within vessels.

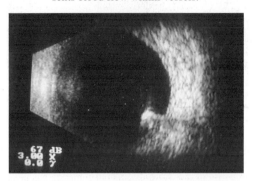

B-scan image of a metallic foreign body located on the surface of the retina. A bright echo is produced by the foreign body with shadowing of the structures posteriorly.

9. How is ocular ultrasound performed?

A standardized examination technique is used for A-scan and B-scan ultrasonography. An immersion technique is used to evaluate the anterior segment. Immersion is accomplished by inserting a small scleral shell between the lids, filling the shell with methylcellulose solution, and placing the probe in the solution. The contact method, in which the probe is placed directly on the globe, is used to evaluate the posterior segment. For contact examination, each quadrant of the globe is scanned systematically. The ultrasound probe positions are chosen to avoid passage of the examining beam or returning echoes through the patient's artifact-inducing lens system. The ultrasound information is most often recorded with a Polaroid photograph of specific "frozen" images that are chosen during the examination, although this technique does not capture the dynamic information obtained during the ultrasound examination.

10. How is ultrasound used in the preoperative cataract evaluation?

The A-scan is used to measure the axial length of the globe, which is required in the formula to calculate the intraocular lens power. The B-scan is useful if the ocular media are opaque to assess for a retinal disorder that may affect visual outcome after cataract surgery.

11. How is ultrasound used to assess intraocular tumors?

Ultrasound may be used for diagnosis, to plan treatment, and to evaluate tumor response to therapy. Specifically the tumor shape, dimensions (such as thickness and basal diameter), and tissue characteristics are evaluated, along with the presence of extraocular extension.

12. What are the characteristic features of a choroidal melanoma on ultrasound?

- Collar-button or mushroom shape
- Low-to-medium internal reflectivity
- Regular internal structure
- Internal blood flow (vascularity)

13. Describe the A-scan pattern of a choroidal melanoma.

The initial echo from the tumor surface on A-scan is a high-amplitude spike secondary to a strong echo from the vitreoretinal interface overlying the tumor. When the acoustic beam passes into the tumor tissue, there is a rapid decline in the amplitude of the echo, which is noted as decreased height of the spike on A-scan (known as low-to-medium internal reflectivity). This is a consequence of tissue homogeneity within the tumor and is revealed on microscopic evaluation as tightly packed, homogeneous small cells.

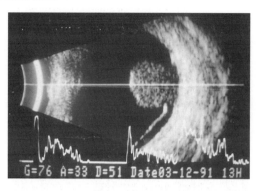

A-scan and B-scan of choroidal melanoma. The B-scan reveals a collar button-shaped mass with a regular internal structure. A serous retinal detachment extends from the margin of the tumor. The A-scan reveals a strong initial echo from the retinal tissue overlying the tumor followed by rapid decline in the A-scan echo amplitude (low internal reflectivity) within the tumor tissue. High reflectivity is noted again at the level of the sclera and orbital fat.

14. What is choroidal excavation?

On B-scan, choroidal excavation refers to a dark appearance in the normally highly reflective choroidal tissue and results from tumor invasion of the choroid. This phenomenon has been described in choroidal melanoma as well as other choroidal disorders.

15. Describe the ultrasound patterns in the differential diagnosis of choroidal melanoma.

Ultrasound is often used in the evaluation of choroidal melanoma, choroidal hemangioma, metastatic choroidal carcinoma, choroidal nevus, choroidal hemorrhage, and a disciform lesion. It should be combined with clinical information because there are more tumor types than differentiating ultrasound patterns.

Lesion	Location	Shape	Internal Reflectivity	Internal Structure	Vascularity
Melanoma	Choroid and/or ciliary body	Dome or collar button	Low to medium	Regular	Yes
Choroidal hemangioma	Choroid, posterior pole	Dome	High	Regular	No
Metastatic carcinoma	Choroid, posterior pole	Diffuse, irregular	Medium to high	Irregular	No
Choroidal nevus	Choroid	Dome or flat	High	Regular	No
Choroidal hemorrhage	Choroid	Dome	Variable	Variable	No
Disciform lesion	Macula	Dome, irregular	High	Variable	No

16. Describe the ultrasound features of a choroidal hemangioma.

Within a choroidal hemangioma, the adjoining cell and tissue layers have marked differences in acoustic impedance (acoustic heterogeneity), which create large echo amplitudes at each interface. The A-scan reveals high internal reflections within the tumor, and lesions appear solid white on the B-scan.

17. Describe the ultrasound features of a retinal detachment.

The B-scan can be used to localize retinal detachment and to determine its configuration. Detached retina produces a bright, continuous, folded appearance on B-scan. When detachment is total or extensive, the retina inserts into both the optic nerve and ora serrata. The A-scan reveals a 100% high spike when the sound beam is directed perpendicular to the detached retina. In an acute rhegmatogenous retinal detachment, there is motion of the detached retina with voluntary eye movement; however, it is less mobile than with a posterior vitreous detachment.

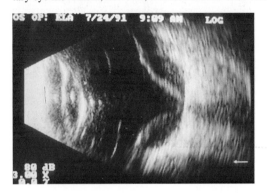

B-scan of a total retinal detachment. An anteroposterior view reveals the characteristic V-shaped appearance with attachment to the optic nerve. A cataract is also present.

18. What features indicate a chronic retinal detachment?

A chronic retinal detachment may show calcification, intraretinal cysts, or cholesterol debris in the subretinal space.

19. Describe the ultrasound features that differentiate retinal detachment, posterior vitreous detachment, and choroidal detachment.

Ultrasound Features	Retinal Detachment	Posterior Vitreous Detachment	Choroidal Detachment
Topographic (B-scan)	Smooth or folded surface Open or closed funnel with insertion at optic nerve Inserts at ora serrata With or without intraretinal cysts	Smooth surface Open funnel with or without disc or fundus insertion Inserts at ora serrata or ciliary body	Smooth, dome, or flat surface No disc insertion Inserts at ora serrata or ciliary body
Quantitative (A-scan)	Steep 100% high spike	Variable spike height that is < 100%	Steeply rising, thick, double-peaked 100% high spike
Mobility after eye movement	Moderate to none	Marked to moderate	Mild to none

20. How is ultrasound used to evaluate patients with proliferative diabetic retinopathy and vitreous hemorrhage?

Ultrasound can assess for the presence of a tractional retinal detachment involving the fovea when visualization is obscured by vitreous hemorrhage. This finding is often an indication for intraocular surgery in diabetics.

21. Describe the ultrasound findings in asteroid hyalosis.

In asteroid hyalosis, calcium soaps in the vitreous produce bright echoes on B-scan that move with the vitreous. An area of clear vitreous gel is typically present between the posterior boundary of the opacities and the posterior hyaloid face. On A-scan, the calcium soaps produce medium-to-high reflective spikes.

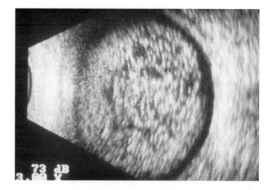

B-scan image of bright echoes in the vitreous in asteroid hyalosis.

22. What is the appearance of calcification on ultrasound?

Intraocular calcification creates a strong acoustic interface, resulting in a high-amplitude A-scan peak as well as white echoes on the B-scan. Behind the area of calcification, there is usually partial or complete shadowing of the sclera and orbital fat.

23. What ocular conditions may demonstrate calcification on ultrasound?

- Tumors (retinoblastoma, choroidal osteoma, optic nerve sheath meningioma, choroidal hemangioma, choroidal melanoma)
- Toxocara granuloma
- Chronic retinal detachment
- Optic nerve head drusen
- Disciform retinal lesion
- Vascular occlusive disease of the optic nerve
- Phthisis bulbi
- Intumescent cataractous lens

24. When is ultrasound used to evaluate ocular trauma?

Ultrasound may be used to evaluate the position of the lens and the status of the retina if visualization is impeded by an opaque cornea, hyphema, or vitreous hemorrhage resulting from trauma. It also may diagnose a posterior rupture site in the globe and assess for an intraocular foreign body.

The globe should be evaluated visually by slit lamp technique before ultrasonography to determine whether ocular integrity has been severely disrupted and whether ultrasound examination is indicated. Radiographs or computed tomography for foreign bodies preferably should be performed before ultrasonography. It is necessary to avoid undue pressure on the globe during the ultrasound evaluation and to use sterile methylcellulose solution to decrease the potential risk of infection.

25. What are the ultrasound findings with an intraocular foreign body?

Ultrasound may diagnose and localize an intraocular foreign body (see figure with question 8), although ultrasound examination alone is not sufficient to exclude a foreign body. It is particularly useful with a nonmetallic intraocular foreign body that may not be visible radiographically. Although computerized tomography is often used for localization, it may not be able to define the exact position of a foreign body that lies close to the ocular wall.

Foreign bodies have high reflectivity when the ultrasound probe beam is perpendicular to a reflective surface of the foreign body. On B-scan, a metallic foreign body produces a bright echo that persists when the gain of the ultrasound output is decreased. Small spherical metallic foreign bodies may demonstrate ringing, which is a string of reflections that extends posterior to the foreign body and is produced by reflections of the acoustic pulses within the foreign body. Shadowing is often present behind a foreign body because of nearly complete reflection of the examining probe beam.

26. List the structures and disorders that can be evaluated by orbital ultrasound.

The orbit, extraocular muscles, and optic nerve can be reassessed for tumors, vascular lesions, infectious and inflammatory processes, effects of trauma, and presence of intraorbital foreign bodies.

27. What are the ultrasound findings in thyroid orbitopathy?

Orbital ultrasound is useful to evaluate exophthalmos related to a number of diseases. In thyroid orbitopathy, thickening of the extraocular muscles has a characteristic appearance that is noted on B-scan as thickening of the muscle belly that spares the tendinous insertion. The internal reflectivity of the thickened muscle is medium to high as a consequence of the tissue interfaces created within the muscle lamella by edema and inflammation. Ultrasound may reveal mild changes in the extraocular muscles before detection of a thyroid disorder on clinical examination.

Other findings may include enlargement of the lacrimal gland, thickening of the periorbital tissues, enlargement of the superior ophthalmic vein, and thickening of the optic nerve sheath if the optic nerve is compressed. Thickening of the muscle tendon and fluid in the episcleral space rarely may be noted with acute thyroid ophthalmopathy.

28. What are the features of phthisis bulbi?

Phthisis bulbi may result from a variety of chronic ocular disorders and is characterized by severe irregular shrinkage of the eye. On ultrasound examination, the globe is often so shrunken that the normal ocular structures cannot be identified and it is not possible to exclude the presence of a small intraocular tumor. There is extensive calcification of the posterior ocular coats, the subretinal space may be filled with dense opacities, and there is often a total, funnel-shaped retinal detachment.

29. What is ultrasound biomicroscopy?

Ultrasound biomicroscopy (UBM) is a new B-scan method that uses high frequencies in the range of 50–100 MHz. The depth of penetration is in the range of 5–7 mm. This technique produces high-resolution images of anterior segment structures and has been useful for characterizing the mechanism of secondary glaucomas.

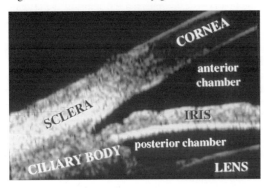

Ultrasound biomicroscopic image of the anterior segment angle structures.

BIBLIOGRAPHY

1. Byrne SF, Green RL: Ultrasound of the Eye and Orbit. St. Louis, Mosby, 1992.
2. Coleman DJ: Reliability of ocular and orbital diagnosis with B-scan ultrasound. II: Orbital diagnosis. Am J Ophthalmol 74:708, 1972.
3. Dallow RL, Hart LJ: Ultrasound diagnosis of the eye and orbit. In Albert DM, Jakobiec FA (eds): Principles and Practice of Ophthalmology: Clinical Practice. Philadelphia, W.B. Saunders, 1994, pp 3543–3554.
4. Fisher YL: Diagnostic ophthalmic ultrasonography. In Tasman W, Jaeger EA (eds): Duane's Clinical Ophthalmology, vol 2. Philadelphia, J.B. Lippincott, 1990.
5. Ossoinig KC: Quantitative echography: The basis of tissue differentiation. J Clin Ultrasound 2:33, 1974.
6. Pavlin CJ, Harasiewicz K, Sherar MD, et al: Clinical use of ultrasound biomicroscopy. Ophthalmology 98:287, 1991.

7. VISUAL FIELDS

David S. Friedman, M.D., M.P.H.

1. What is hemianopia?

Hemianopia is defective vision or blindness in half of the visual field of one or both eyes.

2. Define the terms *homonymous* and *congruous* in relation to visual field defects.

Homonymous: Pertaining to the corresponding vertical halves of the visual fields of both eyes. In plain language, the term is used for defects that occur after neurologic insults that cause loss of a portion of the visual field subsumed by both eyes.

Congruous: Matched visual field defects, indicating a more posterior neurologic lesion.

3. What is a cecocentral lesion?

A lesion involving both the blind spot and the macular area (to the 25° circle). Four primary causes are typically cited; dominant optic atrophy, Leber's optic atrophy, toxic/nutritional optic neuropathy, and congenital pit of the optic nerve with a serous retinal detachment. Optic neuritis also may cause cecocentral lesions.

4. What is meant by a "pie-in-the-sky" lesion?

A "pie-in-the-sky" lesion is a homonymous hemianopia involving the superior quadrant. The term indicates a lesion in the optic radiations through the temporal lobe, but similar defects can be seen with occipital lobe lesions as well.

5. Define scotoma.

An area of lost or depressed vision within the visual field surrounded by an area of less depressed or normal visual field.

6. What is meant by full-threshold testing?

Full-threshold testing refers to static visual field testing in which the exact threshold of the eye is measured at every point tested. This technique differs from suprathreshold testing. In suprathreshold testing, the subject either sees or does not see a test object presented at a fixed intensity. This is a pass/fail approach to testing. Suprathreshold testing strategies are used in screening programs and may miss early defects.

7. Where is the physiologic blind spot located?

In the temporal visual field. The fovea is the center of the visual field. The blind spot is located 15° temporally and just below the horizontal plane. It is marked by a triangle on a Humphrey visual field.

8. How do you know whether the visual field at which you are looking is from the left or right eye?

Hold the field in front of you and note where the blind spot is located. The right eye has the blind spot (and hence, the temporal visual field) on the right and the left eye has the blind spot on the left. If field loss is so great that the blind spot is hard to identify, the top of the printout tells you which eye was tested.

9. What is a Goldmann visual field?

In addition to inventing what is still the most accurate clinical method of measuring intraocular pressure and a lens for viewing the filtering angle (which is still in use today), Hans Goldmann standardized the conditions under which visual fields are taken. The background illumination and the intensity of the light stimulus were made uniform so that tests could be compared over time. The test object is brought into the field of view from the far periphery. Because the object moves, this technique is known as kinetic perimetry. Goldmann visual fields are less sensitive to subtle changes of the field than current static tests (such as the Humphrey and Octopus machines) and therefore are less commonly used today. They also require highly trained personnel to administer the test.

10. What are the causes of a ring scotoma?

Although both severe glaucoma and retinitis pigmentosa can cause a ring scotoma, this defect is often associated with functional visual loss (either hysterical or malingering). Other causes include vitamin A deficiency and other retinal disease that damages the peripheral retina selectively (such as retinitis or choroiditis). Hysteria and malingering can be tested in many ways. For example, a Goldmann visual field can be used to document spiraling (an isopter of greater luminance overlaps one that is dimmer).

11. What are the most common visual field findings in glaucoma?

Glaucoma is a disease characterized by loss of retinal ganglion cells with characteristic optic nerve findings. The classic defects are determined by the anatomy of retinal ganglion cells as they travel to the optic nerve. The axons circle around the fovea in an arc. With damage to the nerve bundles, the classic finding is an arc-shaped defect in the nasal field. Such a defect obeys the horizontal midline (in contrast to neurologic field defects, which obey the vertical midline). In addition to these arcuate defects, generalized depression of the visual field is one of the early findings in glaucoma. The exam of the optic nerve is helpful in making the diagnosis in less clear cases.

12. When has the visual field of a person with glaucoma progressed?

The answer remains controversial. First, do not base a diagnosis of glaucoma on one field. If there is clear optic nerve damage and a corresponding visual field defect, one can make the diagnosis, but the baseline field needs to be repeated because of the general tendency of people to improve after taking the test several times. Persons with glaucoma tend to have more variable fields than normal subjects; thus, a single visual field showing worsening should be confirmed with a repeat field. One study concluded that to be certain of progression, one needs a minimum of 5 years of annual visual fields. Ongoing research is trying to improve our ability to determine which patients are progressing.

13. What are the major causes of bitemporal hemianopia?

Lesions of the chiasm cause bitemporal hemianopia because they damage the crossing nasal nerve fibers. Masses in this area include pituitary tumors, meningiomas, aneurysms, craniopharyngiomas, gliomas, and other less common tumors. In addition, the chiasm may be damaged by trauma (which typically causes a complete bitemporal hemianopia), demyelinating disease, inflammatory diseases such as sarcoidosis, and, rarely, ischemia.

Summary of Nonglaucomatous Visual Field Defects

LESION	VISUAL FIELD
Optic nerve	Central and cecocentral scotomas, or altitudinal defects
Optic chiasm	Anterior: junctional* Body and Posterior: bitemporal hemianopia
Optic tract	Incongruous homonymous hemianopia with or without central scotoma
Optic radiations	Internal capsule: congruous homonymous hemianopia Temporal lobe: superior quadrantanopia Parietal lobe: inferior quadrantanopia
Occipital lobe	Posterior: highly congruous homonymous hemianopia Anterior: Monocular contralateral temporal defect

* Unilateral hemianopia associated with a contralateral superior temporal field defect.

14. What does help to differentiate the various lesions?

1. Monocular defects must be prechiasmal with one exception: the far temporal visual field is seen only by one eye. This means that an anterior occipital infarct can cause a monocular temporal defect.

2. Lesions posterior to the chiasm do not cross the vertical meridian by more than 15°.

3. People with postchiasmal defects typically have normal visual acuity, normal pupils, and a normal exam of the ocular fundus. The major exception to this last rule is the finding of papilledema in patients with space-occupying lesions.

15. What does the future hold for visual field testing?

The three important advances in visual field testing are faster algorithms that decrease test time, short wavelength automated perimetry (SWAP), and frequency-doubling perimetry. The new algorithm uses previous patient responses to help choose the testing threshold and thereby takes less time. Test times are approximately 5 minutes per eye as opposed to 15 minutes with the older algorithms. SWAP may detect field loss earlier than traditional white-on-white perimetry. SWAP uses standard static threshold testing strategies with a blue test object on a yellow background. Early results indicate that visual field defects may be detected several years earlier with SWAP than with standard static testing. Finally, frequency-doubling perimetry is in the early stages of development but may be extremely useful as a screening tool in the future.

BIBLIOGRAPHY

1. Anderson DA: Automated Static Perimetry. St. Louis, Mosby, 1992.
2. Dorland's Illustrated Medical Dictionary, 28th ed. Philadelphia, W.B. Saunders, 1994.
3. Johnson CA, Brandt JD, Khong AM, Adams AJ: Short-wavelength automated perimetry in low-, medium-, and high-risk ocular hypertensive eyes. Arch Ophthalmol 113:70–76, 1995.
4. Johnson CA, Samuels SJ: Screening for glaucomatous visual field loss with frequency-doubling perimetry. Invest Ophthalmol Vis Sci 38:413–425, 1997.
5. Katz J, Tielsch JM, Quigley HA, Sommer A: Automated perimetry detects field loss before manual Goldmann perimetry. Ophthalmology 102:21–26, 1995.
6. Miller NR: Walsh and Hoyt's Clinical Neuro-Ophthalmology, vol 1. Baltimore, Williams & Wilkins, 1982.
7. Smith SD, Katz J, Quigley HA: Analysis of progressive changes in automated visual fields in glaucoma. Invest Ophthalmol Vis Sci 37:1419–1428, 1996.

II. Cornea and External Diseases

8. THE RED EYE

Janice A. Gault, M.D.

1. Name the main causes of a red eye.
- Conjunctivitis
- Scleritis
- Anterior uveitis
- Episcleritis
- Corneal disease and trauma
- Acute glaucoma

2. A 40-year-old woman complains of watery, itchy eyes with swollen lids. How should you proceed?

In the differential diagnosis of a red eye, the history is often helpful. By asking more questions, you find that she has been mowing the grass; subsequently, her hayfever worsened and her eyes flared. Examination reveals red edematous lids, chemosis, conjunctival papillae, and mucous strands in the cul-de-sac. A preauricular node is not palpable. Appropriate treatment includes systemic medications such as lovatidine (Claritin) or diphenhydramine (Benadryl), a topical mast-cell inhibitor, and/or an antihistamine.

A patient who is allergic to a medication used in or around the eyes presents in a similar fashion. Typical offenders include aminoglycosides, sulfa medications, atropine, epinephrine agents, apraclonidine, trifluorothymidine (Viroptic), pilocarpine, and any ophthalmic medication with preservatives. Immediate cessation of the offending agent as well as cool compresses and preservative-free artificial tears or a topical antiallergy medication are appropriate. Impress on the patient that lid rubbing will worsen the condition. If the lid reaction is severe, an ophthalmic steroid cream may be prescribed. Some patients are affected severely enough to develop an ectropion of their lower lids.

If the patient states that her child came home from school recently with "pink eye," examination may reveal tarsal conjunctival follicles as well as a preauricular node. In more severe cases, the patient may have membranes or pseudomembranes. Often, the condition may begin in one eye and spread to the other. Viral conjunctivitis may precede, accompany, or follow an upper respiratory infection. This condition is contagious, and patients need to be warned not to leave any contaminated material in a place where others may touch it. Frequent handwashing is crucial. The physician's exam room needs to be washed down thoroughly, because an epidemic may occur among other patients as well as staff. Patients should not return to work until the eyes stop weeping, often as long as 2 weeks. The condition typically worsens in the first week before improving over the course of 2–3 weeks. Treatment is mainly supportive with artificial tears and cool compresses. Only in select cases should steroid therapy be used. Examples include subepithelial infiltrates that reduce vision and membranes or pseudomembranes. Steroids may help in the short term but often increase the duration of the disease.

3. A 25-year-old man states that his eyes have been dripping with discharge over the past 8 hours. You notice significant purulent discharge, a preauricular node, and marked chemosis. What is the next step?

This condition is an emergency. The most likely diagnosis is gonococcal conjunctivitis. An immediate Gram stain and conjunctival scrapings for culture and sensitivities are imperative. Cultures should be done on blood agar, on chocolate agar at 37°C and 10% CO_2, and a Thayer-Martin plate.

4. What are you looking for on the Gram stain?

Gram-negative intracellular diplococci.

5. How should the patient be treated?

1. Ceftriaxone, 1 gm IM in a single dose. However, if corneal involvement exists or you are unable to visualize the cornea because of chemosis and lid swelling, the patient should be hospitalized and treated with ceftriaxone, 1 gm IV every 12–24 hours. *Neisseria gonorrhoeae* can perforate an intact cornea quickly.

2. Topical bacitracin or erythromycin ointment 4 times/day or ciprofloxacin drops every 2 hours.

3. Eye irrigation with saline 4 times/day until the discharge is gone.

4. Tetracycline or doxycycline for 2–3 weeks for chlamydial infection, which often coexists. Use erythromycin if the patient is pregnant or breast feeding because of the risk of teeth staining.

5. Referral of the patient and sexual partners to family doctors for evaluation of other sexually transmitted diseases.

6. A 35-year-old man complains of pain in his left eye for several days, watery discharge, and blurred vision. He thinks he has had the same symptoms before. He admits to stress on the job as well as a recent cold sore. What do you expect to see?

Herpes simplex. With fluorescein staining of the eye, you can see a dendritic ulcer with terminal bulbs. It is placed centrally, accounting for the decrease in vision. The patient may also have some anterior chamber cell and flare. He needs a topical antiviral such as trifluorothymidine (Viroptic) and a cycloplegic drop if photophobia and anterior chamber reaction are significant.

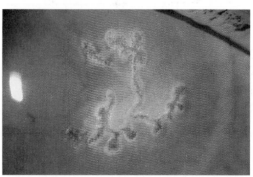

A dendrite typical of herpes simplex keratitis with epithelial ulceration, raised edges, and terminal bulbs. (From Tasman W, Jaeger EA: Wills Eye Hospital Atlas of Clinical Ophthalmology. Philadelphia, Lippincott-Raven, 1995, with permission.) (See Fig. 1, Color Plates.)

7. An 80-year-old woman complains of red eyes that constantly tear and burn. She also feels foreign body sensation and reports that her vision is not as clear as before. The vision varies with tear blink. She has noticed this condition over the past several years. What may you find?

On exam, you may find a poor tear film filled with debris, a low tear meniscus, superficial punctate keratopathy inferiorly or throughout the cornea, and, if severe, mucus filaments adherent to the cornea. A normal meniscus is 1 mm in height in a convex shape. A Shirmer test can quantify her tearing. Rose bengal stains the cornea and conjunctiva (see figure, top of next page). Make sure that she can close her eyes completely, because lagophthalmos may cause similar symptoms. The condition may be due to an eyelid deformity from scarring, tumor, or Bell's palsy. Patients may have trouble closing their eyes after ptosis surgery.

Treatment for dry eye is aimed at increasing tear film with lubricants such as artificial tears and ointments as well as keeping the tears in the eye longer by using punctal plus if frequent installation is not enough. Mucus strands can be debrided, and acetylcysteine may help to prevent recurrence.

8. What may cause dry eye syndrome?

Causes include collagen vascular diseases (rheumatoid arthritis and Sjögren's syndrome are common), conjunctival scarring, vitamin A deficiency, infiltration of the lacrimal glands by sarcoid or tumor, and medications such as oral contraceptives, antihistamines, beta blockers, and phenothiazines. Dry eye syndrome also may be idiopathic and occur in any age group, but it is more common in women and elderly people. Referral to an internist is appropriate if history and symptoms suggest an undiagnosed collagen vascular disease.

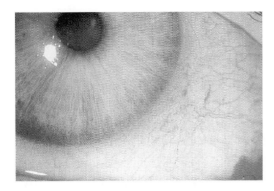

Rose bengal will stain devitalized epithelial cells and mucus in dry eye syndrome. (From Tasman W, Jaeger EA: Wills Eye Hospital Atlas of Clinical Ophthalmology. Philadelphia, Lippincott-Raven, 1995, with permission.)

9. What else may cause superficial punctate keratopathy (SPK)?

Blepharitis, trauma from eye rubbing, exposure, topical drug toxicity, ultraviolet burns (welder's flash, snow blindness), foreign body under the upper lid, mild chemical injury, trichiasis, floppy lid syndrome, entropion, and ectropion may cause SPK. Treatment consists of lubrication and eliminating the cause.

10. An 83-year-old man has crusty lids and red eyes, and complains of "sand in my eyes." What is your diagnosis?

A common scenario indeed. Blepharitis manifests with crusty, red, thickened eyelid margins with prominent blood vessels. Inspissated oil glands at the lid margins cause meibomianitis. Patients often have both and complain of red, tearing eyes. The lids may be significantly swollen. Patients often have trouble opening their eyes in the morning because of the amount of crusting. SPK is common.

This chronic condition requires indefinite treatment. Warm compresses 4 times/day for 10 minutes at a time, baby shampoo on a washcloth to scrub the eyelid margins twice a day, and artificial tears as needed will help. It may take a week or two of compliance before improvement is seen. Once the condition is under better control, the regimen can be reduced to once a day or as needed. However, when the condition flares, the regimen needs to be increased. In severe cases, a topical antibiotic/steroid combination may be helpful in the short term, but make sure that the patient understands the risks of long-term use of steroids (e.g., cataracts, glaucoma, increased risk of infection).

Patients also may have trichiasis or misdirected lashes that scratch the cornea and conjunctiva. If this condition is found, the lashes can be epilated. If they become a recurring problem, electrolysis or cryotherapy may provide a more permanent solution.

11. A 45-year-old man with red, weepy eyes complains of foreign body sensation, which has been occurring for a while. Of note, you realize he has a bulbous nose and telangiectasias across both cheeks. What is your diagnosis? How do you treat?

Acne rosacea is a disease of the eyes and the skin. Pustules, papules, telangiectasias, and erythema develop on the nose, cheeks, and forehead. Rhinophyma occurs in the later stages of the disease. Telangiectasias of the eyelid margin and chalazia are common as are blepharitis and meibomianitis. Dry eyes, SPK, phylectenules, and staphylococcal hypersensitivity may occur. In severe cases, the cornea may develop vascularization and even perforate.

Treatment for blepharitis and meibomianitis with warm compresses and lid scrubs may be all that is necessary. If the patient does not respond, tetracycline or doxycycline for several weeks may relieve the symptoms. However, some patients require a low dose indefinitely. Erythromycin should be substituted in pregnant or nursing women and children. A low-dose antibiotic/steroid combination may be useful if SPK or staphylococcal hypersensitivity is a problem; staphylococcal exotoxins may be the cause. However, patients also develop infected corneal ulcers; thus, scrapings for smears and cultures may be necessary before steroids are used.

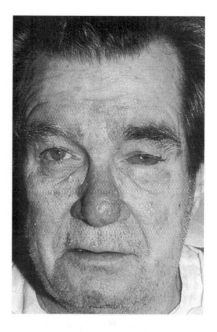

Blepharitis as seen in a patient with acne rosacea. Note the telangiectasis of the nose and cheeks. (From Tasman W, Jaeger EA: Wills Eye Hospital Atlas of Clinical Ophthalmology. Philadelphia, Lippincott-Raven, 1995, with permission.)

12. An 18-year-old contact lens wearer comes in with her hand over her right eye. She noticed that her eye was somewhat red and irritated 2 days ago but believes that it has gotten worse even though she took out her lens at that time. What are you concerned about?

Whenever a contact lens wearer complains of a red, irritated eye that does not improve over a few hours, a corneal ulcer is high on the differential. After a corneal anesthetic such as proparacaine is instilled, the patient feels some relief and can tolerate examination. You notice a corneal infiltrate with an overlying epithelial defect and anterior chamber cell and flare. See the chapter on corneal infections for the necessary work-up and treatment.

13. What else is in the differential diagnosis of a red eye in a contact lens wearer?

1. Hypersensitivity reactions to preservatives in solution. The patient may develop an allergy or may not be rinsing the enzyme off completely before placing the lens in the eye.

2. Giant papillary conjunctivitis. Patients have large conjunctival papillae on upper lid eversion. Patients may need to discontinue lens wear for several weeks, change to a disposable lens regimen, and/or use topical medications such as nonsteroidal antiinflammatory medications, mast cell inhibitors, or antihistamines. Increased enzyme use and discontinuation of overnight wear also help.

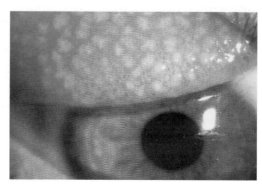

A typical case of giant papillary conjunctivitis in a contact lens wearer. (From Tasman W, Jaeger EA: Wills Eye Hospital Atlas of Clinical Ophthalmology. Philadelphia, Lippincott-Raven, 1995, with permission.) (See Fig. 2, Color Plates.)

3. Contact lens deposits. Old lenses should be replaced.

4. Tight lens syndrome. Lenses shrink with age. On exam, the patient may have significant chemosis around the lens, and the lens will not move with a blink. In severe cases, a sterile hypopyon can develop.

5. Corneal abrasion.

14. A young mother enters with her infant child. Her left eye is tearing profusely, and she has trouble keeping it open. She states that she was changing the child's diaper when he scratched her eye with his fingernail. What treatment do you recommend?

At the slit lamp, you see a fairly large central corneal abrasion with no sign of an infiltrate. The upper lid is everted, and no foreign body is seen. The abrasion will heal fairly quickly regardless of treatment; the goals are comfort and prevention of infection. Some patients desire a pressure patch, but they should not be used in patients who wear contact lenses or who have had trauma from a fingernail or vegetable matter (e.g., a dirty nail or tree branch). Such injuries have a higher chance of contamination and need to be observed for the development of a corneal ulcer. Patching may increase the rate of infection. A cycloplegic drop, such as cyclopentolate 2%, may relieve the discomfort of ciliary spasm. An antibiotic such as erythromycin or trimethoprim/polymyxin (Polytrim) 4 times/day is a reasonable choice. If the infection is considered "dirty," tobramycin is a better choice for *Pseudomonas* sp. coverage. A topical antiinflammatory decreases pain, and some evidence suggests that it may promote healing.

If the abrasion is large, central, or in a contact lens wearer, the patient should return the next day to make sure that no infection is developing and that the lesion is healing. A contact lens wearer can resume lenses after the defect has healed and the eye feels normal for 3 or 4 days. Make sure that the lens does not have a tear or significant deposits, which may have contributed to the abrasion.

15. The same woman returns 3 months later complaining that she awoke in the morning with severe pain, redness, and tearing in the left eye. It feels like the original scratch. She denies rubbing her eye or any other trauma. What may have happened?

Patients who have had a corneal abrasion from a sharp object such as a paper edge or a fingernail may develop recurrent corneal erosions. Recurrent erosions also may be seen in patients who have corneal dystrophy, such as Meesmann's, map-dot-fingerprint, Reis-Buckler, lattice, macular, or granular dystrophy. Typically, patients awaken with severe pain and tearing, or symptoms develop after eye rubbing. On examination, an abrasion may be seen in the area of previous injury, or the epithelium may have healed the defect but appear irregular. Sometimes no abnormalities can be seen, and the diagnosis must be made from the history. Look carefully for any signs of dystrophy, especially in the other eye.

Treatment consists of antibiotics, a cycloplegic, and a pressure patch for 24 hours when the defect is present. After healing, lubrication is crucial. If the eye is dry and the lid becomes stuck to the abnormal epithelium, the cycle will begin again. Artificial tears during the day and lubricating ointment at night will help. Some recommend a hypertonic solution of 5% sodium chloride, which theoretically draws out the water from the cornea and promotes epithelial adhesion to its basement membrane. If the corneal epithelium is loose and heaped upon itself, this treatment may allow it to heal. If such treatment does not prevent further erosions, an extended-wear bandage soft contact lens worn for several months may help. Some patients require anterior stromal puncture, which causes small permanent corneal scars that prevent further erosions. Others have found excimer laser a promising treatment.

16. A car mechanic complains of a painful red eye. He was fixing a muffler at the time of the onset of pain. What are your concerns?

Most likely, he has a foreign body in his cornea or conjunctiva. It is important to find out what he was doing at the time of the injury. He states that he was hammering metal without safety glasses. This report increases your concern that he may have a ruptured globe. A metal piece that breaks off would travel at a high rate of speed.

On exam, he has 20/20 vision in both eyes. You see no foreign bodies in the conjunctiva or the cornea. You evert the upper lid and find nothing. The intraocular pressure is 2 mmHg. The other eye has a pressure of 15 mmHg. A conjunctival defect with subconjunctival hemorrhage makes it impossible to determine whether a scleral laceration is present.

17. What do you do now?

First, put a shield over the eye to prevent further damage to the globe. It is best to examine and treat in the controlled setting of the operating room. The pupil should be dilated to determine whether the foreign body can be seen with the indirect ophthalmoscope. The patient should have nothing else by mouth. A computed tomography (CT) scan of the orbits is necessary to screen for foreign bodies in the eye or orbit. Always evaluate the patient systemically to make sure no other injuries are missed.

18. How do you proceed if, instead of a potential ruptured globe, you find a superficial metallic foreign body at 4:00 on the cornea.

Document visual acuity. Sometimes an infiltrate may be found around the foreign body, especially if it is over 24 hours old. Usually, the infiltrate is sterile. Apply a topical anesthetic (proparacaine), and remove the foreign body with a 25-gauge needle or a foreign body spud at the slit lamp. A rust ring may have formed, depending on how long the metal has been present. Often it can be removed with the same instruments. It is sometimes safer to leave a rust ring if it is deep or in the center of the visual axis. The rust ring will eventually migrate to the corneal surface, where it is easier and safer to remove. Dilate the pupil, and make sure that the vitreous and retina are normal. The history of hammering makes a dilated exam imperative.

Treatment consists of a cycloplegic, an antibiotic ointment or drug, and optional pressure patching. Large or central defects need follow-up to make sure that healing occurs without infection. An antibiotic such as erythromycin or trimethoprim/polymyxin is appropriate for the next 3–4 days.

19. A lifeguard states that his eye has been red for a long time. He has a wing-shaped fold of fibrovascular tissue nasally in both eyes that extends onto the cornea. Should he be worried?

The lesion is a pterygium. A similar lesion called a pingueculum involves the conjunctiva but not the cornea. Both are usually bilateral. They are thought to result from damage due to chronic ultraviolet exposure or chronic irritation from wind and dust. They may be associated with dellen, an area of corneal thinning secondary to drying because the area adjacent to raised areas may not receive adequate lubrication. It is necessary to rule out conjunctival intraepithelial neoplasia, which is unilateral, often elevated, and not in a wing-shaped configuration.

Counsel the lifeguard to wear ultraviolet blocking sunglasses and to use artificial tears frequently, especially on sunny, windy days. Surgical removal of a pterygium is indicated if it interferes with contact lens wear, causes significant irritation, or involves the visual axis. Because the lesion may recur quite aggressively, surgery is deferred if possible.

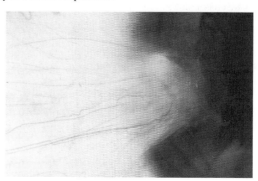

An early pterygium. It can be observed that it is not in the visual axis and is not inflamed. (From Tasman W, Jaeger EA: Wills Eye Hospital Atlas of Clinical Ophthalmology. Philadelphia, Lippincott-Raven, 1995, with permission.)

20. An unfortunate victim of domestic abuse had lye thrown in his face. What should you do?

Even before you check vision, quickly check pH and then begin copious irrigation with saline or Ringer's lactated solution for at least 30 minutes. An eyelid speculum and a topical anesthetic will help. Make sure to irrigate the fornices. Stop irrigation only when pH of 7.0 is reached. If it is not reached after a significant time, check for particulate matter that may trap the chemical.

21. What is his prognosis?

Acids tend to have a better outcome than alkalis. Acids precipitate proteins, which limit penetration. Alkalis (lye, cement, plaster) penetrate more deeply. A mild burn may have only SPK or sloughing of part or all of the epithelium. No perilimbal ischemia is seen. Patients need a cycloplegic, antibiotic ointment, and pressure patching. Check intraocular pressure, which may be elevated by damage to the trabecular meshwork.

A moderate-to-severe burn has perilimbal blanching and corneal edema or opacification with a poor view of the anterior chamber. A significant anterior chamber reaction may be seen. The intraocular pressure may be elevated and the retina may be necrotic at the point where the alkali penetrated the sclera. The patient may need hospital admission to monitor intraocular pressure and corneal status. A topical antibiotic, cycloplegic, and pressure patching are used. Steroids may be used if the anterior chamber reaction or corneal inflammation is severe. However, they cannot be used for more than 7 days because they promote corneal melting. Collagenase inhibitors may help in a melt. Patients require long-term care.

22. A young boy presents with purulent discharge over the past few days. His mother thinks that he needs antibiotics. Do you agree?

Yes. Purulent discharge signals bacterial conjunctivitis as opposed to the watery discharge of viral conjunctivitis. Patients usually have a conjunctival papillary reaction and no preauricular node. Gram stain and conjunctival swab for culture and sensitivities should be done if the conjunctivitis is severe.

23. What are the common organisms? How should you treat?

Staphylococcus aureus, *Streptococcus pneumoniae*, and *Haemophilus influenzae* are common; *H. influenzae* is especially common in children. Topical antibiotics such as trimethoprim/polymyxin (polytrim) or ciprofloxacin or erythromycin 4 times/day for 5–7 days is appropriate. *H. influenzae* should be treated with oral amoxicillin/clavulanate because of the possibility of systemic involvement, such as otitis media, pneumonia, or meningitis.

24. A 27-year-old woman complains of red, irritated eyes with watery discharge over the past 6 weeks. A follicular conjunctivitis and palpable preauricular node are present. What is the differential diagnosis?

Conjunctivitis lasting longer than 4 weeks is considered chronic. The differential for chronic conjunctivitis includes chlamydial inclusion conjunctivitis, ocular toxicity, Parinaud's oculoglandular conjunctivitis, trachoma, molluscum contagiosum, and silent dacryocystitis.

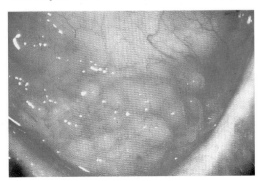

Chronic follicular conjunctivitis. (From Tasman W, Jaeger EA: Wills Eye Hospital Atlas of Clinical Ophthalmology. Philadelphia, Lippincott-Raven, 1995, with permission.)

25. How do you proceed?

History is important. On questioning, the patient reports a recent vaginal discharge. Chlamydial infection becomes high on the list. Such patients also may have white peripheral subepithelial infiltrates and a superior corneal pannus. Stringy, mucous discharge is common. Obtain a chlamydial immunofluorescence test and/or a chlamydial culture of the conjunctiva. Giemsa stain will show basophilic intracytoplasmic inclusion bodies in epithelial cells as well as polymorphonuclear leukocytes. Tetracycline, doxycycline, or erythromycin should be taken orally for 3 weeks by the patient and her sexual partners. Topical ocular erythromycin, tetracycline, or sulfacetamide ointment is used at the same time. Counseling and evaluation for other sexually transmitted diseases should be done by the family physician.

26. How do you diagnose the other causes of chronic conjunctivitis?

1. **Toxic conjunctivitis** is common with many drops (see question 2 for offending agents). Treat with preservative-free artificial tears.

2. **Parinaud's oculoglandular conjunctivitis** presents with a mucopurulent discharge and foreign body sensation. Granulomatous nodules on the palpebral conjunctiva and swollen lymph nodes are necessary for the diagnosis. Fever and rash also may occur. The etiology includes cat scratch disease (most common), tularemia (contact with rabbits or ticks), tuberculosis, and syphilis.

3. **Trachoma** occurs in underprivileged countries with poor sanitation. It is also caused by chlamydial infection. Patients develop superior tarsal follicles and severe corneal pannus, which, if untreated, leads to significant dry eye, trichiasis, and scarring. Patients may become functionally blind. Diagnosis and treatment are the same as for chlamydial inclusion conjunctivitis.

4. **Molluscum contagiosum** develops a chronic follicular conjunctivitis from a reaction to toxic rival products. On the lid or lid margin, multiple dome-shaped, umbilicated nodules are present. These lesions must be removed by excision, incision and curettage, or cryosurgery to resolve the conjunctivitis.

5. **Dacryocystitis** is an inflammation of the lacrimal sac. Patients usually present with pain, erythema, and swelling over the inner aspect of the lower lid. They also may have a fever. But a red eye may be the only sign. Pressure over the lacrimal sac may elicit discharge and a complaint of tenderness. Treatment is systemic antibiotics, warm compresses with massage over the inner canthus, and topical antibiotics. Watch patients closely because cellulitis can occasionally develop.

27. A 40-year-old woman presents with a bright red eye that she noticed on awakening in the morning. On examination, she has a subconjunctival hemorrhage. What questions are important to ask?

You need to know whether this is her first episode. Does she have a history of easy bruising or poor clotting? Is she taking any medications that may increase bleeding time, such as coumadin or aspirin? Has she been rubbing her eye or had any injury to her eye? Has she done any heavy lifting or straining? Has she been sneezing or vomiting—anything that may cause a Valsalva maneuver?

28. She answers no to the above questions and states that this is her first episode. Should she be worried?

No. Reassure her that the symptoms will resolve within 2 weeks. Artificial tears will make her more comfortable. Tell her to return if she has further episodes.

29. With further thought, she remembers two other hemorrhages in her left eye and reports that her menses have been much heavier recently. What now?

At this point, referral to an internist for a complete blood count with differential, blood pressure check, prothrombin time, partial thromboplastin time, and bleeding time is appropriate.

30. A 60-year-old woman complains that her eyes have been red and burning over the past several weeks. She also has some tearing and photophobia. On exam, you notice mild conjunctival injection and a slightly low tear meniscus. Should you think of anything else?

Make sure to elevate the upper eyelid. Superior limbic keratoconjunctivitis is a thickening and inflammation of the superior bulbar conjunctiva. Sometimes a superior corneal micropannus, superior palpebral papillae, and corneal filaments can be found. Fifty percent of patients have associated dysthyroid disease. Artificial tears and ointments are all that are necessary for mild disease. Silver nitrate solution (**not** cautery sticks) may be applied to the superior tarsal and bulbar conjunctiva; mechanical scraping, cryotherapy, cautery, or surgical resection or recession of the superior bulbar conjunctiva may be necessary for more severe disease.

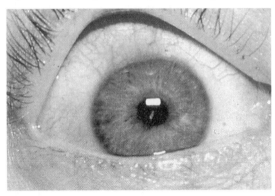

Elevating the upper lid reveals superior limbic keratoconjunctivitis. (From American Academy of Ophthalmology: Basic and Clinical Science Course, Section 8, with permission.) (See Fig. 3, Color Plates.)

31. A 22-year-old woman presents with mild redness in the temporal quadrant of her left eye for about 1 week. She notices no discomfort. On exam, she has normal vision. Large episcleral vessels beneath the conjunctiva are engorged in the area. They can be easily moved with a cotton swab, and no tenderness is present. The cornea and anterior chamber are clear. The sclera appears to be uninvolved. What is the diagnosis?

You must distinguish between episcleritis and scleritis. A drop of 2.5% phenylephrine blanches the episcleral vessels but leaves any injected vessels of the sclera untouched. Look for any discharge or conjunctival follicles and papillae to rule out conjunctivitis.

Episcleritis is usually idiopathic. It may be diffuse or sectorial, unilateral or bilateral. Sometimes a nodule may be seen. Rarely, it is associated with collagen-vascular disease, gout, herpes zoster, syphilis, or Lyme disease. Usually artificial tears and/or a topical vasoconstrictor/antihistamine drop, such as naphazoline/pheniramine, will suffice. If the patient is unresponsive, a mild steroid drop should help. Rarely, oral nonsteroidal antiinflammatory drugs are necessary. Warn the patient that episcleritis may recur.

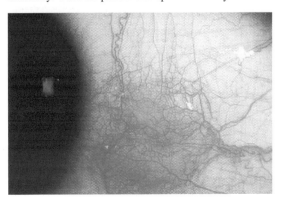

A slightly tender and mobile elevated nodule with epithelial injection is typical for nodular episcleritis. (From Tasman W, Jaeger EA: Wills Eye Hospital Atlas of Clinical Ophthalmology. Philadelphia, Lippincott-Raven, 1995, with permission.)

32. The same patient returns 2 months later. Her left eye is still red, but it is now diffuse. She denies arthritis, rash, venereal disease, tick exposure, or other medical problems. She has been using a vasoconstrictor/antihistamine drop since her last visit. She began using it 4 times/day, then increased the frequency because her eye continued to be red unless she used it. She now applies drops every 1–2 hours. Does this make a difference?

Counsel patients not to use a vasoconstrictor for longer than 2 weeks and no more than 4 times/day. Just as vasoconstrictor nose sprays produce dependence so that patients are congested unless they use them, so do eyedrops. She should stop the drop immediately. Her left eye will be very red for a time until dependence resolves.

33. A 65-year-old woman with rheumatoid arthritis states that her left eye has been red and painful for a couple of weeks. The pain is severe and radiates to her forehead and jaw and has awakened her at night. It has worsened slowly. Her vision is decreasing. She thinks that she has had a similar condition before. On exam, the conjunctival, episcleral, and scleral vessels are injected temporally. The scleral vessels do not move, and the area is very tender. A scleral nodule is present. The sclera appears bluish in this area, adjacent to which is a peripheral keratitis with a mild anterior chamber reaction. The intraocular pressure is 24 mmHg in the affected eye and 16 mmHg in the unaffected eye. What may she have?

Nodular anterior scleritis. The inflamed blood vessels are much deeper than those seen in conjunctivitis or episcleritis. In addition, the cornea and anterior chamber are involved. The deep, boring pain is typical with scleritis.

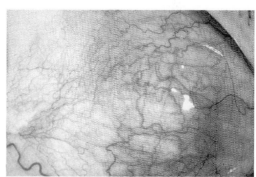

Nodular scleritis is painful with a nonmobile nodule associated with swelling of the episclera and sclera. (From Tasman W, Jaeger EA: Wills Eye Hospital Atlas of Clinical Ophthalmology. Philadelphia, Lippincott-Raven, with permission.)

34. How else may scleritis present?

1. Diffuse anterior scleritis.

2. Necrotizing anterior scleritis with inflammation. The pain is severe, and the choroid is visible through the transparent sclera. The mortality rate is high due to systemic disease.

3. Necrotizing anterior scleritis without inflammation (scleromalacia perforans [see figure, top of next page]). Such patients have almost a complete lack of symptoms, and most have rheumatoid arthritis.

4. Posterior scleritis. It may mimic an amelanotic choroidal mass, exudative retinal detachment, retinal hemorrhage, choroidal folds, or choroidal detachment. Restricted extraocular movements, proptosis, pain, and tenderness may also occur. Rarely is it related to a systemic disease.

35. What percentage of patients with scleritis have systemic disease? What diseases are associated with scleritis?

Fifty percent. The connective tissue diseases, such as rheumatoid arthritis, ankylosing spondylitis, systemic lupus erythematosus, polyarteritis nodosa, and Wegener's granulomatosis, are common associations. Herpes zoster ophthalmicus, syphilis, and gout also may cause scleritis. Less frequently, scleritis may be associated with tuberculosis, sarcoidosis, or a foreign body.

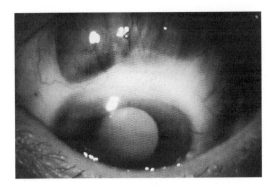

Scleromalacia perforans is a noninflammatory form of necrotizing scleritis. (From Tasman W, Jaeger EA: Wills Eye Hospital Atlas of Clinical Ophthalmology. Philadelphia, Lippincott-Raven, 1995, with permission.) (See Fig. 4, Color Plates.)

36. What work-up is appropriate for a patient with scleritis?

Any avascular areas of the scleritis must be identified. The severity of the disease is increased with more thinning. The risk of a melt is much higher. A dilated exam evaluates posterior segment involvement. Patients should be referred to an internist or a rheumatologist for a complete physical exam, complete blood count, erythrocyte sedimentation rate (ESR), uric acid level, rapid plasmin reagin test (RPR), fluorescent treponemal antibody, absorbed test (FTA-ABS), rheumatoid factor and antinuclear antibody tests (ANA), and fasting blood sugar. If history or symptoms warrant, a purified protein derivative test (PPD) with anergy panel, a chest radiograph, sacroiliac radiograph, and/or B-scan ultrasonography to detect posterior scleritis should be ordered.

37. How should you treat the patient?

An oral nonsteroidal antiinflammatory drug—such as ibuprofen, 400–600 mg 4 times/day, or indomethacin, 25 mg 3 times/day—coupled with an antacid or H_2 blocker such as ranitidine is a good initial choice. If the patient is nonresponsive, oral steroids are the next step. In diseases such as systemic vasculitis, polyarteritis nodosa, and Wegener's granulomatosis, an immunosuppressive agent such as cyclophosphamide may be necessary. Decreased pain is an indication of successful treatment, although the clinical picture may not be significantly different quickly.

Scleromalacia perforans does not have ocular treatment. Immunosuppression for the underlying systemic disease may be necessary.

38. What about topical steroids or a subconjunctival steroid injection?

Topical steroids are not usually effective. Subconjunctival steroids are contraindicated because they may lead to scleral thinning and perforation.

39. A 35-year-old man presents with severe photophobia, pain, and decreased vision in his right eye for two days. This condition has occurred several times before. He says that it is helped by using drops. On examination, his vision is 20/50 in the right eye and 20/20 in the left eye. His pupil is poorly reactive on the right and miotic. The left eye is normal, and no afferent pupillary defect is present. The right eye is diffusely injected, especially around the limbus. The anterior chamber is deep, but 2+ cell and flare are present with a few fine keratic precipitates. The left eye is clear. The right eye has an intraocular pressure of 5 mmHg; the left is 15 mmHg. Dilated exam is normal. What are the diagnosis and treatment?

The diagnosis is acute, nongranulomatous anterior uveitis. A cycloplegic drop such as cyclopentolate, 1–2% 3 times/day, for mild inflammation and scopolamine 0.25% or atropine 1% 3 times/day for more severe inflammation will relax the ciliary spasm, making the patient more comfortable as well as preventing formation of synechiae in the angle and on the pupillary margin. Formation of synechiae increases the long-term risk of angle closure glaucoma. A steroid drop every 1–6 hours, depending on the severity of the anterior chamber inflammation, is started. If no response occurs, subconjunctival injection or oral steroids may be necessary. Rarely, systemic immunosuppressive agents are necessary.

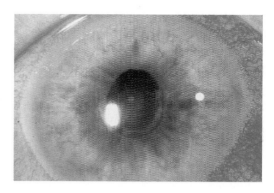

Significant ciliary injection in a patient with acute iritis. Note the dilated iris vessels and the peripheral anterior synechiae. (From Tasman W, Jaeger EA: Wills Eye Hospital Atlas of Clinical Ophthalomology. Philadelphia, Lippincott-Raven, 1995, with permission.)

40. The patient returns after 3 days of prednisolone acetate 1% every 3 hours and cyclopentolate 2% 3 times/day. His eye is more comfortable, and the anterior chamber reaction has decreased to 1+. His intraocular pressure has increased to 25 mmHg in the right eye. It is 15 mmHg in the left eye. Why would the pressure increase? How do you treat it?

The differential of increased intraocular pressure in this situation includes:

1. Steroid response. Decreasing steroids lowers the pressure if steroids are the cause.

2. Cellular blockage of the trabecular meshwork from the inflammatory cells. Increasing the steroids lowers the pressure if cellular blockage is the cause.

3. Synechiae formation causing an element of secondary angle closure or blocking the meshwork. Gonioscopy determines whether the angle was open. Increased steroids may melt the synechiae.

4. Neovascularization of the iris blocking the meshwork or closing the angle. Gonioscopy helps to identify the vessels.

Gonioscopy reveals a clean, open angle. The inflammation has decreased since his last visit. Appropriate treatment is to decrease the steroids to 4 times/day and add an antiglaucoma medication, such as a beta blocker or apraclonidine, until you see the patient again.

41. Is systemic evaluation needed?

A first episode of unilateral nongranulomatous uveitis without history, symptoms, or signs of systemic disease does not need systemic work-up. When the uveitis is bilateral, granulomatous, or recurrent and the history and examination are unremarkable, a nonspecific work-up is enough: complete blood count, ESR, ANA, RPR, FTA-ABS, PPD and anergy panel, and a chest radiograph to rule out sarcoid and tuberculosis. In endemic areas, a Lyme titer is recommended. An HLA-B27 test also may be done.

42. The patient states that he has noticed some lower back pain over the past few months. How may this direct your testing?

Ankylosing spondylitis may present with the patient's symptoms. Sacroiliac spine radiographs show sclerosis and narrowing of the sacroiliac joints. ESR and an HLA-B27 test also should be done. A high incidence of heart block and aortic insufficiency is found in such patients.

43. What if the patient reports urethral pain?

Reiter's syndrome is a possibility. Conjunctival, urethral, and prostatic cultures are indicated. Joint radiographs and an HLA-B27 test should be performed. Urethritis is treated with tetracycline, doxycycline, or erythromycin.

44. What if the patient reports frequent mouth and genital ulcerations?

Behçet's disease may present with ulcerations as well as an acute hypopyon, erythema nodosum, and retinal vasculitis and hemorrhages. Episodes are often recurrent.

45. What other diseases may present as an acute nongranulomatous anterior uveitis?

Inflammatory bowel disease, psoriatic arthritis, glaucomatocyclitic crisis, lens-induced uveitis, herpes simplex, herpes zoster, UGH syndrome (uveitis, glaucoma, hyphema), Lyme disease, mumps, influenza, adenovirus, and measles may have a nongranulomatous anterior uveitis as part of their presentation. Rarely, pars planitis may present similarly; however, it usually occurs as a complaint of floaters without a red eye in a young person. Of course, any granulomatous disease may present as a nongranulomatous uveitis, including sarcoid, syphilis, tuberculosis, and sympathetic ophthalmia.

46. What diseases may mimic uveitis?

All patients should be evaluated fully to rule out rhegmatogenous retinal detachment or posterior segment tumor such as retinoblastoma or malignant melanoma. An intraocular foreign body or endophthalmitis also may present similarly.

47. A 68-year-old Asian American presents with an acutely painful red left eye that developed after a recent anxiety attack. She has blurred vision and sees halos around lights. She has vomited twice. On exam, she has a fixed, mid-dilated pupil and conjunctival injection. The cornea is cloudy. What are you concerned about?

Angle closure glaucoma. When the pressure rises quickly in the eye, severe pain and nausea with decreased vision develop. Asian Americans are at increased risk because of their shallow anterior chambers. Examination of the angle of the affected eye may be facilitated by glycerin to clear the corneal edema. If the shallow angle cannot be visualized, the other eye may reveal a narrow angle. For further information about diagnosis and treatment, see chapter 17.

BIBLIOGRAPHY

1. Cullom RD, Chang B: The Wills Eye Manual: Office and Emergency Room Diagnosis and Treatment of Eye Disease, 3rd ed. Philadelphia, J.B. Lippincott, 1994.
2. Vaughn D, Asbury T, Tabbara KF: General Ophthalmology, 14th ed. Norwalk, CT, Appleton & Lange, 1995.
3. Tasman W, Jaeger EA: Wills Eye Hospital Atlas of Clinical Ophthalmology. Philadelphia, Lippincott-Raven, 1995.

9. CORNEAL INFECTIONS

Terry Kim, M.D., Richard C. Rodman, M.D., and Elisabeth J. Cohen, M.D.

1. What is a corneal ulcer?

Infections of the cornea involve the epithelium and/or stroma. Some infections may occur strictly within the epithelium (i.e., herpes simplex epithelial keratitis), whereas others manifest as an infiltrate in the corneal stroma. The term corneal ulcer refers to the loss of stroma associated with an overlying epithelial defect (that stains with fluorescein). A corneal ulcer is usually considered infectious when accompanied by a stromal infiltrate, but may also be caused by noninfectious (or sterile) etiologies.

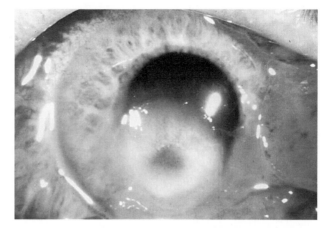

Central pseudomonas corneal ulcer.

2. Which clinical features distinguish an infectious versus a sterile corneal ulcer?

Infectious corneal ulcers caused by bacterial, fungal, viral, and parasitic microorganisms elicit an inflammatory response that can manifest with conjunctival injection, a visible corneal infiltrate, surrounding corneal edema, and floating cells and protein in the anterior chamber (termed **cell** and **flare**) that can deposit on the endothelium of the cornea (termed **keratic precipitates**). If the anterior chamber inflammation is severe enough, these inflammatory cells can layer out to form a sterile hypopyon. Patients are usually symptomatic, with acute redness, pain, decreased vision, and/or photophobia (light sensitivity). Bacterial corneal ulcers may also be associated with a mucopurulent discharge.

Sterile corneal ulcers are not due to infection with microorganisms and therefore can present quite differently, with a relatively quiet, noninjected conjunctiva, minimal or absent corneal infiltrate and/or epithelial defect, and a quiet anterior chamber (see figure on next page). Patients may notice decreased vision depending on the location of the ulcer but often do not complain of significant redness, pain, or photophobia. The large variety of etiologies of sterile corneal ulcers include dry eyes (keratoconjunctivitis sicca), neutrophic keratopathy (i.e., from previous herpes simplex or zoster corneal infections), exposure keratopathy (i.e., Graves' ophthalmopathy or cranial nerve VII palsy), and autoimmune disorders (i.e., rheumatoid arthritis, systemic lupus erythematosus, Wegener's granulomatosis). Sterile infiltrates may also present in the cornea as a result of immunologic phenomena elicited by staphylococcal hypersensitivity or hypoxia (i.e., from contact lens wear). These are usually located in the peripheral cornea owing to the presence of leukocytes in the vascular limbus (junction between sclera and cornea).

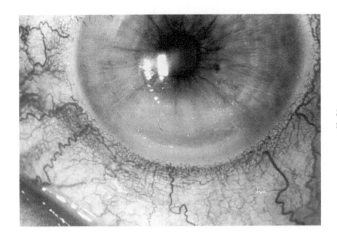

Sterile corneal ulcer caused by
rheumatoid arthritis.

3. What conditions predispose to corneal infections?

The corneal epithelium serves as a protective barrier, and any condition ultimately causing
an alteration or reduction of epithelial integrity can predispose to corneal infections. Epithelial
defects commonly precede infections and are produced by many factors. Trauma and contact
lens wear are important risk factors for infection. Structural eyelid abnormalities such as ectro-
pion/entropion, trichiasis, and lagophthalmos can lead to an exposed and/or disrupted epithelium.
Tear-film abnormalities contribute to insufficient lubrication of the corneal epithelium, which
causes accelerated epithelial drying and breakdown. Other conditions that directly affect normal
epithelial structure and function include physical/chemical trauma, recurrent erosion syndrome,
contact lens wear, topical medication toxicity, and corneal edema (i.e., bullous keratopathy).
Immunosuppressed states occurring both locally (i.e., topical corticosteroid use) and systemically (i.e., systemic corticosteroid or other immunosuppressive therapy, diabetes mellitus, severe
malnutrition, chronic alcoholism, HIV/AIDS, malignancy, old age) can also induce a predisposition to infection.

4. How can a contact lens wearer reduce the risk of infection?

The major risk factor identified for corneal infection with contact lens use is the overnight
wear of contact lenses both approved and not approved for extended wear. Patients need to
know that disposable contact lenses are not any safer than conventional contact lenses. Extended wear of conventional and disposable lenses is associated with 5- to 10-fold increase in
risk of infection. Proper contact lens cleaning and disinfection prior to reinsertion are also of
crucial importance in reducing the incidence of contact lens-related corneal infections. Use of
homemade saline solutions increases the risk of infection. Contact lens wearers who develop
ulcers often have a history of sleeping in their lenses and/or reinserting their lenses without
proper cleaning and disinfection. Careful instructions should be given to every contact lens
wearer regarding recommended wearing time, proper cleaning and disinfecting regimens, the
signs and symptoms (i.e., pain or blurred vision) that require immediate care, and regular
follow-up exams.

5. Describe ways to differentiate between various types of corneal infections (bacterial, viral, fungal, etc.).

A careful history is frequently helpful in pointing toward a general category of infectious microorganism. For example, a history of trauma with any vegetable or plant matter should always
alert the physician to the possibility of a fungal keratitis or infection caused by unusual bacteria.
A history of oral and eyelid vesicles or blisters or repeated problems in only one eye should suggest the potential for herpes simplex keratitis. A history of contact lens wear should be a warning

for possible pseudomonas or acanthamoeba infection. The various etiologies of infectious corneal ulcers may be difficult to differentiate by clinical exam alone. Bacterial infections can vary in presentation depending on the specific bacteria and the severity of infection. Gram-positive organisms tend to produce a focal, discrete infiltrate, whereas gram-negative organisms can cause a rapidly spreading diffuse infiltrate, but exceptions always occur. Streptococcal infections can be as suppurative as pseudomonas infections or associated with only minimal inflammation. Generally, bacterial infections produce a whitish infiltrate and surrounding corneal edema with a variable amount of mucopurulent discharge and anterior chamber inflammation. A fungal infiltrate caused by a filamentous organism commonly has a feathery, irregular border and is sometimes associated with satellite lesions (see figure). Herpes keratitis frequently manifests as a characteristic dendritic defect in the epithelium. Acanthamoeba keratitis can present after weeks of symptoms as a ring infiltrate and is often accompanied by extreme pain out of proportion to the findings.

The definitive diagnosis is obtained from smears and cultures of corneal scrapings. Bacterial organisms can be subclassified according to whether there are gram-positive or gram-negative cocci or bacilli on Gram's stain. Fungal elements can present in the form of yeasts or hyphae with Giemsa, Gomori methenamine silver, or calcofluor white stains. The cysts and trophozoites of acanthamoeba are evident with Giemsa, calcofluor white, or periodic acid-Schiff staining of a corneal scraping or biopsy.

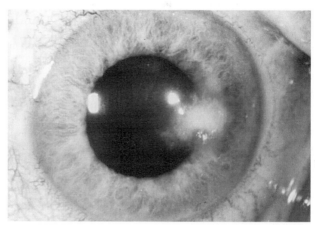

Infectious ulcer caused by a filamentous fungus. Note the indistinct, feathery borders.

6. How and when should smears and cultures be performed?

Corneal scrapings for smears and cultures should be obtained on most corneal ulcers suspected to be infectious. Small corneal infiltrates (less than 1 mm in diameter) do not necessarily have to undergo scraping prior to the initiation of intensive empiric broad-spectrum antibiotic therapy. Corneal infections that do not improve on therapy should undergo scraping or rescraping, and documentation of current antibiotic medication should be given to the laboratory.

Corneal smears and cultures should be performed at the slit lamp after the patient has been given topical anesthetic drops. To obtain the corneal scrapings, use a sterile Kimura spatula, which should be resterilized over a flame between each scraping. Alternatively, sterile calcium alginate swabs can be used. Separate slides should be used for routine smears for Gram's stain and for Giemsa or calcofluor white stains. Specimens for routine culture should be plated on blood (for bacteria) and chocolate (for *Hemophilus* and *Neisseria* species) agar, Sabaroud's dextrose agar without cycloheximide (for fungi) kept at room temperature, and thioglycolate broth (for anaerobic bacteria). Optional stains include calcofluor white (for acanthamoeba) and acid-fast stain (for atypical mycobacteria and *Nocardia* species). Optional culture media include nonnutrient agar with *E. coli* overlay (for acanthamoeba) and Lowenstein-Jensen medium (for atypical mycobacteria and *Nocardia* species).

7. What is the diagnostic yield for smears and cultures performed prior to the initiation of therapy?

Although Gram's stain smears may provide early insight into the causative organism, they may be negative (with a highly variable positivity range of 0 to 57%) and even misleading and should be used cautiously before altering empiric broad-spectrum therapy. If evidence of fungal or acanthamoeba infection is found on smears, therapy is changed to cover these organisms. On the other hand, cultures grow organisms in approximately 50 to 75% of suspected infectious ulcers. Traditional recommendations mandate that cultures be performed prior to starting antibiotics because the yield will be higher at that time. However, clinical evidence suggests that the yield is not significantly diminished by antibiotic treatment if the infection is not responding.

8. What is the recommended initial therapy for suspected infectious ulcers? How does one determine whether single-agent, broad-spectrum antibiotics or combination fortified antibiotics should be used?

This is a controversial and evolving area. In general, initial therapy for corneal ulcers must cover a broad range of gram-positive and gram-negative bacteria and be administered frequently (every 15 to 30 minutes). A multicentered study has demonstrated that ofloxacin and combined fortified cefazolin and tobramycin have equal efficacy, with less toxicity in the fluoroquinolone group. Previously, another study provided evidence that topical ciprofloxacin was as effective as fortified antibiotics. However, a gap in the gram-positive coverage of fluoroquinolones (specifically, streptococcal species) has been identified, as well as cases of fluoroquinolone "failures" of gram-positive and negative infections caused by sensitive organisms that subsequently responded to combination fortified antibiotic therapy. It is our practice to treat small, peripheral ulcers with a single fluoroquinolone antibiotic and to use combination fortified antibiotics for more severe sight-threatening infections.

9. How does the presence of a hypopyon affect management?

The presence of a hypopyon is indicative of an infection severe enough to cause a marked anterior chamber response. Therefore, the treatment should be intense, including hospitalization for frequent combined fortified antibiotics in most cases. Hypopyons associated with corneal ulcers are sterile and do not require evaluation and treatment for endophthalmitis.

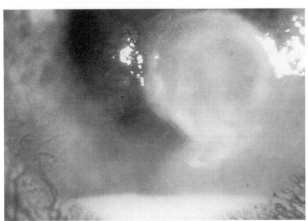

Hypopyon associated with an infectious corneal ulcer.

10. When should an anterior chamber and/or vitreous tap be performed?

Whenever endophthalmitis is suspected. Endophthalmitis must be considered when there is severe inflammation after intraocular surgery or perforating trauma. Once diagnosed, topical antibiotics are inadequate and intravenous antibiotics are unnecessary; antibiotics must be injected directly into the vitreous cavity after taking samples for culture (with vitrectomy indicated in severe cases). Endophthalmitis secondary to infectious keratitis in the absence of perforation is uncommon, and a sterile inflammatory response in the vitreous may be present that resolves with the clearing of the corneal infection.

11. When should patients with corneal ulcers be hospitalized?

1. If the patient lacks the ability or support to administer drops as frequently as every 30 minutes around-the-clock

2. If the patient lives too far away to be followed on a daily basis

3. Any condition requiring intravenous antibiotics or possible surgery (i.e., *Neisseria* infections involving the cornea and perforated corneal ulcers)

12. When are systemic medications indicated?

Systemic antibiotics are seldom indicated in bacterial corneal ulcers. However, parenteral antibiotics play an important role in the treatment of aggressive infections from *Neisseria* and *Hemophilus* species with corneal involvement. They are also used for a perforated ulcer (antibiotics usually given intravenously) and ulcers with impending or existing scleral involvement (oral antibiotics such as ciprofloxacin usually suffice).

Systemic oral antifungal agents are used in cases in which the fungal infiltrate involves deep corneal stroma or in cases that worsen on topical antifungal therapy alone. Oral antifungal agents are also recommended in the treatment of acanthamoeba keratitis. Oral antiviral agents (i.e., acyclovir) are the primary mode of therapy for patients with ocular herpes zoster and are also used by some physicians for primary herpes simplex infection. Overt primary herpes simplex infection is decidedly uncommon. Finally, oral pain medications may be necessary in patients experiencing extreme pain from a severe corneal infection.

13. Other than antibiotics, what adjunctive therapy may be necessary in the treatment of corneal ulcers?

Topical cycloplegic agents are often indicated in the treatment of corneal ulcers that are associated with photophobia due to anterior chamber inflammation. They accomplish several objectives: decreasing pain/photophobia by decreasing ciliary spasm, decreasing inflammation by stabilizing the blood-aqueous barrier inside the eye, and dilating the pupil to prevent scar formation between the iris and the anterior surface of the lens (termed **posterior synechiae**).

If inflammation in the anterior chamber is severe enough, the intraocular pressure may rise, often necessitating the use of antiglaucoma medications. Frequently, topical antiglaucoma medications such as beta-blockers or carbonic anhydrase inhibitors (pilocarpine should be avoided because of the phenomenon of blood-aqueous breakdown with subsequent increase in anterior chamber inflammation) suffice, and systemic medications are rarely necessary.

In the case of impending or frank perforated corneal ulcer, tissue glue such as cyanoacrylate can be useful in temporarily and sometimes permanently sealing the open wound. This will avoid the need for penetrating keratoplasty in the setting of active infection and inflammation.

14. How should the smear and culture results be used to modify treatment?

Smears and cultures play a valuable role in the treatment of corneal infections. The smears may provide a quick means of telling the clinician the general type of infection (i.e., bacterial, fungal, etc.) and can help start the appropriate empiric therapy. Descriptive information from the smears can be used to guide empiric therapy by providing more specific information on the microorganism (e.g., topical ciprofloxacin or tobramycin may be used with the finding of a gram-negative rod, and topical natamycin may be initiated with the finding of a filamentous fungus). However, one must not rely too heavily on smear results, because their correlation with culture results is low as result of contamination by normal flora and improper staining/ processing technique. We recommend broad-spectrum antibiotic coverage until culture results are available.

Cultures give tremendous information to the clinician; they not only identify the pathogen but also determine sensitivities to various antibiotics. For patients with bacterial infections who are undergoing broad-spectrum empiric therapy with more than one antibiotic, the identification of the organism will help to target therapy and eliminate the extraneous medication (e.g., an infection found to be caused by a pseudomonas species will lead the physician to discontinue fortified cefazolin and continue or even increase the frequency of fortified tobramycin). Sensitivities can be useful when an infection does not seem to be improving on the current regimen (to which the organism may show resistance on testing) and can offer other antibiotics with good in vitro efficacy. However, antibiotic therapy should not be changed in the face of clinical improvement despite conflicts in sensitivity reports. The value of sensitivities in ocular infections is problematic because they are based on drug levels attainable in the serum and not the more relevant corneal drug levels.

15. What are the important immediate and delayed sequelae of corneal ulcers?
The immediate concern with corneal ulcers is progressive thinning and perforation. Management and prognosis change considerably with perforation, and the concern for intraocular infection (i.e., endophthalmitis) rises dramatically. Perforated corneal ulcers can result in the loss of the eye. The delayed sequelae of corneal ulcers deal mainly with corneal scarring, which can severely limit visual acuity and function.

16. How should impending and frank corneal perforations be managed?
Any corneal infection associated with marked thinning or perforation should be protected with an eye shield without a patch. When the cornea becomes thinned to the point of imminent or existent corneal perforation, certain steps need to be taken. If the affected area is small, cyanoacrylate glue can be used to help seal the defect. However, most cases of perforation will eventually need patch grafting or corneal transplantation if the eye has visual potential.

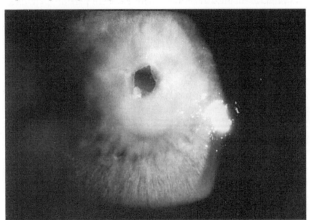

Perforated corneal ulcer.

17. What steps should be taken when a corneal ulcer does not respond to empiric therapy?
Reassess the situation. Is compliance a problem? Hospitalization eliminates this issue. If a culture has not been performed, this should be done so that therapy may be culture-directed. If the empiric therapy is a fluoroquinolone, fortified antibiotics may be better, especially when streptococcal species or other gram-positive organisms are involved. Consider toxicity from the antibiotics themselves, which may prevent the healing of an ulcer. Think also of the possibility of unusual organisms that would not be covered by broad-spectrum antibiotics: a fungal or mixed bacterial/fungal infection, a viral process with bacterial superinfection, or a protozoan such as acanthamoeba.

18. When should a corneal biopsy be considered?
Whenever an ulcer is failing intensive antibiotic therapy and the etiology remains unclear owing to negative cultures. Acanthamoeba is particularly difficult to grow in culture, and the infection may be deep. If this organism is suspected, a corneal biopsy is the best opportunity to identify cysts (more commonly) or trophozoites in the tissue.

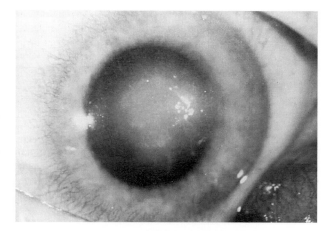

Central acanthamoeba ulcer.

19. What is the role of topical corticosteroids in the treatment of corneal ulcers?

The role of topical corticosteroids as an adjunctive therapy for corneal ulcers is controversial. Some advocate that corticosteroids help to reduce inflammation and decrease corneal scarring, whereas others fear that corticosteroids predispose to recrudescent infection and progressive thinning leading to perforation. Corticosteroids should not be used in the initial treatment of corneal ulcers and can be used in conjunction with antibiotics with extreme caution only after clinical improvement has been demonstrated with appropriate antibiotics.

20. How are staphylococcal hypersensitivity infiltrates diagnosed and managed?

Corneal infiltrates due to staphylococcal hypersensitivity may be multiple, stain minimally or not at all with fluorescein, are located in the peripheral cornea separated from the limbus by a clear area, and are not associated with anterior chamber inflammation. They accompany staphylococcal blepharitis and meibomitis and represent an immunologic reaction to staphylococcal antigens. Mild cases of staphylococcal hypersensitivity should be treated with warm compresses and lid hygiene scrubs along with an antibiotic ointment. In more severe cases, combined antibiotic-steroid eyedrops or ointments can be added along with oral doxycycline to prevent recurrences. If concerned about an infectious etiology, treat the infiltrate(s) initially with intensive antibiotics.

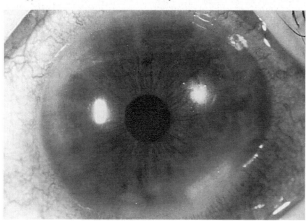

Staphylococcal hypersensitivity infiltrate located in the inferior peripheral cornea. Note its marginal location and clear separation from the limbus.

21. What is appropriate therapy for small peripheral infiltrates in a contact lens wearer?

It is important to remember that small infiltrates in a contact lens wearer may be sterile or infectious. Sterile infiltrates are associated with acute and chronic hypoxia as well as hypersensitivity or toxic reactions to preservatives in contact lens solutions. They are usually located in the peripheral subepithelium with an overlying intact epithelium and are associated with a quiet anterior chamber, minimal pain, and no discharge. Infectious infiltrates may be located anywhere in the cornea and present with an overlying epithelial defect and variable anterior chamber reaction. When in doubt, infiltrates in a contact lens wearer should be presumed to be infectious.

Patients with infiltrates should first stop all contact lens wear. One can forego scraping and treat presumed infectious infiltrates frequently (every 30 to 60 minutes) with a single broad-spectrum antibiotic (i.e., ciprofloxacin or ofloxacin) after a loading dose and then an antibiotic ointment (i.e., tobramycin) at bedtime. Patients should be followed closely and undergo scraping if the epithelial defect and infiltrate do not improve. Corneal abrasions in contact lens wearers should be treated with antibiotic ointment. Patching abrasions in contact lens wearers is to be avoided because of the risk of infection.

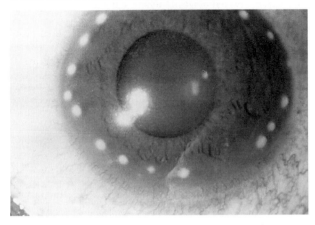

Small peripheral infiltrates caused by a sterile reaction to contact lens solution.

22. When should a gonococcal infection be suspected? What additional workup and treatment should be initiated?

A gonococcal infection should be suspected when an acute onset of marked conjunctival injection is associated with severe mucopurulent discharge. Other signs that may accompany gonococcal conjunctivitis/keratitis are marked chemosis and preauricular adenopathy. Infiltrates begin in the superior cornea and can progress rapidly and perforate within 48 hours.

Workup should include conjunctival scrapings for immediate Gram's stain (look for gram-negative intracellular diplococci) and culture (using chocolate agar media promptly incubated in a CO_2-enriched environment). If Gram's stain is positive or if the diagnosis is highly suspected,

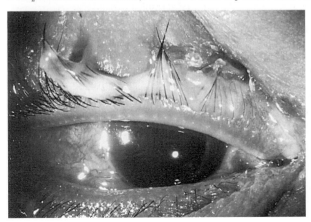

Gonococcal conjunctivitis with marked conjunctival injection and copious mucopurulent discharge on the eyelid margins.

treatment should be initiated with frequent irrigation with saline, a 1-g intramuscular dose of ceftriaxone, frequent topical bacitracin ointment or ciprofloxacin drops, and oral tetracycline or erythromycin. If the cornea is involved or if compliance is problematic, the patient should be hospitalized for parenteral ceftriaxone therapy and close follow-up.

23. Why do herpetic infections occur?

There are two major groups of herpetic ocular disease: herpes simplex and herpes zoster ophthalmicus. Herpes simplex keratitis is usually caused by the type 1 virus (this is not a sexually transmitted disease and one should tell this to the patient). Neonatal ocular infection is caused by the type 2 virus after passing through an infected birth canal. Herpes simplex virus type 1 is usually spread by adults who shed the virus asymptomatically from an oral "cold sore" to children. The first contact of an individual with the virus is referred to as primary infection, which is usually inapparent. A follicular conjunctivitis, corneal dendritic ulcers, cutaneous vesicles, and preauricular adenopathy may be seen.

Herpes zoster ophthalmicus represents reactivation of the varicella zoster virus (see figure). The initial contact with the virus causes chickenpox. Recrudescence of the disease may lead to herpes zoster ophthalmicus when the first division of cranial nerve V is involved. It remains latent in the trigeminal ganglion. Nerve damage in a dermatomal distribution may lead to severe pain, which is referred to as postherpetic neuralgia. Associated keratitis, uveitis, and glaucoma may be severe, chronic, and difficult to treat.

24. Why is herpes a recurrent disease?

After primary contact with the herpes simplex virus (HSV), access is gained to the central nervous system. The virus becomes latent in the trigeminal ganglia (HSV type 1) or in the spinal ganglia (HSV type 2). Recurrent attacks occur when the virus travels peripherally via sensory nerves to infect target tissues such as the eye. These attacks may be triggered by any of the following stressors: fever, ultraviolet light exposure, trauma, stress, menses, and immunosuppression. The most impressive example of this pathway of recrudescence is the dermatomal involvement of the zoster virus.

25. Give some nonocular signs suggestive of a herpetic corneal infection.

Some nonspecific signs of primary herpetic corneal infection include fever, malaise, and lymphadenopathy (particularly preauricular adenopathy on the involved side). The vesicular skin rash of herpes zoster infections characteristically involves the dermatome of the first division of cranial nerve V on one side, does not cross the midline, and progresses to scarring. The presence of this rash on the tip of the nose (referred to as Hutchinson's sign) is a useful sign indicating probable ocular involvement, because both areas are innervated by the nasociliary nerve. Patients with herpes simplex keratitis also get dermatologic manifestations of infection. They can present with vesicular lesions in the perioral and periocular region that resolve without scarring.

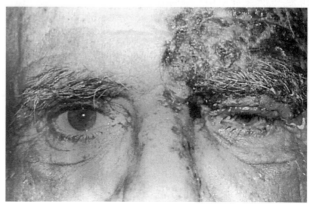

Characteristic appearance and location of herpes zoster skin lesions. (From Tasman W, Jaeger EA (eds): The Wills Eye Hospital Atlas of Clinical Ophthalmology. Philadelphia, Lippincott-Raven, 1996, p 17, with permission.)

26. Are there differences between corneal infections caused by herpes simplex and herpes zoster viruses?

Although corneal infections from herpes simplex and herpes zoster can present in a similar clinical fashion, there are subtle features that can help differentiate between the two. Herpes simplex keratitis is a recurrent condition, whereas herpes zoster ophthalmicus results in chronic disease. The corneal dendrites of herpes simplex infections are epithelial ulcers whose edges stain brightly with fluorescein and have terminal bulbs. Herpes zoster dendrites are raised lesions, do not have terminal bulbs, and do not stain well with fluorescein.

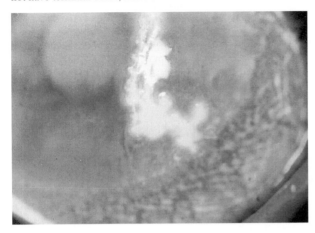

Classic herpes simplex dendrite staining brightly with fluorescein.

27. What are the noninfectious manifestations of a herpetic keratitis?

Patients with herpetic keratitis can present with ophthalmic findings that are not directly caused by the viral infection itself but instead relate to the immunologic response to the infection. Examples of this phenomenon include chronic keratouveitis (where large keratic precipitates are associated with corneal edema) and disciform and necrotizing keratitis (in which stromal infiltration with leukocytes and neovascularization can occur with an intact epithelium).

Corneal scarring is a nonspecific sign of previous herpetic keratitis that can be visually debilitating and potentially necessitate penetrating keratoplasty. Neurotrophic corneal ulcers represent a sterile process that occurs because of previous neural involvement with the herpes virus and may sometimes require tarsorrhaphy (suturing the eyelids closed) for healing.

28. How should these infections be treated?

Herpes simplex epithelial keratitis and conjunctivitis should be treated with frequent topical antiviral agents (i.e., trifluorothymidine [Viroptic] drops or vidarabine [Vira-A] ointment). Zovirax ointment can be added for skin involvement but cannot be used in or near the eye. Disciform stromal keratitis should be managed with topical corticosteroids and prophylactic antiviral agents.

All herpes zoster infections regardless of ocular involvement are treated primarily with oral acyclovir (800 mg PO 5 times a day for 7 to 10 days). Alternative antiviral agents include famcyclovir. Skin lesions should also receive antibiotic ointment (i.e., bacitracin) and warm compresses, and topical medications should be added according to the presence and severity of ocular involvement (i.e., conjunctivitis, uveitis, glaucoma, etc.). Keratouveitis usually develops after the skin rash.

29. What is the role of topical corticosteroids in herpes simplex keratitis?

Although topical corticosteroids are contraindicated in the presence of active epithelial disease, their use in treating herpes simplex stromal keratitis is beneficial. The Herpetic Eye Disease Study has documented that topical steroids and prophylactic antivirals are safe and effective in the treatment of stromal keratitis.

30. When should oral acyclovir be used in herpes simplex keratitis? In herpes zoster keratitis?

Oral acyclovir should always be used to treat acute herpes zoster ophthalmicus but is only indicated in primary herpes simplex keratitis. Its use to reduce the frequency of recurrent herpes simplex keratitis is currently under investigation in a multicentered randomized trial of the Herpetic Eye Disease Study. It is important to remember that acyclovir is contraindicated during pregnancy and in patients with renal disease.

CONCLUSION

Corneal infections have many causes as well as variable manifestations that require different treatment. Corneal infections can result in loss of vision due to scarring and even loss of the eye due to perforation. Early, correct diagnosis and therapy are necessary to achieve optimal outcome in the management of corneal infections.

BIBLIOGRAPHY

1. Arffa RC: Grayson's Diseases of the Cornea, 3rd ed. St. Louis, Mosby, 1991.
2. Cohen EJ, Fulton JC, Hoffman CJ, et al: Trends in contact lens-associated corneal ulcers. Cornea (in press).
3. Cohen EJ, Parlato CJ, Arentsen JJ, et al: Medical and surgical treatment of acanthamoeba keratitis. Am J Ophthalmol 103:615–625, 1987.
4. Cullom RD Jr, Chang B: The Wills Eye Manual: Office and Emergency Room Diagnosis and Treatment of Eye Disease, 2nd ed. Philadelphia, J.B. Lippincott, 1994.
5. Leibowitz HM: Clinical evaluation of ciprofloxacin 0.3% ophthalmic solution for treatment of bacterial keratitis. Am J Ophthalmol 112:34S–47S, 1991.
6. Liesegang T: Diagnosis and therapy of herpes zoster ophthalmicus. Ophthalmology 98:1216–1229, 1991.
7. McDonnell PJ, Nobe J, Gauderman WJ, et al: Community care of corneal ulcers. Am J Ophthalmol 114:531–538, 1992.
8. McLeod SD, Kolahdouz-Isfahani A, Rostamian K, et al: The role of smears, cultures, and antibiotic sensitivity testing in the management of suspected infectious keratitis. Ophthalmology 103:23–38, 1996.
9. O'Brien TP, Maguire MG, Fink NE, et al: Efficacy of ofloxacin vs cefazolin and tobramycin in the therapy of bacterial keratitis: Report from the Bacterial Keratitis Research Group. Arch Ophthalmol 113:1257–1265, 1995.
10. Smolin G, Thoft RA: The Cornea: Scientific Foundations and Clinical Practice, 3rd ed. Boston, Little, Brown, 1994.
11. Stein RM, Clinch TE, Cohen EJ, et al: Infected vs sterile corneal infiltrates in contact lens wearers. Am J Ophthalmol 105:632–636, 1988.
12. Wilhelmus KR, Gee L, Hauck WW, et al: Herpetic Eye Disease Study: A controlled trial of topical corticosteroids for herpes simplex stromal keratitis. Ophthalmology 101:1883–1895, 1994.

10. OPHTHALMIA NEONATORUM

Janine G. Tabas, M.D.

1. How does ophthalmia neonatorum typically present?

Inflammation of the conjunctiva within the first month of life is classified as ophthalmia neonatorum (neonatal conjunctivitis). A purulent or mucoid discharge is present from one or both eyes. Besides conjunctival injection, edema and erythema of the lids are often present.

2. What is the usual means of transmission for neonatal conjunctivitis?

Conjunctivitis is usually transmitted to the newborn by passage through the mother's infected cervix at the time of delivery and reflects the sexually transmitted diseases prevalent in the community. It may be spread, however, by people handling the baby soon after birth.

3. What is the most common cause of neonatal conjunctivitis?

Neonatal conjunctivitis is the most common ocular disease of newborns and is most often caused by *Chlamydia trachomatis* (8.2/1000 live births). One hundred years ago *Neisseria gonorrhoeae* was the leading cause of blindness in infants. Today gonococcal conjunctivitis is less often seen in industrialized nations (0.3/1000 live births) because of neonatal ocular prophylaxis and better prenatal screening.

4. List the common causes of ophthalmia neonatorum, their usual clinical presentations, and their approximate times of onset after birth.

Type	Time of Onset	Typical Characteristics
Chemical (e.g., silver nitrate drops)	Within hours of instillation	Self-limiting, mild, serious discharge (occasionally purulent) Lasts 24–36 hours
Chlamydia trachomatis	5–14 days	Mild-to-moderate, thick, purulent discharge (severity is variable) Erythematous conjunctiva, with palpebral more than bulbar involvement
Neisseria gonorrhoeae	24–48 hr	Hyperacute, copious, purulent discharge Lid swelling and chemosis common
Bacterial (nongonococcal)*	After 5 days	Variable presentation, depending on organism
Herpetic	Within 2 wk	Conjunctiva only mildly injected Serosanguineous discharge Vesicular rash on lids sometimes seen Most have concomitant systemic herpetic disease

* *Staphylococcus aureus, S. epidermidis, Streptococcus pneumoniae, S. viridans, Haemophilus influenzae, Escherichia coli, Pseudomonas aeruginosa.*

5. What other diagnostic tool is used to differentiate the various causes of neonatal conjunctivitis?

In most cases one cannot rely solely on clinical characteristics and time of onset for accurate diagnosis; therefore, initial therapy is also based on the results of Gram and Giemsa stains performed immediately on conjunctival swabs and scrapings. Their classic characteristics are as follows:

Cause	Stain	Findings
Chemical	Gram	Polymorphonuclear neutrophils (PMNs)
Chlamydial	Giemsa	Basophilic intracytoplasmic inclusion bodies in conjunctival epithelial cells
Gonococcal	Gram	Gram-negative intracellular diplococci in PMNs
Bacteria	Gram	Gram-positive or gram-negative organisms
Herpes simplex	Giemsa	Multinucleated giant cells, lymphocytes, plasma cells

The above findings, although classic, are not seen in all cases. Specimens are also sent for culture and sensitivity testing and antigen detection tests. Treatment regimens are adjusted accordingly once the results are known, and clinical response is observed.

6. Is a follicular reaction in the conjunctiva more indicative of a chlamydial or gonococcal infection?

Neither. Follicular reactions are not seen in the neonate because of the immaturity of the immune system.

7. Why is Crede prophylaxis (2% silver nitrate drops) no longer the standard agent of choice for routine neonatal conjunctivitis prevention?

Crede prophylaxis is no longer the favored agent because of its high incidence of associated chemical conjunctivitis.

8. What is currently used for neonatal prophylaxis?

The American Academy of Pediatrics endorses the use of 1% tetracycline or 0.5% erythromycin ointment for neonatal prophylaxis. This is aimed primarily at preventing gonococcal conjunctivitis, which can have devastating ocular consequences. It is also effective for chlamydial infection.

9. What is the differential diagnosis of neonatal conjunctivitis?

1. Birth trauma (usually evident by history)

2. Foreign body/corneal abrasion (usually diagnosed by a combination of history and exam with flourescein)

3. Congenital glaucoma (Accompanying early signs are tearing, photophobia, blepharospasm, and fussiness. Later signs include corneal edema and corneal enlargement. Intraocular pressure is elevated.)

4. Nasolacrimal duct obstruction (Occurs in 6% of neonates and is usually associated with edema of the inner canthus and matting of the eyelids. Tearing is common, and the conjunctiva is usually not affected.)

5. Dacryocystitis (infection of the lacrimal sac, with erythema and swelling of the inner canthus and nasal conjunctival injection. Purulent drainage can often be expressed from the punctum.)

10. When is systemic treatment indicated for neonatal conjunctivitis? Why?

Systemic treatment is necessary for all cases of chlamydial, gonococcal, and herpetic conjunctivitis because of the potential for serious disseminated disease. A complete systemic examination is performed at the time of diagnosis to determine the extent of disease.

11. List the potential ocular and systemic sequelae of untreated neonatal conjunctivitis.

Type	Ocular	Systemic
Chemical	None (a self-limited entity)	None
Chlamydial	Chronic infection may cause corneal scarring and symblepharon (adhesion of eyelid to eye)	Pneumonitis and otitis media

(Table continued on following page.)

Type	Ocular	Systemic
Gonococcal	Corneal ulceration, perforation, and endophthalmitis (may occur within 24 hr of onset)	Meningitis, arthritis, and sepsis
Bacterial	*Pseudomonas* sp. may cause corneal ulcer, perforation, and endophthalmitis	Usually none
Herpetic	Recurrences throughout life may cause corneal scarring and profound amblyopia. Chorioretinitis and cataracts also may develop.	Meningitis and disseminated CNS disease (mortality rate can be as high as 85%)

12. What is the treatment for chlamydial conjunctivitis?

Oral erythromycin syrup is given for 2–3 weeks (50 mg/kg/day in 4 divided doses) along with erythromycin or sulfa ointment to the eye 4 times/day. The mother and her sexual partner also are treated with oral tetracycline, 250–500 mg 4 times/day, or doxycycline, 100 mg 2 times/day, for 7 days for presumed systemic disease, even if asymptomatic. Tetracycline cannot be used in children or breast-feeding mothers because it will stain developing teeth.

13. What is the treatment for gonococcal conjunctivitis?

Because of the high incidence of penicillin-resistant organisms, the Centers for Disease Control recommends treatment with penicillinase-resistant antibiotics. Intravenous ceftriaxone (a third-generation cephalosporin) is started immediately and is given for 7 days at a dose of 25–50 mg/kg/day. The intravenous form can be changed to an oral equivalent after significant improvement is noted to complete a 7-day course. A single 125-mg intramuscular dose of ceftriaxone or a 100-mg/kg intramuscular dose of cefotaxime given immediately after diagnosis is an accepted alternative treatment. Bacitracin ointment may be administered topically 4 times/day, and saline lavage is used hourly until the discharge is eliminated. Because of the high incidence of concomitant chlamydial infection in women who contract gonorrhea, the infant, mother, and her sexual partner are also treated systemically for chlamydia as outlined above. It is reasonable to test for other sexually transmitted diseases.

14. What is the treatment for bacterial conjunctivitis?

Erythromycin or gentamicin ointment is applied 4 times/day for 2 weeks for gram-positive or gram-negative conjunctival swab results, respectively. Antibiotic choice may be altered later once culture and sensitivity results are known. In cases of corneal involvement, as seen with virulent organisms such as *Pseudomonas* sp., fortified topical antibiotics are administered and are often supplemented by systemic treatment.

15. What is the treatment for herpes simplex viral conjunctivitis?

Intravenous acyclovir, 10 mg/kg, is given every 8 hours for 10 days, along with vidarabine 3% ointment (Vira-A), 5 times/day, or trifluorothymidine 1% (viroptic), every 2 hours, for 1 week.

16. How can the incidence of ophthalmia neonatorum be reduced in future generations?

The population most at risk for contracting neonatal conjunctivitis is infants born to mothers without adequate prenatal care or mothers involved with substance abuse. Because of its high association with serious systemic disease, neonatal conjunctivitis is still an important public health issue worldwide. Although not universally accepted, some countries (e.g., Sweden and England) have abandoned the use of routine prophylaxis after birth in favor of careful screening for sexually transmitted diseases and better prenatal care.

BIBLIOGRAPHY

1. Albert DM, Jakobiec FA: Principles and Practice of Ophthalmology. Philadelphia, W.B. Saunders, 1994.
2. Chandler JW: Controversies in ocular prophylaxis of newborns. Arch Ophthalmol 107:814–815, 1989.
3. Cullom R, Chang B: The Wills Eye Manual—Office and Emergency Room Diagnosis and Treatment of Eye Disease. Philadelphia, J.B. Lippincott, 1994.
4. Hammerschlag M: Neonatal conjunctivitis. Pediatr Ann 22:346–351, 1993.
5. Laga M, Naamara W, Brunham R, et al: Single-dose therapy of gonococcal ophthalmia neonatorum with ceftriaxone. N Engl J Med 315:1382–1385, 1986.
6. O'Hara M: Ophthalmia Neonatorum. Pediatr Clin North Am 40:715–725, 1993.
7. Weiss A: Chronic conjunctivitis in infants and children. Pediatr Ann 22:366–374, 1993.

11. TOPICAL ANTIBIOTICS AND STEROIDS

Stephen Y. Lee, M.D.

1. You are an antibiotic or steroid eye drop just placed in the conjunctival fornix. Discuss the barriers to your journey into the eye.

Many eye drop dispensers deliver a 50-μl eye drop. However, only 20% of this volume is retained by the conjunctival cul-de-sac in most patients, and the excess immediately flows over the eyelids. Of the portion that remains, approximately 80% drains through the lacrimal system. In addition, because of the 15% per minute tear turnover rate, almost all of the topically applied medication disappears from the conjunctival cul-de-sac in about 5 minutes. Irritating drugs produce reflex tearing and may be cleared more quickly.

During this critical 5 minutes, the topically applied drug faces numerous tissue obstacles. Nonproductive absorption by the conjunctiva quickly disperses the medication systemically via the conjunctival vasculature. The small portion that penetrates the episclera faces the relative impermeability of the sclera and the tight junctions of the retinal pigment epithelium. The cornea poses three different barriers to entry. The corneal epithelium and the endothelium possess tight junctions that force the drugs to pass through the cellular membranes and limit passage of hydrophilic drugs. The corneal stroma is water-rich and limits movement of lipophilic drugs. Even after entry into the anterior chamber, the lens effectively limits most drug penetration, and very little enters the posterior segment of the eye through topical administration.

Such formidable barriers seem insurmountable, but inflammation and infection render these barriers less effective, and modifications of the drug and/or its vehicle can facilitate entry into the eye. In addition, the desired site of action may be the ocular surface and not inside the eye.

2. Given the above barriers, how would you increase delivery of topical antibiotics or steroids to the desired site of action?

The patient can perform punctal occlusion to decrease the amount of drainage through the lacrimal system by 65% and leave more drugs for intraocular absorption. Of course, frequent instillation also increases drug absorption, but the practical limit is probably every 5 minutes because the subsequent eye drop can wash out the previous eye drop before intraocular absorption.

Changing the characteristics of the drug and/or its vehicle also improves delivery. Increasing the concentration of the drug may be limited by the solubility of the drug in the vehicle, and the high tonicity of higher concentrations triggers reflex tearing that quickly clears the drug from the ocular surface. Also, increasing lipid solubility of the drug appears to promote corneal passage despite the dual barrier characteristic of the cornea. In addition, adding surfactants that disturb the corneal epithelium dramatically increases drug entry.

3. Name the three different formulations of topical medications and the advantages and the disadvantages of each.

Ophthalmic preparations can be made as eye drops, suspensions, or ointments. Eye drops are easily instilled, but contact time is minimal, requiring frequent administration. In addition, the "pulse" nature of absorption invites transient overdose and toxicity. Suspensions allow longer contact time, but the particulate nature of the preparation may be irritating and trigger reflex tearing. Suspensions settle to the bottom of the bottle and need to be shaken before instilling the eye drop. Patients also may complain of accumulation of the precipitates or forget to shake the bottle before administering the eye drop. Ointments increase the contact time further, requiring the least frequent instillation, but leave a film over the eye that blurs vision. In addition, water-soluble drugs do not dissolve in the ointment vehicle and are present as crystals. Crystals are trapped in the ointment vehicle until the crystals on the surface of the ointment contact the ocular surface after the ointment vehicle melts with exposure to body temperature. This type of absorption allows entry of constant but low amounts of the drug.

Other delivery systems such as soft contact lenses, soluble ocular inserts, or implantable devices are also options.

4. A 60-year-old man complains of crusting of the eyelids in the morning and chronic foreign body sensation. Examination reveals moderate blepharitis with numerous collarettes around the eyelashes. What would you recommend?

Blepharitis often responds well to just warm compresses, but supplemental antibiotic ointments applied to the eyelash base or conjunctiva may be helpful, especially when numerous collarettes are seen around the eyelashes. Frequently used antibiotic ointments include erythromycin, bacitracin, and polysporin. Erythromycin is a macrolide antibiotic that inhibits bacterial protein synthesis by binding to 50S ribosomal unit. It has a broad spectrum of coverage but suffers from poor intraocular absorption and is most appropriate for blepharitis and mild conjunctivitis. Bacitracin is composed of numerous polypeptides that inhibit bacterial cell wall synthesis. Polysporin combines bacitracin and polymyxin B, which are peptides that act like detergents to lyse bacterial cell membranes, and offers better coverage of gram-negative bacteria.

5. A 30-year-old woman with "cold" symptoms presents with redness and mucous discharge in both eyes. The ocular symptoms began in the right eye 1 week ago but now involve both eyes despite treatment of the right eye with sulfacetamide 4 times/day, as prescribed by her family physician. Examination reveals bilateral follicular conjunctivitis with preauricular adenopathy. What would you recommend?

History and examination are consistent with viral conjunctivitis. Artificial tears and cool compresses may provide comfort. Topical antibiotics are not required, but 1-week follow-up is advisable to look for potential membranous conjunctivitis, which may require topical steroids. Sulfacetamide is a bacteriostatic structural analog of p-amino-benzoic acid and inhibits synthesis of folic acid. It has a broad spectrum of coverage and good corneal penetration and becomes more effective when combined with trimethoprim, which blocks a successive step in bacterial folate metabolism. It appears to be used often by nonophthalmologists for initial treatment of red eyes; it is fine for mild bacterial conjunctivitis but is not required for viral conjunctivitis.

6. A 55-year-old woman complains of discharge and redness of her right eye for 4 weeks. Her family physician told her that she had "pink eye" and prescribed erythromycin ointment, then sulfacetamide, and then ciprofloxacin, but the symptoms have not improved. Examination reveals diffuse papillary conjunctivitis with purulent discharge. There is no preauricular adenopathy or previous history of "cold" symptoms. What should you do?

The patient has chronic bacterial conjunctivitis. Topical therapy usually brings prompt relief, and you should make sure that she uses the medications properly. Assuming that she is getting the medications into the eye in a proper dosing regimen, conjunctival cultures can be performed to look for resistant or unusual bacteria. Chronic dacryocystitis should be investigated by applying firm pressure below the medial canthal tendon in an attempt to produce a diagnostic purulent discharge through the lacrimal punctum. An abscess in the nasolacrimal sac may provide a source of bacteria resistant to topical antibiotics.

7. A 25-year-old man holding a towel over his right eye complains of copious discharge that began in the morning. Examination reveals diffuse conjunctival hyperemia and chemosis with thick purulent discharge. A prominent preauricular adenopathy is also present. What should you do?

Hyperacute bacterial conjunctivitis in sexually active patients should prompt a conjunctival smear and culture to look for gonococcal conjunctivitis. Although rare, gonococcal conjunctivitis requires immediate systemic antibiotics with topical antibiotics as an adjunctive treatment only.

8. A 26-year-old physician in a general surgery residency with a doctorate in pharmacology presents with foreign body sensation and photophobia in both eyes after sleeping with soft contact lenses during his call night. A midperipheral 2-mm corneal ulcer with surrounding corneal stromal edema is present with scant anterior chamber reaction. What should you do?

The chances of developing a corneal ulcer increase by a factor of ten when the patient sleeps with contact lenses. In addition, corneal cultures are recommended, although some ophthalmologists may manage small corneal ulcers without cultures (controversial).

Initial therapy should cover a broad spectrum of bacteria. Traditionally, fortified cephalosporin and aminoglycoside have been used, but some believe that fluoroquinolones offer similar efficacy with less toxicity (controversial). In addition, fortified topical antibiotics are not universally available and need to be refrigerated.

Fluoroquinolones inhibit bacterial DNA synthesis by binding to DNA gyrase and inhibiting the supercoiling of bacterial DNA. They offer a superb spectrum of coverage in in vitro studies, even against methicillin-resistant *Staphylococcus aureus*, if administered early in the course of infection. It appears to be highly effective for most corneal ulcers, especially contact lens-induced corneal ulcers, but large clinical series with attention to resistance and treatment failure have not been completed.

Aminoglycosides bind to bacterial ribosomal subunits and interfere with protein synthesis. They offer a broad spectrum of coverage but require transport into the bacteria, which may be reduced in anaerobic environments of an abscess. Coadministration of antibiotics that alter bacterial cell wall structure improves aminoglycoside penetration into bacteria and produces a synergistic effect.

Cephalosporins are beta-lactam antibiotics synthesized or derived from compounds isolated from the fungus *Cephalosporium acremonium*. They inhibit bacterial transpeptidase, which is critical for bacterial cell wall synthesis. In general, later generations provide broader coverage with better gram-negative but poorer gram-positive activity. Cephazolin is a first-generation cephalosporin that is traditionally combined with an aminoglycoside for the initial treatment of a corneal ulcer. It covers gram-positive and some gram-negative organisms but misses *Pseudomonas* sp. and, therefore, requires the addition of an aminoglycoside for initial broad-spectrum coverage.

9. After corneal cultures are done, the patient is instructed to take ciprofloxacin every hour around the clock. Next day, he is in worse pain, and the corneal ulcer has enlarged to 3 mm with tenacious purulent discharge. What is your next step?

Make sure the eye drops are getting into the eye. Ask the patient to demonstrate eye drop administration. Several eye drops fall on the floor, then on his cheeks, and finally he announces success when the eye drops fall on his closed eyelids. Often, antibiotic failure is due to improper administration. Patients should be observed taking their eye drops, and a friend or family member may need to administer the eye drops to be sure that the medications are getting to the source of infection, especially when frequent instillation is required. Indeed, some patients require hospitalization to receive intensive eye drop administration.

In addition, the patient should have taken the drug more often. Manufacturer's recommended dose of ciprofloxacin for corneal ulcers is two drops every 15 minutes for the first 6 hours followed by 2 drops every half hour for the remainder of the first day. Frequent dosing of ciprofloxacin may produce a white precipitate over the ulcer , but this precipitate does not appear to impede the bactericidal activity and usually resolves when the dose is tapered.

10. The patient now prefers a "proven" treatment regimen with a long history and requests topical fortified antibiotics. However, he recalls that minimal bactericidal concentration for most pathogenic bacteria is far below that provided by the fortified antibiotics and accuses you of wasting money and drugs. Is he right?

No. In vitro and in vivo results in other sites of the body may not be applicable to the eye. Indeed, in the vitreous, the dose-response relationship has been demonstrated up to 100 times the in vitro minimal bactericidal concentration.

11. The patient reminds you that he is penicillin-allergic and does not enjoy anaphylaxis. What antibiotics should you choose. How do you begin therapy?

Penicillin is often not used in ophthalmology because of poor penetration into the blood ocular barrier and active transport out of the eye by the organic acid transport system of the ciliary body. However, inflammation improves ocular penetration. Penicillin inhibits bacterial transpeptidase and prevents bacterial cell wall synthesis. Varieties of modification of the original compound have produced varying spectrums of activity. Penicillin G and V are still highly effective for many gram-positive and gram-negative bacteria, but many strains of *Staphylococcus aureus* and *epidermidis* are now resistant. Penicillinase-resistant penicillins such as methicillin are useful for penicillinase-producing staphylococci. Broad-spectrum penicillins, ampicillin and amoxicillin, have better gram-negative coverage, and semisynthetic penicillins such as carbenicillin and ticarcillin extend coverage to *Pseudomonas, Enterobacter,* and *Proteus* spp.

Immediate allergic response to penicillin, such as hives or anaphylaxis, is a strong contraindication for its use, and there is 10% cross-reactivity with cephalosporins. Therefore, for patients with penicillin allergy, cefazolin should be replaced with vancomycin. Vancomycin is a complex glycopeptide that inhibits bacterial cell wall synthesis with principally gram-positive coverage, including methicillin-resistant *S. aureus* and *Streptococcus faecalis*, which is a frequent bacterial pathogen in infections of filtering blebs.

As mentioned above, an aminoglycoside is synergistic with cell wall-inhibiting antibiotics, and the patient should be started on fortified vancomycin and tobramycin, alternating every 5 minutes times 4 doses, followed by alternation every half hour. Actual dosing may vary in different institutions.

12. Next morning the ulcer looks worse with 4 mm corneal infiltrate and purulent material overlying the ulcer. The corneal culture confirms *Pseudomonas aeruginosa*. Why did the patient not improve?

Pseudomonas corneal ulcers sometimes require double coverage. Fortified ticarcillin should be added in a nonpenicillin-allergic patient. In this case, ciprofloxacin could be resumed.

13. Next day, the ulcer looks stable, but the patient complains of persistent and perhaps worsening pain. Examination reveals diffuse punctate corneal epithelial defects, inferior conjunctival erythema, and swollen lower eyelids. What should you do?

Toxicity is often less severe with topical administration; indeed, some common topical antibiotics such as neomycin and polymyxin cannot be given intravenously because of systemic toxicity. However, intensive regimens of potent antibiotics often produce surface toxicity with prominent involvement of lower more than upper conjunctiva. Occasionally, only analgesics and cool compresses can be offered if the infection is not under control. Fortified vancomycin may be decreased because tobramycin and ciprofloxacin are more important for *Pseudomonas* ulcer, and the ulcer appears to be stabilizing.

14. The patient slowly improves, but significant corneal scar remains. He would like binocular vision for his surgical career and asks you to get rid of his corneal scar. How do you respond?

Read on to learn about topical steroids. Often, inflammatory scars fade well with topical steroids. When and how much and how long to use topical steroids is controversial, but a trial of topical steroids is certainly warranted before considering surgical options.

15. Review the currently available topical antibiotics in generic and brand names.

Generic Name	Brand Name	Preparation
Aminoglycosides		
Gentamicin	Genoptic S.O.P.	Ointment or solution 0.3%
Tobramycin	Tobrex	Ointment or solution 0.3%

(Table continued on following page.)

Generic Name	Brand Name	Preparation
Bacitracin	AK-tracin	Ointment 500 U/gm
Chloramphenicol	Chloromycetin Ocu-chlor Chloroptic	0.5% ointment, 1.0% solution
Ciprofloxacin	Ciloxan	0.3% solution
Erythromycin	AK-mycin Ilotycin	0.5% ointment

Bacitracin, neomycin,
  and polymyxin B
	Neosporin	400 U/g, 3.5 mg/gm,
		  10,000 U/gm

Sulfisoxazole	Gantrisin	4% solution
Sulfacetamide	Bleph-10 Vasosulf Sodium Sulfamyd	10% solution 10% solution 10% ointment
Tetracycline	Achromycin	1% solution or ointment
Polymyxin and bacitracin	Polysporin	10,000 U/gm, 500 U/gm
Trimethoprim and polymyxin B	Polytrim	0.1%/10,000 U/ml

16. How do topical steroids work?

The specific mechanisms of action of steroids are incompletely understood. At a molecular level, inhibition of arachidonic acid release from phospholipids may be the most important effect. Arachidonic acid is converted to prostaglandins and related compounds that are potent mediators of inflammation. At a cellular level, steroids must be carried to the cytoplasm, where they bind to soluble receptors and then enter the nucleus to alter transcription of various proteins involved in immune regulation and inflammation. At the tissue level, steroids suppress the cardinal signs of inflammation such as edema, heat, pain, and redness through a variety of mechanisms. They cause vasoconstriction and decrease vascular permeability to inflammatory cells. Cellular and intracellular membranes are stabilized to inhibit release of inflammatory mediators such as histamine. Neutrophilic leucocytosis is inhibited, and macrophage recruitment and migration are also decreased. Overall, steroids are potent antiinflammatory and immune-suppressing agents with wide-ranging ophthalmic applications, but their adverse effects as well as their benefits should be understood.

17. Since steroids are not cures, what general categories of disorders warrant ophthalmic use of topical steroids?

Abelson and Butrus identify three broad categories of disorders that warrant steroid use: postsurgical, immune hyperreactivity, and combined immune and infectious processes. Remarkably, postoperative use of steroids has not been evaluated in a well-controlled, double-blinded study. Although their use in this setting is almost universal, some ophthalmologists report adequate control of postoperative inflammation with topical nonsteroidals for various ophthalmic procedures (controversial). The second category includes various uveitides, allergic and vernal conjunctivitis, corneal graft rejections, and other processes in which the immune system activity is harmful to the host tissue. The last category includes viral and bacterial corneal ulcers, especially herpes simplex and herpes zoster, in which control of infectious process must be balanced with control of inflammation that may scar delicate ocular tissue.

18. The physician with the residual corneal scar wants to minimize his corneal scar but is concerned about potential side effects of topical steroids. How do you advise him?

Exacerbation of the existing infection with reactivation of dormant organisms or inhibition of wound healing is the most immediate concern. Other well-known adverse effects include glaucoma and cataracts, but numerous other side effects have been observed, including blepharoptosis, eyelid skin or scleral atrophy, and mydriasis.

Systemic absorption may be significant, and punctal occlusion should be encouraged. A 6-week regimen of topical 0.1% dexamethasone sodium phosphate has been shown to suppress the adrenal cortex, and some patients with systemic hay fever improve with topical ocular steroids. Of course, all of these effects are more frequent with intensive and chronic use of steroids.

19. After a lengthy discussion, the patient agrees to try topical steroids. However, given his interest in pharmacology, he requests a brief discussion of the pharmacokinetics of a few of the available topical steroids.

Topical steroids may be prepared as solutions, suspensions, or ointments. Phosphate preparations may be prepared as solutions because they are highly water-soluble in the aqueous vehicles but penetrate less well into intact corneal epithelium than acetate or alcohol suspensions, which have biphasic solubility. Nevertheless, 1% prednisolone phosphate achieves a significant corneal level of 10 μg/gm within 30 minutes after instillation, which improves to 235 μg/gm when the corneal epithelium is removed. Dexamethasone phosphate enters the cornea and anterior chamber within 10 minutes, reaches a maximum in 30–60 minutes, and slowly disappears over the next few to 24 hours.

20. The patient also requests that the most potent steroid be used with rapid taper so that the overall course may be shortened. Which steroid do you choose?

Antiinflammatory effects of topical steroids differ depending on the clinical setting and method of measurement. However, certain generalizations can be made:

1. Higher concentrations and more frequent instillations, up to every 5 minutes, increase concentrations of steroids in the cornea and aqueous.

2. With corneal epithelium intact, prednisolone acetate suspension > dexamethasone alcohol solution > prednisolone sodium phosphate solution > dexamethasone phosphate ointment.

3. With corneal epithelial defects, prednisolone sodium phosphate solution > dexamethasone phosphate solution > prednisolone acetate suspension.

21. The patient is started on 1% prednisolone acetate 4 times/day. His scar is beginning to recede, but he returns 2 days later with complaints of a white precipitate that forms in his conjunctiva and insists on a change of medication to prevent this annoying build-up. Which steroid do you choose now?

Suspensions leave a milky precipitate that some patients find unpleasant. In addition, despite shaking the bottles before instillation, a variable amount of the suspension may be delivered if particles are not evenly distributed. Therefore, some ophthalmologists prefer phosphate solutions despite lower potency with intact epithelium. A change to 1% prednisolone phosphate is reasonable if patient compliance is improved.

22. On day 10 of steroid therapy, the corneal scar is receding rapidly, but the patient complains of foreign body sensation. Examination reveals large corneal epithelial dendrites. What should you do?

Steroids do not cause herpetic keratitis but may promote herpetic keratitis when viral shedding is timed with the presence of steroids on the ocular surface. Often the dendrites are large and numerous in the presence of steroids, and steroids should be stopped or rapidly tapered. Of course, full dose of trifluridine should be begun.

23. Fortunately, the dendrite heals rapidly and the previous corneal scar has faded significantly with return to 20/20 vision in that eye. Four years have passed, and the patient is now seeking employment. Opportunities are scarce, and his only job offer is from a large organized health company that hopes to use him as a pharmacist as well as a physician as a cost-saving measure. Understandably, he is stressed. Now he notices extreme photophobia

and redness of his eye. **Examination reveals corneal stromal edema and focal keratic precipitates consistent with herpes simplex keratouveitis. What should you do?**

Many stimuli, including stress, promote recurrence of herpetic keratitis. Other stimuli include menses, sun exposure, and fever. If the inflammation is severe or central vision is threatened, steroids should be given with trifluridine coverage to decrease corneal scarring and intraocular inflammation. One regimen may be trifluridine and 1% prednisolone acetate, both 4 times/day. Other regimens may be acceptable, but an easily remembered regimen is to add trifluridine drop for drop with the topical steroids. Antiviral coverage is probably unnecessary below 1 drop per day of 1% prednisolone acetate.

24. Two days later, only marginal improvement is noted, but intraocular pressure is 35 mmHg. What happened?

Significant steroid-induced rises in intraocular pressure have been demonstrated in up to 6% of patients after 6 weeks of topical dexamethasone, and patients with glaucoma or family history of glaucoma are particularly susceptible. The mechanism appears to be decreased aqueous outflow, perhaps as a result of deposition of mucopolysaccharides in the trabecular meshwork. The extent of intraocular pressure rise varies with type and dose of steroids. Usually, steroids with greater anti-inflammatory potency elicit greater elevation of intraocular pressure. For example, steroids with low intraocular bioavailability and potency, such as fluorometholone, cause lower rises in intraocular pressure after a greater duration of therapy than more potent steroids such as dexamethasone. Rimexolone claims to be the exception. It appears to have similar suppression of anterior chamber cell and flare as 1% prednisolone acetate with intraocular pressure elevation similar to fluorometholone. Regardless, the elevated intraocular pressure subsides, usually within 2 weeks, by decreasing or discontinuing steroid therapy, but topical aqueous suppressants may be needed in some patients.

However, steroid-induced rises in intraocular pressure rarely occur in less than 2 weeks and certainly not after 2 days of steroid therapy. Patients with intraocular inflammations, especially in herpetic keratouveitis, may have increased intraocular pressure as a result of intraocular inflammation. Therefore, in the present patient, the topical steroids should be increased and not decreased.

25. The frequency of prednisolone acetate administration was increased to every 3 hr while awake, and timolol, 2 times/day, was added. One week later intraocular pressure is normal, and intraocular inflammation has subsided. Prednisolone acetate is tapered to 2 times/day. The patient returns 2 days later with recurrence of pain and photophobia and return of intraocular inflammation. What happened?

You tapered the steroids too quickly. A useful rule is to decrease steroids by no more than half of the previous dose, especially in herpetic keratouveitis, in which rebound inflammation is frequent. Make sure that the patient is still taking the eye drops. Sometimes patients abruptly stop the eye drops when they feel better and then suffer rebound inflammation.

26. Review the commonly available topical steroids and their generic and brand names.

Generic Name	Brand Name	Preparation
Dexamethasone sodium phosphate	AK-Dex AK-Dex	0.05% ointment 0.1% solution
Fluorometholone	FML forte FML liquifilm, Fluor-op FML S.O.P.	0.25% suspension 0.1% suspension 0.1% ointment
Prednisolone acetate	Predforte, Econopred plus Predmild, Econopred	1% suspension 0.125% suspension
Prednisolone sodium phosphate	Inflamase forte, AK-pred 1% Inflamase mild, AK-pred 0.125%	1% solution 0.125% solution
Rimexolone	Vexol	1% suspension

BIBLIOGRAPHY

1. Abelson MB, Butrus S: Corticosteroids in ophthalmic practice. In Jakobiec FA, Albert D (eds): Principles and Practice of Ophthalmology, vol 6. Philadelphia, W.B. Saunders, 1994, pp 1013–1022.
2. Axelrod J, Glew R, Barza M, et al: Antibacterials. In Jakobiec FA, Albert D (eds): Principles and Practice of Ophthalmology, vol 6. Philadelphia, W.B. Saunders, 1994, pp 940–960.
3. Baum JL: Initial therapy of suspected microbial corneal ulcers. I: Broad antibiotic therapy based on prevalence of organisms. Surv Ophthalmol 24:97–105, 1979.
4. Callegan MC, Engel LS, Hill JM, et al: Ciprofloxacin versus tobramycin for the treatment of staphylo-coccal keratitis. Inv Ophthalmol Vis Sci 35:1033–1037, 1994.
5. Foster CS, Alter G, Debarge LR, et al: Efficacy and safety of rimexolone 1% ophthalmic suspension vs. 1% prednisolone acetate in the treatment of uveitis. Am J Ophthalmol 122:171–182, 1996.
6. Leibowitz HM, Bartlett JD, Rich R, et al: Intraocular pressure-raising potential of 1% rimexolone in pa-tients responding to corticosteroids. Arch Ophthalmol 114:933–937, 1996.
7. Tripathi RC, Tripathi BJ, Li J, et al: Ocular pharmacology. In Basic and Clinical Science Course, sect 2. San Francisco, American Academy of Ophthalmology, 1995, pp 312–354.
8. Ueno N, Refojo MF, Abelson M: Pharmacokinetics. In Jakobiec FA, Albert D (eds): Principles and Practice of Ophthalmology, vol 6. Philadelphia, W.B. Saunders, 1994, pp 916–928.

12. DRY EYES

Peter R. Laibson, M.D.

1. What is the definition of a dry eye?

A dry eye, or keratoconjunctivitis sicca, is a condition in which the precorneal tear film is deficient and cannot fulfill its normal function of lubricating the anterior surface of the cornea. The resulting changes in ocular surface are associated with ocular discomfort.

2. What is the precorneal tear film?

The precorneal tear film is a thin fluid layer measuring approximately 7 microns in thickness. It is present on the front surface of the cornea adjacent to the corneal epithelium.

3. Discuss the types of dry eye conditions.

There are basically two types of dry eye conditions: (1) the tear-deficient dry eye, in which the fluid component of the tear film is decreased or insufficient, and (2) the evaporative type of dry eye, in which other problems may be related to the tear film, such as eyelid problems, difficulty with contact lenses that ride on the tear film, or corneal surface changes.

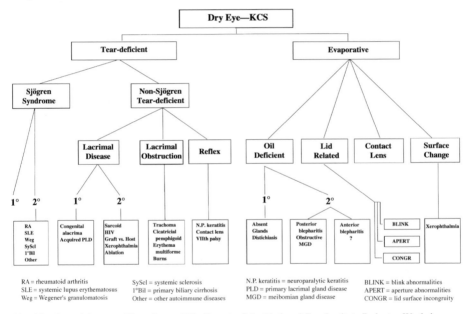

Classification of dry eye. (From Lemp MA: Report of the National Eye Institute/Industry Workshop on Clinical Trials in Dry Eyes. CLAO J 21(4):221–232, 1996, with permission.)

4. What are the components of the precorneal tear film?

The precorneal tear film consists of three components. The outer layer exposed to the air is a thin lipid layer derived from the meibomian glands, the openings of which are along the margin of the upper and lower lids. The middle layer of the tear film, the thickest section, is composed of aqueous tears derived from the main and accessory lacrimal glands. The innermost layer is a mucin layer attached to the outer epithelial cell surface (the villus surface). This mucus gel is responsible for the aqueous layer remaining intact on the corneal surface. The mucin is mainly derived from conjunctival goblet cells but can be produced by corneal and conjunctival epithelial cells.

5. How does the precorneal tear film maintain its position on the corneal epithelial surface?

Hydrodynamic factors such as mechanical spreading during the blink, tear clearance during the blink, and tear film corneal surface tension aid in maintaining the precorneal tear film on the corneal surface.

6. What are the symptoms of a dry eye condition?

The symptoms of dry eye are related to a decreased presence or lowered volume of the precorneal tear film. Symptoms consist of irritation, foreign body sensation, a sensation of sand in the eye, and light sensitivity. These symptoms are usually prevalent more in the afternoon or evening than in the morning on awakening. Patients in a dry or dusty environment or an environment that has air pollutants are more symptomatic than patients with dry eye who are not exposed to ocular irritants.

7. What conditions are seen in conjunction with keratoconjunctivitis sicca?

Patients with dry eye conditions frequently have eyelid inflammation and blepharitis, which may or may not be due to staphylococcal infection of the meibomian glands. Another associated condition is seborrheic blepharitis, which often occurs with keratoconjunctivitis sicca. Patients with collagen vascular disorders are more likely to have keratoconjunctivitis sicca than patients without these disorders.

8. What is Sjögren's syndrome? How is it related to a dry eye condition?

Sjögren's syndrome is a triad of symptoms: dry eyes, dry mouth (xerostomia), and a collagen vascular disorder, usually rheumatoid arthritis. Other collagen vascular disorders include systemic lupus erythematosus, Wegener's granulomatosis, scleroderma, systemic sclerosis, primary biliary cirrhosis, and other autoimmune diseases.

9. What medications can worsen or even create a dry eye condition?

Many topical or systemic medications may exacerbate a dry eye condition. Topical eye drops may worsen dry eyes because the medication or the preservative in the eye drop may cause toxicity to the corneal epithelial cells. The aminoglycoside antibiotics (e.g., neosporin and gentamicin), some beta blockers, and even artificial tears with preservatives may worsen a dry eye state. Any topical eye drop with preservatives can alter the ocular surface.

Numerous systemic medications may decrease tear film production and exacerbate dry eye symptoms. Atropine and scopolamine may decrease tear production. Estrogens, antihypertensive medications, antidepressant drugs, marijuana, morphine, and numerous other medications used systemically may decrease tear film production and exacerbate a dry eye condition.

10. Are women or men more likely to develop dry eyes?

Women are more likely than men to develop dry eyes later in life, probably in relation to the varying estrogen levels in postmenopausal women, in whom dry eyes are most frequently seen.

11. At what age do people get keratoconjunctivitis sicca?

Keratoconjunctivitis sicca may be seen at all ages but is much more common after 60 years of age, particularly in women. Keratoconjunctivitis sicca may be seen in infants and young children, although it is rare in infants and uncommon in young children. It may be prevalent in people in their 20s and 30s, but unless it is suspected, it may be overlooked because most people with dry eye conditions are older. Younger patients who develop keratoconjunctivitis sicca may later develop collagen vascular disorders. The dry eye may be the earliest manifestation of a collagen vascular disorder.

12. What are the most common signs of dry eye disorder?

Most often the early stages relate to ocular symptoms rather than signs of dry eye. When signs of dry eye occur, they include a decreased tear film meniscus and debris in the precorneal tear film. Intermittent conjunctival injection and superficial punctate keratitis, as well as superficial punctate conjunctivitis, may be seen. Later patients may develop filamentary keratitis with their dry eye problems. Blepharitis is often an accompanying symptoms of keratoconjunctivitis sicca.

13. What conjunctival disorders may cause a dry eye problem?

Patients with evaporative dry eyes may have conjunctival scarring, which decreases or eliminates the conjunctival goblet cells responsible for the inner layer of the tear film (the mucus layer). Conjunctival scarring diseases include cicatricial ocular phemphigoid, severe scarring from the end stages of erythema multiforme (Stevens-Johnson syndrome); chemical burns, particularly alkali burns of the conjunctiva; and the unusual circumstances of conjunctival scarring from graft vs. host disease in patients with bone marrow transplantation. Patients with other conjunctival disorders that accompany conditions such as aniridia also may have dry eyes.

14. How is keratoconjunctivitis sicca diagnosed?

Patients who have symptoms of dry eye need to show objective evidence of keratoconjunctivitis sicca for proper diagnosis and institution of therapy. The first signs of dry eye may be seen at the slit lamp, including a decreased tear film meniscus with excessive debris and mucus in the tear film. This sign indicates that the volume of the tear film is decreased. Superficial punctate corneal gray spots and conjunctival injection may be seen. Dry eye condition is often accompanied by eyelid inflammation due either to seborrheic or staphylococcal blepharitis.

15. What objective tests help to make a diagnosis of keratitis sicca?

The ophthalmologist has several means available in the office to help make the diagnosis of a dry eye state. Fluorescein staining of the corneal epithelium and the conjunctival epithelium, usually in the exposed interpalpebral fissure or the lower one-third of the cornea, may be evident. The earliest staining may be along the limbus, between 3:00 and 5:00 o'clock and between 7:00 and 9:00 o'clock. There also may be punctate conjunctival epithelial staining in the exposed inter palpebral fissure. Usually the corneal epithelium and the conjunctival epithelium in the upper half of the cornea are spared in the early stages of dry eye problem. Rose bengal stains epithelial cells that are degenerated but still in place and may show earlier staining than fluorescein. Rose bengal is not as readily available as fluorescein dye and may cause irritation when it is used in the relatively undiluted form.

16. How can tear film stability help to diagnose dry eyes?

Once fluorescein is placed on the corneal surface, the tear film assumes a fine, uniform dark green-black appearance as the dye disperses. Where the tear film is insufficient, the uniform dark green-black color may break up rapidly, indicating the presence of a relative dry eye condition. The normal tear film break-up time is 10 seconds or more, but it decreases with age. Although the fluorescein test is variable, a tear film break-up time of 1–3 seconds may indicate that the tear volume is decreased and a dry eye state exists.

17. What is the Schirmer test? How can it be used to diagnose dry eyes?

In the Schirmer test filter paper strips with a notched end are placed over the lid margin. They absorb the precorneal tear film and fluid in the lacrimal lake over a defined period, usually 5 minutes. If a patient has moderate-to-severe dry eyes, the amount of tears absorbed by the filter paper may register 0 (no tear absorption). In patients with severe dry eye conditions, with little tear film present, the Schirmer test is usually 0 or in the very low numbers. A normal Schirmer test wets the filter paper for a distance of 10 mm, usually over a 5-minute period.

The Schirmer test may be done with or without topical anesthesia. When a patient is suspected of having a dry eye condition, the irritation of the Schirmer strip may cause reflex tearing and mask the presence of dry eyes. For this reason, a topical anesthetic drop is placed in the eye a few minutes before the Schirmer test strip is placed over the lid margin. This technique eliminates the reflex tearing from irritation of the Schirmer strip and theoretically measures the basic tear level.

The Schirmer test without anesthesia evaluates the precorneal tear film without placement of excessive fluid, as when an anesthetic drop is applied. If the Schirmer test without anesthesia registers less than 10, the result can be considered positive in patients who are younger than 60. In patients over 60, a Schirmer tear test in the 5–10 mm range may even be considered normal. Patients who are young and have decreased wetting of the tear strip without anesthesia can be assumed to have some form of dry eye condition. With use of the slit lamp examination, fluorescein or rose bengal dye, tear film break-up time, and Schirmer test, along with the patient's symptoms, most dry eye conditions can be evaluated and followed.

18. What is the treatment for dry eyes?

Tear replacement therapy is the first choice for patients with dry eyes. Artificial tears are used infrequently or frequently, depending on the patient's symptoms. The lacrisert is a solid form of artificial tears; when placed in the lower cul-de-sac, it melts over a period of 12 hours and replaces tears. Although seldom used, the lacrisert is effective in a small number of patients. Medication to stimulate tear production is not available for humans, although pilocarpine has been effective in dogs. The use of cyclosporine in drop form to help reverse loss of lacrimal gland tissue from immune causes is currently under investigation.

19. How should artificial tears be used?

The frequency of drops depends on the patient's signs and symptoms. With minimal superficial punctate keratitis and mild signs of dry eye, use of artificial tears 4–8 times/day is usually sufficient to relieve symptoms. Since the symptoms may be intermittent, patients may increase or decrease tear use depending on eye symptoms. For patients with moderate and severe dry eyes, artificial tears must be used every 2 hours, every hour, or sometimes even every 15 minutes for certain periods of the day when symptoms are greater. Patients comment that symptoms may be increased on a dry day with air pollutants such as cigarette smoke or chemicals where the patient works.

20. Should artificial tears be used with or without preservatives?

Artificial tears with preservatives have the advantage that a larger bottle can be bought and the drops used over a period of days, weeks, and perhaps up to a month if the patient is careful when instilling the drops so that the lid margin is not touched with the dropper tip. Most drops without preservatives become contaminated quickly because the tip of the applicator sucks up tear fluid, which may contain bacteria. Patients frequently are sensitive to preservatives in artificial tears as well as to the tears themselves. Patients who are sensitive to preservatives or who must use artificial tears frequently often benefit by using tears without preservatives. The disadvantage of nonpreserved tears is that they are unit dose-packaged and must be discarded at the end of the day. They are somewhat more expensive than large bottles of artificial tears, but their comfort and safety may compensate.

21. How can tears be preserved in the eye?

If patients do not blink properly, if they blink infrequently, or if their blink excursion is too short, they should be instructed in the proper blink. Lubricating ointments at bedtime may be used to decrease evaporation if the patient sleeps with eyes slightly opened.

The main form of tear preservation is punctal occlusion. Lateral canthoplasty or narrowing the interpalpebral fissure also preserves tears in some patients.

22. When should the puncta be closed in patients with dry eye symptoms?

Patients who must use artificial tears every 2 hours or more may benefit from closing the punctum first in the lower lid and then in the upper lid to prevent loss of tears through the lacrimal system.

First, the lower puncta should be closed on a temporary basis by using a punctal plug. Plugs come in several sizes, ranging from 0.5 mm–0.8 mm. Most patients are comfortable with a 0.5- or 0.6-mm plug. The plug is easily inserted with the applicator and causes little discomfort. The plugs in the lower lids usually stay in place from 1 to 4 or 5 months. If the patient is comfortable during that time, the punctum can be closed on a permanent basis by using cautery.

23. When are the upper puncta closed?

If the patient has plugs in the lower puncta and symptoms continue, particularly if accompanied by superficial punctate keratitis and rose bengal staining, the upper puncta may be closed. I usually close the upper puncta either temporarily with punctal plugs or permanently with cautery. Approximately 10–20% of the fluid from the precorneal tear film is lost through the upper puncta and the rest through the lower puncta. Thus, it is important to close the lower puncta first.

24. Can you close the puncta with means other than cautery?

Argon laser, excimer laser, surgical closure with suture, and cyanoacolaid adhesives have been used to close the puncta permanently. The least expensive and most effective way of closing a punctum on a permanent basis is heat cautery.

25. What other surgical means are available for treating dry eye condition?

Lateral tarsorrhaphy is used in patients with wide interpalpebral fissures, exposure (such as in Graves' disease), or infrequent, poor blinking. This procedure narrows the palpebral fissure, decreases evaporation, and maintains the ocular surface.

Parotid duct transfer, which allows saliva to act as an ocular lubricant, has been used in the past, but it is a difficult procedure and not highly effective.

BIBLIOGRAPHY

1. Chow CYC, Gibard JP: Tear film. In Krachmer JH, Mannis MJ, Holland EJ (eds): Cornea, vol 1. St. Louis, Mosby, 1997, pp 49–60.
2. Fox RI: Systemic diseases associated with dry eye. Int Ophthalmol Clin 34:71–87, 1994.
3. Laibovitz RA, Solch S, Andriano K, et al: Pilot trial of cyclosporine 1% ophthalmic ointment in the treatment of keratoconjunctivitis sicca. Cornea 12(4):315–323, 1993.
4. Lemp MA: Report of the National Eye Institute/Industry Workshop on Clinical Trials in Dry Eyes. CLAO J 21(4):221–232, 1996.

13. CORNEAL DYSTROPHIES

Sadeer B. Hannush, M.D., and Lorena Riveroll, M.D.

1. What are corneal dystrophies?

Corneal dystrophies are bilateral, inherited, noninflammatory, commonly progressive alterations of the cornea that are usually not associated with any other systemic condition. Most corneal dystrophies are autosomal dominant disorders occurring after birth. Because each dystrophy may exhibit a spectrum of clinical manifestations, examining multiple family members frequently aids in establishing the diagnosis.

2. How do degenerations differ from dystrophies?

In contrast to dystrophies, degenerations are unilateral or bilateral aging changes that are not inherited. They are also not associated with systemic disease.

3. Discuss the general anatomic classification of corneal dystrophies.

1. **Anterior membrane dystrophies** include disorders affecting the corneal epithelium, epithelial basement membrane, and Bowman's layer.

2. **Stromal dystrophies** occur anywhere in the stromal layer of the cornea between Bowman's layer and Descemet's membrane.

3. **Posterior membrane dystrophies** are primarily abnormalities of the endothelium and Descemet's membrane.

4. Describe the inheritance patterns of anterior membrane dystrophies.

All anterior membrane dystrophies are autosomal dominant. Examples are Meesmann's juvenile epithelial dystrophy, epithelial basement membrane dystrophy, and corneal dystrophies of Bowman's layer.

5. Which is the most common anterior membrane dystrophy? Which is strictly epithelial?

Epithelial basement membrane dystrophy is by far the most common anterior membrane dystrophy. In fact, it has the highest prevalence of all of the corneal dystrophies. Areas of extra basement membrane result in maplike and/or fingerprint changes as well as intraepithelial microcysts. Five percent of otherwise normal corneas have been observed to have such changes.

Second in prevalence are the corneal dystrophies of Bowman's layer (CDBs): true Reis-Bücklers (CDB-1) and Thiel-Behnke honeycomb-shaped dystrophy (CDB-II). These disorders consist of gray reticular opacities beneath the epithelium.

Meesmann's dystrophy is the rarest of the three. This disorder, noted in the first few years of life, presents as a bilaterally symmetric pattern of microcysts or vesicles seen strictly in the epithelial layer of the cornea, usually in the interpalpebral fissure.

6. What are the most common presenting symptoms of anterior membrane dystrophies?

First are the symptoms associated with corneal erosions—pain, foreign body sensation, photophobia, and tearing, especially with opening of the lids during sleep or awakening in the morning. Erosions are most common in the setting of epithelial basement membrane dystrophy. The second symptom is blurred vision secondary to both corneal opacification and irregularity of the surface, most frequently seen in the dystrophies of Bowman's layer.

7. Discuss treatment options for recurrent corneal erosions associated with anterior membrane dystrophies.

The conservative approach includes the generous use of lubricant eye drops during the day and ointments at night. Some physicians advocate the use of topical steroids to stabilize the basement membrane, and others advocate hypertonic saline, especially in ointment form at night to dehdydrate the epithelium and aid in its attachment to the underlying layers. Patching, either conventional or with collagen or bandage contact lenses, hypothetically decreases the mechanical effect of lid movement on the already denuded corneal surface. Recalcitrant cases may require surgical intervention.

8. Discuss the role of surgery in the treatment of anterior membrane dystrophies.

In the setting of recalcitrant corneal erosions mechanical debridement of the loose epithelium or anterior stromal puncture, together with the use of a bandage lens, may aid in reepithelialization of the surface and adherence of the epithelium to the underlying layers. Mechanical debridement also may be used to remove an irregular epithelial basement membrane if an associated visual decline is noted. For the Bowman's layer dystrophies a more aggressive superficial or lamellar keratectomy may be required. Lamellar and penetrating keratoplasties also have been used.

9. Do lasers have a role?

The yttrium-aluminum-garnet (YAG) laser has been used instead of a needle to accomplish anterior stromal puncture but does not offer a clear advantage. The excimer laser has been used for treatment of recurrent erosions associated with basement membrane dystrophies and for removal of deeper layers in conditions such as Reis-Bücklers and Thiel-Behnke dystrophies. Although in the first instance the excimer laser may not offer a clear advantage over debridement, in the second it has supplanted lamellar keratectomy as the treatment of choice.

10. Describe the inheritance patterns of the stromal dystrophies.

1. **Autosomal dominant:** granular (Groenouw type I), lattice, Avellino granular-lattice, Schnyder's crystalline, fleck, central cloudy of François, pre-Descemet, congenital hereditary (stromal), and posterior amorphous dystrophies.

2. **Autosomal recessive:** macular (Groenouw type II) and possibly gelatinous droplike dystrophies.

11. Match the stromal dystrophy with the histochemical stain for the accumulated substance.

1. **Granular:** Masson trichrome stains hyaline
2. **Lattice:** Congo red stains amyloid (amyloid deposits exhibit polarized light birefringence and dichroism)
3. **Macular:** Alcian blue stains mucopolysaccharides (glycosaminoglycans)
Lattice and macular dystrophies also stain with periodic acid-Schiff stain.

12. Describe the clinical features of the three major stromal dystrophies.

Feature	Granular Dystrophy	Lattice Dystrophy	Macular Dystrophy
Age of onset			
Deposits	First decade	First decade	First decade
Symptoms	Third decade or none	Second decade	First decade
Decreased vision	Fourth or fifth decade	Second or third decade	First or second decade
Erosions	Uncommon	Frequent	Common
Corneal thickness	Normal	Normal	Thinned
Opacities	Discrete with sharp borders and clear intervening stroma early but becoming hazy later, not extending to limbus	Refractile lines and subepithelial spots, diffuse central haze, not extending to limbus except in advanced cases	Indistinct margins with hazy stroma between, extending to limbus; central lesions more anterior and peripheral lesions more posterior

13. Is lattice dystrophy associated with systemic amyloidosis?

There are three types of lattice dystrophy. Only type II (Meretoja's syndrome or familial amyloid polyneuropathy type IV), which has less corneal involvement than types I or III, is associated with systemic findings, including blepharochalasis, bilateral facial nerve palsies, peripheral neuropathy, and systemic amyloidosis.

14. What is the differential diagnosis of corneal stromal crystals? What systemic findings are associated with Schnyder's crystalline dystrophy?

The differential diagnosis of corneal stromal crystals includes Bietti's peripheral crystalline dystrophy, cystinosis, and dysproteinemias, such as multiple myeloma, Waldenstrom's macroglobulinemia, and benign monoclonal gammopathy.

Schnyder's dystrophy is strongly associated with hypercholesterolemia with or without hypertriglyceridemia. There is no direct association with primary hyperlipidemias, and serum lipid levels do not correlate with the density of the corneal opacities. The dystrophy more likely represents a localized defect in cholesterol metabolism. Of importance, not all patients with Schnyder's dystrophy have clinical evidence of corneal crystalline deposits.

15. How does central dystrophy of François differ from posterior crocodile shagreen?

Although some physicians have argued that location of the lesions differs in the two conditions, the lesions are clinically the same. It is generally accepted that the polygonal "cracked-ice" lesions of the dystrophy are more central, deeper, and, by definition, bilateral with an inheritance pattern. On the other hand, posterior crocodile shagreen is more commonly peripheral and anterior stromal and is classified as degeneration. Of importance, both conditions are associated with normal corneal thickness but not with recurrent erosions or significant visual compromise.

16. What characterizes Avellino dystrophy?

Avellino dystrophy also has been called granular-lattice dystrophy. The granular deposits occur in the anterior stroma early in the progression of the condition, followed later by lattice lesions in the mid to posterior stroma and finally by anterior stromal haze. More patients with Avellino dystrophy experience recurrent erosions than patients with typical granular dystrophy. Recently, the disease-causing genes of lattice dystrophy type I, granular dystrophy, Avellino dystrophy, and Reis-Bücklers dystrophy were mapped to chromosome 5q, suggesting one of the following possibilities:

1. A corneal gene family exists in this region; or
2. These corneal dystrophies represent allelic heterogeneity (i.e., different mutations within the same gene manifest as different phenotypes); or
3. They are the same disease.

17. How are stromal dystrophies treated?

To the extent that some dystrophies, such as lattice and Avellino, are associated with recurrent erosions, they are treated as discussed earlier. When the lesions obscure vision and are restricted to the anterior one-third of the stroma, they are usually amenable to surgical lamellar or phototherapeutic keratectomy (PTK) with the excimer laser. If the lesions are deeper, lamellar or penetrating keratoplasty is necessary.

18. Is penetrating keratoplasty a definitive treatment?

In most instances, penetrating keratoplasty for stromal dystrophies is associated with recurrence of the pathology in the graft as early as 1 year after surgery. The recurrent pathology is sometimes milder than in the original cornea but requires regrafting not infrequently.

19. Name the three posterior membrane dystrophies.

1. Posterior polymorphous dystrophy (PPMD)
2. Fuchs' dystrophy
3. Congenital hereditary endothelial dystrophy (CHED)

20. What is their common clinical manifestation?

All three essentially share the pathway of corneal edema and increased thickness, resulting in visual compromise.

21. Describe the inheritance patterns of the three posterior membrane dystrophies.

Posterior polymorphous and Fuchs' dystrophies have an autosomal dominant inheritance pattern. Two forms of congenital hereditary endothelial dystrophy exist. The autosomal dominant form presents in early childhood and is slowly progressive and frequently symptomatic. The autosomal recessive form presents at birth and is nonprogressive, but it is associated with significant visual compromise and nystagmus.

22. Describe the main clinical characteristics of the three posterior membrane dystrophies.

Feature	PPMD	Fuchs' Dystrophy	CHED
Onset	Second to third decades, rarely at birth	Fifth to sixth decades	Birth to first decade
Corneal findings	Vesicles, diffuse opacities, and corneal edema	Guttae, stromal thickening, epithelial edema, and subepithelial fibrosis	Endothelium rarely visible with marked corneal thickening and opacification
Other ocular abnormalities	Peripheral synechiae, iris atrophy/corectopia, and glaucoma	Narrow angles and glaucoma	None
Differential diagnosis	ICE syndrome, early-onset CHED	Pseudoguttae, Chandler's syndrome, herpes simplex keratitis, aphakic or pseudophakic bullous keratopathy, and other guttate conditions	Congenital glaucoma, metabolic opacification, Peters' anomaly, forceps injury, early-onset PPMD, and infectious etiologies

ICE = iridocorneal endothelial.

23. How does Fuchs' dystrophy differ from cornea guttata?

Cornea guttata basically refers to a pattern of corneal guttae that are usually found on the central cornea, sometimes coalesce, produce a beaten metal appearance, and are associated with increased pigmentation. This condition does not affect vision significantly. In 1910 Fuchs described a more severe form of the condition associated with stromal thickening and epithelial edema with secondary visual compromise. They represent different stages of the same dystrophy.

24. Describe the work-up of a patient with Fuchs' dystrophy.

1. History: previous intraocular surgery?
2. Biomicroscopic examination: endothelial guttae, increased stromal thickness, and epithelial edema with possible subepithelial bullae
3. Intraocular pressure measurement
4. Ultrasound or optical pachymetry
5. Specular microscopy to evaluate number, size, and shape of endothelial cells

25. What overlapping features are seen in PPMD and ICE syndromes?

Abnormal corneal endothelium, peripheral anterior synechiae, corectopia, and glaucoma.

26. What is unique about the CHED cornea?

Markedly increased corneal thickness, unlike any other corneal dystrophy.

27. Discuss management and prognosis of posterior membrane dystrophies.

Conservative management has a small role, especially in the earlier stages of Fuchs' dystrophy. Topical hypertonic saline solution, dehydration of the cornea with a blow-dryer, and reduction of intraocular pressure may decrease corneal edema and improve vision. Bandage contact lenses may be used in the setting of recurrent erosions or subepithelial bullae. However, when vision is significantly compromised by Fuchs' or other posterior membrane dystrophies, the definitive solution is penetrating keratoplasty. Penetrating keratoplasty has the best prognosis in Fuchs' dystrophy, especially in the absence of glaucoma; a fairly good prognosis in PPMD in the absence of glaucoma; and a guarded prognosis in CHED, especially in the early pediatric age group.

28. Can PPMD recur in the graft?

Recurrence of PPMD has been reported.

29. Discuss considerations for combined cataract extraction and corneal transplantation in patients with Fuchs' dystrophy.

1. **First scenario: visually significant cataract and borderline corneal function.** The decision whether to perform corneal transplantation at the time of cataract extraction may be based on a number of factors, including appearance of the corneal endothelium by specular microscopy, corneal thickness, visual variation throughout the day, and postoperative visual requirements of the patient. Patients with no evidence of frank stromal edema, including absence of morning blur and a stable central corneal thickness less than 620 μ, are likely to tolerate cataract extraction alone. The risk of corneal decompensation is outweighed by the advantage of rapid visual rehabilitation from cataract surgery alone. On the other hand, in patients with frank stromal edema, central corneal thickness greater than 650 μ, or an increase of more than 10% in corneal thickness in the morning compared with later in the day, the cornea is unlikely to tolerate routine cataract extraction. The patient will benefit from a triple procedure (i.e., cataract extraction with implant combined with penetrating keratoplasty).

2. **Second scenario: corneal edema requiring corneal transplantation and mild-to-moderate cataract.** One must weigh the added intraoperative risk of cataract surgery and the unpredictability of refractive error after a combined procedure against the risk of graft failure from secondary cataract extraction. Several retrospective studies indicate that most patients undergoing corneal transplantation alone eventually require cataract extraction. The incidence of corneal decompensation after secondary cataract surgery is small. As such, to avoid increased costs and delay in visual rehabilitation, the triple procedure is recommended for patients with Fuchs' endothelial dystrophy and visually significant cataract over nonsimultaneous surgery.

30. What controversy surrounds the dystrophies affecting Bowman's layer?

Until recently there has been some confusion over dystrophies affecting Bowman's layer because they present with two different sets of characteristics but historically have been lumped under Reis-Bücklers dystrophy. The first was described by Reis in 1917 and later by Bücklers in 1949, and the second by Thiel and Behnke in 1967. Küchle et al. recently divided the Bowman's membrane dystrophies into two classifications: corneal dystrophy of Bowman's layer type I and type II. Type I is synonymous with Reis-Bücklers original dystrophy and equivalent to what also has been described as superficial variant of granular dystrophy. Type II is honeycomb-shaped and should be known as Thiel-Behnke corneal dystrophy. The two dystrophies have slightly different characteristics on light microscopy. Transmission electron microscopy, on the other hand, differentiates them unequivocally.

31. Corneal dystrophy trivia:

1. The apostrophe in Fuchs' dystrophy is after the "s," not before.

2. In cornea guttata, guttata is the adjective describing the cornea. The actual excrescences of Descemet's membrane between the endothelial cells are corneal guttae, not corneal guttata.

3. Although keratoconus is usually bilateral and may have an inheritance pattern, it is considered an ectasia, not a dystrophy.

BIBLIOGRAPHY

1. Adamis AP, Filatov V, Tripathi BJ, Tripathi RC: Fuchs' endothelial dystrophy of the cornea. Surv Ophthalmol 38:149–168, 1993.
2. Arffa RC: Grayson's Diseases of the Cornea, 4th ed. St. Louis, Mosby, 1997.
3. Casey TA, Sharif KW: A Color Atlas of Corneal Dystrophies and Degenerations. London, Wolfe Publishing, 1991.
4. Cullom RD, Chang B (eds): The Wills Eye Manual: Wills Eye Hospital Office and Emergency Room Diagnosis and Treatment of Eye Disease, 2nd ed. Philadelphia, J.B. Lippincott, 1994.
5. Krachmer JH, Mannis MJ, Holland EJ: Cornea. St. Louis, Mosby, 1997.
6. Krachmer JH, Palay DA: Cornea Color Atlas. St. Louis, Mosby, 1997.
7. Küchle M, Green WR, Volcker HE, Barraquer J: Reevaluation of corneal dystrophies of Bowman's layer and the anterior stroma (Reis-Bücklers and Thiel-Behnke types): A light and electron microscopic study of eight corneas and review of the literature. Cornea 14:333–354, 1995.
8. Piñeros OE, Cohen EJ, Rapuano CJ, Laibson PR: Triple versus nonsimultaneous procedures in Fuchs' dystrophy and cataract. Arch Ophthalmol 114:535–525, 1996.
9. Small KW, Mullen L, Barletta J, et al: Mapping of Reis-Bücklers' corneal dystrophy to chromosome 5q. Am J Ophthalmol 121:384–390, 1996.
10. Stone EM: Three autosomal dominant corneal dystrophies mapped to chromosome 5q. Nature Genetics 6:47–51, 1994.
11. Waring GO, Rodriguez MM, Laibson RR: Corneal dystrophies. I: Dystrophies of epithelium, Bowman's layer and stroma. Surv Ophthalmol 23:71–122, 1978.
12. Waring GO, Rodriguez MM, Laibson RR: Corneal dystrophies. II: Endothelial dystrophies. Surv Ophthalmol 23:147–168, 1978.

14. KERATOCONUS

Irving Raber, M.D.

1. What is keratoconus?

Keratoconus is a noninflammatory ectatic disorder of the cornea that leads to variable visual impairment. The cornea becomes steepened and thinned, thereby inducing myopia and irregular astigmatism. In advanced stages the cornea assumes a conical shape; hence the term keratoconus. The condition is usually bilateral, although frequently asymmetric.

2. Who gets keratoconus?

It is difficult to estimate the incidence of keratoconus because the diagnosis is easily overlooked, especially in the early stages. The reported incidence ranges from 400–600 per 100,000. There does not appear to be a sexual predilection. Some studies report a female predominance, whereas other studies report a male predominance. There is no known racial predilection.

3. What is the cause of keratoconus?

The cause of keratoconus is unknown. Various biochemical abnormalities have been documented in keratoconic corneas, including reduced collagen content, decreased or altered keratin sulfate molecules, reduced total protein and increased nonproteinaceous material, and increased collagenolytic and gelatinolytic activity associated with reduced matrix metalloproteinase inhibitor levels. Several studies have shown that the enzyme and proteinase inhibitor abnormalities are most prominent in the epithelial layer of the cornea, which suggests that the basic defect in keratoconus may reside in the epithelium and its interaction with the stroma. Eye rubbing has been implicated as a cause of keratoconus. When asked, patients with keratoconus will frequently admit to excessive eye rubbing.

4. What is the relationship between contact lens wear and keratoconus?

The relationship between contact lens wear and keratoconus is controversial. Circumstantial evidence suggests that contact lens wear may lead to the development of keratoconus, especially long-term wearing of rigid contact lenses. Such patients tend to present at an older age and have a flatter corneal curvature than typical patients with keratoconus. In addition, the so-called contact lens-induced cones tend to be more centrally located in the cornea than the more characteristic cones, which are decentered inferiorly.

In the syndrome known as contact lens warpage, contact lens wear induces irregular astigmatism without slit lamp features of keratoconus. Discontinuing lens wear for weeks to months eliminates the irregular astigmatism and allows the cornea to resume its normal shape, whereas in the so-called contact lens-induced keratoconus the changes are permanent and do not resolve when contact lens wear is discontinued.

Some contact lens practitioners are of the opinion that contact lenses can be used to flatten the cornea and reverse, or at least retard, further progression of keratoconus. However, I believe that corneal flattening induced by contact lens wear in patients with keratoconus is temporary and that the cornea reverts to its precontact lens shape once lens wear is discontinued.

5. Is keratoconus hereditary?

The role of heredity in keratoconus has not been clearly defined. The vast majority of cases occur sporadically with no familial history. However, some cases of keratoconus are transmitted within families. One study using corneal topography to diagnose subclinical cases of keratoconus

documented evidence of familial transmission in 7 of 12 families (58.3%) of patients with keratoconus and no known family history of corneal or ocular disease. The authors postulate autosomal dominant inheritance with incomplete penetrance as the mode of transmission.

6. What systemic conditions are associated with keratoconus?

There is a definite relationship between atopy and keratoconus. The prevalence of atopic diseases such as asthma, eczema, atopic keratoconjunctivitis, and hay fever is higher in patients with
keratoconus than in normal controls. Atopic patients are bothered by ocular itching, and excessive eye rubbing also may contribute to the development of keratoconus.

There is an association between Down's syndrome and keratoconus. Approximately 5% of
patients with Down's syndrome manifest signs of keratoconus. The incidence of acute hydrops in
Down's syndrome is definitely higher than in non-Down's syndrome. As in atopic subjects, patients with Down's syndrome tend to be vigorous eye rubbers, which may explain, at least in part,
the relationship with keratoconus.

Keratoconus is also associated with various connective tissue disorders, such as Ehlers-
Danlos syndrome, osteogenesis imperfecta, and Marfan's syndrome. Reports of an association
between keratoconus, mitral valve prolapse, and joint hypermobility are conflicting. One study
has reported an association between keratoconus and false chordae tendineae in the left ventricle.
The relationship between various connective tissue diseases and keratoconus suggests a common
defect in the synthesis of connective tissue.

7. What ocular conditions are associated with keratoconus?

Keratoconus has been described in association with various ocular diseases, including retinitis pigmentosa, Leber's congenital amaurosis, vernal conjunctivitis, floppy eyelid syndrome,
corneal endothelial dystrophy, and posterior polymorphous corneal dystrophy.

8. What are the symptoms of keratoconus?

The characteristic onset of keratoconus is in the late teens or early 20s. Symptoms usually begin as blurred vision with shadowing around images. Vision becomes progressively
more blurred and distorted with associated glare, halos around lights, light sensitivity, and
ocular irritation.

9. How is the diagnosis of keratoconus made?

Corneal topography can document the presence of keratoconus even before keratometric
or slit lamp findings become apparent. In the early stages of keratoconus, the patient presents
with myopic astigmatism. An irregular light reflex with scissoring on retinoscopy can be appreciated through the dilated pupil. As the disease progresses, the cornea steepens and thins with irregularity of the mires on keratometry and development of obvious keratoconus on slit lamp
examination.

10. What are the topographic signs of keratoconus?

The characteristic sign of keratoconus on topography is inferior midperipheral steepening.
Numerous studies have tried to develop quantitative topographic parameters to define keratoconus. In one recent study, central corneal power > 47.20 diopters combined with steepening of
the inferior cornea compared with the superior cornea of > 1.20 diopters detected 98% of patients
with keratoconus. However, it may be difficult to make a definitive diagnosis of keratoconus
based on topographic findings alone. This is of particular importance in patients seeking refractive surgery because the results of the surgery are poorly predictable in patients with keratoconus. Patients with apparently normal corneas may have inferior midperipheral steepening
> 1.20 diopters but normal central corneal powers in the range of 43–45 diopters. It is difficult to
know whether such patients represent a form fruste of keratoconus and, as such, should be dis-
suaded from considering refractive surgery. Each case must be analyzed on an individual basis.

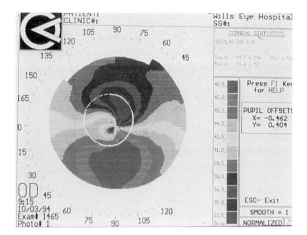

Computed topographic map demonstrating asymmetric inferior steepening.
(See Fig. 5, Color Plates.)

11. What are the slit lamp findings of keratoconus?

The earliest slit lamp signs of keratoconus are apical thinning and steepening, usually located inferior to the center of the pupil. As the keratoconus progresses, the thinning and ectasia
become more prominent with the development of apical scarring that begins in the anterior
stroma and then appears in the deeper layers of the stroma. Fine linear striae become apparent in
the deep stroma just anterior to Descemet's membrane, usually oriented vertically or obliquely.
They are thought to represent stress lines in the posterior stroma and are known as Vogt's striae.
They can be made to disappear when the intraocular pressure is transiently raised by applying external pressure to the globe. Moreover, in some mild cases of keratoconus, the pressure from
rigid gas permeable contact lens wear can induce the formation of such striae, which disappear
when the lens is removed. A Fleischer ring is commonly seen outlining the base of the cone, the
result of hemosiderin pigment deposition within the deeper layers of the corneal epithelium. A
Fleischer ring may outline the cone only partially but, as the ectasia progresses, tends to become
a complete circle with more dense accumulation of pigmentation that is best appreciated while
viewing the cobalt blue filter on the slit lamp. Subepithelial fibrillary lines have been described in
a concentric circular fashion just inside the Fleischer ring. The source of these fibrils is unknown
but has been postulated as epithelial nerve filaments. Anterior clear spaces thought to represent
breaks in Bowman's membrane are sometimes seen within the thin portion of the conical protrusion. Prominent corneal nerves are reportedly more common in keratoconic corneas. In the more
advanced stages, when the eye is rotated downward, the corneal ectasia causes protrusion of the
lower lid, which is known as Munson's sign.

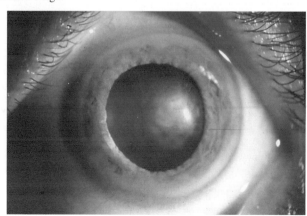

Apical scarring.

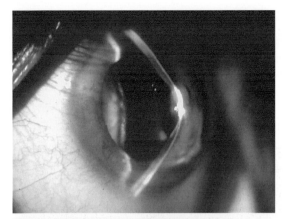

Apical thinning and scarring demonstrated in slit beam.

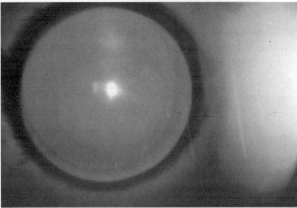

Fleischer ring seen in diffuse
cobalt blue illumination. (See
Fig. 6, Color Plates.)

12. How does keratoconus progress?

The onset of keratoconus characteristically occurs in the the mid to late teens, progressing slowly for several years before stabilizing. However, delayed onset or late progression of kerato-conus is not uncommon. As the disease progresses, the corneal thinning and ectasia become more prominent with increasing apical scarring. Two types of cones have been described: (1) a small round or nipple-shaped cone that tends to be more central in location and (2) an oval or sagging cone that is usually larger and displaced inferiorly with the thinning extending close to the infe-rior limbus. Progression of keratoconus tends to manifest as increased thinning and protrusion, although enlargement of the cone also occurs with extension peripherally.

13. What is acute hydrops?

Acute hydrops occurs in the more advanced cases of keratoconus. Ruptures in Descemet's membrane allow aqueous to enter into the corneal stroma, resulting in marked thickening and opacification of the cornea that is usually restricted to the cone. The involved stroma becomes massively thickened with large, fluid-filled clefts, overlying epithelial edema, and bulla forma-tion. Rarely a fistulous tract may develop with resultant leakage of aqueous through the fluid-filled stroma and epithelium on the corneal surface. The corneal edema gradually resolves over weeks to months as endothelial cells adjacent to the rupture in Descemet's membrane enlarge and migrate across the defect, laying down new Descemet's membrane. With healing, scarring tends to flatten the cornea, thereby facilitating the possibility of subsequent contact lens fitting. Some corneas with acute hydrops tend to develop stromal neovascularization that increases the potential risk of graft rejection if corneal transplantation becomes necessary. Acute hydrops is more common in patients with Down's syndrome and vernal keratoconjunctivitis, presumably related to the repeated trauma of eye rubbing in these patients.

Most cases of acute hydrops resolve spontaneously, requiring supportive treatment with topical hyperosmotic agents such as 5% sodium chloride drops and/or ointment to promote corneal deturgescence. Some patients with acute hydrops complain of severe photophobia and benefit from the use of topical steroids and/or cycloplegic agents. In addition, topical steroids should be instituted in patients with signs of corneal neovascularization. Once the hydrops has resolved, the patient can then try to resume contact lens wear if the central cornea has not become excessively scarred. Otherwise the only alternative is a corneal transplant.

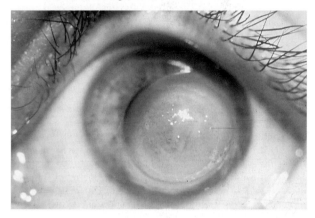

Acute hydrops.

14. What is the histopathology of keratoconus?

Most histopathologic studies of keratoconic corneas are performed on advanced cases that require penetrating keratoplasty. In addition, most patients were previous long-term contact lens wearers, which also may affect the histopathologic findings.

Changes have been described in every layer of the cornea. The stroma of the cone is thinner than the surrounding cornea. The apical epithelium tends to be flattened and thinned with scattered fragmentation and dehiscence of the epithelial basement membrane. Iron can be demonstrated in the epithelial cells outlining the cone, corresponding to the Fleischer ring.

Among the most characteristic histologic changes of keratoconus are breaks in Bowman's membrane that are sometimes filled with epithelium and/or stromal collagen. Ultimately, the anterior corneal stroma may become replaced with irregularly arranged connective tissue.

Descemet's membrane is normal unless acute hydrops has occurred. Depending on the stage of the reparative process, breaks in Descemet's membrane with curled edges subsequently become covered by adjacent endothelial cells that slide over and lay down new membrane. The corneal endothelial cells tend to be normal, although they may exhibit increased pleomorphism.

15. How is keratoconus treated?

Mild cases of keratoconus can be successfully managed with spectacles. However, as the keratoconus progresses and the amount of irregular astigmatism increases, patients become unable to obtain satisfactory vision with spectacle correction. Contact lenses can then be used to neutralize the irregular astigmatism, thereby offering significant visual improvement over spectacles. As the cornea becomes more distorted and ectatic, contact lens fitting becomes more difficult and vision deteriorates, ultimately necessitating surgical intervention.

16. What types of contact lenses are used to treat keratoconus?

Conventional spherical myopic soft contact lenses may be used successfully in mild cases of keratoconus with minimal manifest astigmatism. Toric soft contact lenses also may be used in some patients without excessive amounts of irregular astigmatism. The vast majority of patients with keratoconus are managed with rigid gas-permeable contact lenses. Fitting such lenses over a distorted ectatic cornea is difficult. Numerous lens designs are available for fitting patients with keratoconus, including varying diameters of spherical lenses, aspheric lenses, toric lenses, and lenses with multiple curvatures on the posterior surface, such as the Soper cone lens. The Soper cone lenses have a steeper central curve to vault the apex of the cone and a flatter peripheral curve to align with the more normal peripheral cornea. Computed topography is used by some contact lens practitioners to help fit these challenging patients.

Large gas-permeable scleral contact lenses are sometimes used to manage patients with prominent ectatic cones who cannot be fit with more conventional gas-permeable lenses and for whatever reason are not considered good candidates for corneal transplantation. A piggyback system is another option available for treating patients with keratoconus: a gas-permeable contact lens is fitted on top of a soft contact lens. This system is expensive and time-consuming for both practitioner and patient but can be helpful in managing select cases that have failed more conventional contact lens fitting. Another specialized lens design incorporates a rigid gas-permeable center with a soft peripheral skirt to reduce the edge awareness of conventional gas-permeable lenses. Moreover, such "saturn-style" lenses may actually center better and offer a more stable fit by virtue of their large diameter, which extends beyond the limbus.

17. What are the surgical options for treating keratoconus?

Surgical intervention is reserved for patients with keratoconus who cannot be successfully fit with contact lenses or who fail to obtain satisfactory vision with contact lenses. Atopic patients with keratoconus tend to come to surgery much more frequently than nonallergic patients because the allergic diathesis tends to interfere with contact lens tolerance.

Penetrating keratoplasty (full-thickness corneal transplantation) is the most common surgical technique used to rehabilitate patients with keratoconus. The surgical procedure requires excision of the entire cone, frequently determined by the outline of the Fleischer ring. If the cone extends close to the limbus (usually inferiorly), a large corneal graft is needed. Usually the grafted tissue is centered on the pupil, but when the cone is eccentric, an eccentric graft is used to encompass the entire cone, taking care to leave the optical zone free of sutures. Increasing graft size with proximity to the limbal blood vessel reduces the "immune privilege" of the usually avascular cornea, thereby increasing the risk of immunologic reaction.

Lamellar (partial-thickness) keratoplasty may be used in patients with keratoconus, although the procedure is technically more difficult and in the hands of most surgeons achieves a slightly poorer visual outcome than a full-thickness procedure. However, a lamellar graft has the advantage of being an extraocular procedure that avoids the risk of endothelial rejection. Most cases of lamellar keratoplasty are performed as tectonic procedures for large cones in which the thinning extends out to the limbus. If a satisfactory visual result is not obtained, a smaller central full-thickness corneal transplant can subsequently be performed within the confines of the lamellar graft, thereby avoiding the increased risk of immunologic rejection with large full-thickness corneal transplants.

Epikeratophakia is a type of onlay lamellar procedure using a freeze-dried donor cornea that is sewn on top of a deepithelialized host cornea. The purpose of this procedure is to flatten the cornea with the hope of offering improved spectacle-corrected visual acuity and/or better contact lens fitting. After initial enthusiasm in the late 1980s, the procedure has been abandoned by most surgeons because of complications and poor visual results. However, in select cases in which a full-thickness corneal transplant is contraindicated, such as patients with Down's syndrome who may aggressively rub their eyes and dehisce a full-thickness wound or patients at high risk for immune rejection (i.e., multiple graft failures in the other eye), partial-thickness procedures such as lamellar grafts or epikeratophakia are worthy of consideration.

Thermokeratoplasty is a technique whereby heating the cornea to 90–120° C causes shrinkage of corneal collagen fibers with resulting flattening of the cornea. This procedure has been abandoned for the most part because of unpredictable results, induced scarring, and the potential for recurrent corneal erosions because of damage to the epithelial basement membrane complex. However, when the apex of the cone spares the visual axis, thermokeratoplasty may be used to flatten the cornea, thereby allowing more favorable spectacle-corrected visual acuity and/or contact lens fitting. In addition, thermokeratoplasty may be helpful in promoting resolution of acute hydrops.

Some patients with keratoconus develop an elevated subepithelial scar at the apex of the cone as the result of chronic apical irritation from contact lens wear. Corneal epithelial breakdown may develop over the scar, thereby interfering with contact lens wear. These scars can be removed manually with a blade or with the excimer laser, thereby allowing resumption of contact lens wear and sparing the patient an otherwise needed corneal transplant.

18. What are the results of corneal transplant in patients with keratoconus?

As mentioned previously, most corneal surgery for keratoconus involves penetrating keratoplasty. The results of such surgery are excellent with clear grafts in approximately 90% of patients, most of whom obtain visual acuity of 20/40 or better. The most frequent problem arising in patients with keratoconus who undergo corneal transplantation is high postkeratoplasty astigmatism. However, the astigmatism following corneal transplant surgery tends to be regular as opposed to the irregular astigmatism of the original disorder. This difference allows most patients to achieve satisfactory visual results with spectacle correction, even if they have a large amount of astigmatism that most patients without keratoconus would not be able to tolerate in spectacles. Because keratoconus tends to be asymmetric, many patients undergoing corneal transplantation in one eye manage with a contact lens in the lesser involved eye and thus prefer to wear a contact lens in the operated eye as well. The contact lens tends to neutralize most of the astigmatism in the corneal transplant. A small percentage of patients may not be able to tolerate a large degree of astigmatism in spectacles. If they cannot be fit with a contact lens, they ultimately require keratorefractive surgery to reduce the astigmatic error.

It usually takes up to a full year or more for the corneal transplant wound to heal. If the patient is seeing well with the sutures in place, the sutures (most commonly 10-0 nylon) are left undisturbed and tend to disintegrate spontaneously over a few years. Sometimes disintegrating sutures erode through the corneal epithelium and cause a foreign body sensation. If they are not removed from the surface of the cornea, they may cause secondary infection. After sutures disintegrate and/or are removed, a significant change in the refractive error is frequently notable. All graft sutures should have disintegrated or be removed before keratorefractive surgery is contemplated.

Graft rejection occurs in approximately 25% of patients with keratoconus who undergo penetrating keratoplasty. Most rejections can be reversed with appropriate local steroid therapy if they are caught early. Irreversible rejection leads to permanent corneal clouding that requires repeat penetrating keratoplasty. A repeat graft has a reasonably good prognosis, although the success rate is lower than the primary graft and tends to diminish with each successive transplant if multiple graft failures occur.

BIBLIOGRAPHY

1. Bran AJ: Keratoconus. Cornea 7(3):163, 1988.
2. Krachmer JH, Feder RS, Belin MW: Keratoconus and related noninflammatory thinning disorders. Surv Ophthalmol 28:293, 1984.
3. Lawless M, Coster DJ, Phillips AJ, Loane M: Keratoconus: Diagnosis and management. Aust N Z J Ophthalmol 17:33, 1989.
4. Macsai MS, Valery GA, Krackmer JH: Development of keratoconus after contact lens wear: Patient characteristics. Arch Ophthalmol 108:534, 1990.
5. Maeda N, Klyce SD, Smolek MD: Comparison of methods for detecting keratoconus using video keratography. Arch Ophthalmol 113:870, 1995.
6. Tuft SJ, Moodaley LC, Gregory WM, et al: Prognostic factors for the progression of keratoconus. Ophthalmology 101:439, 1994.

15. REFRACTIVE SURGERY

*Richard C. Rodman, M.D., Terry Kim, M.D., René Dinh, M.D.,
and Christopher J. Rapuano, M.D.*

1. What are the refractive components of the eye?

The cornea and the lens refract incident light so that it is focused on the fovea, the center of the retina. The cornea contributes approximately 44 diopters compared with only 18 diopters from the lens. In addition, anterior chamber depth and axial length of the eye contribute to refractive status.

2. What are the different types of refractive errors?

Myopia, or nearsightedness, exists when the refractive elements of the eye place the image in front of the retina. **Hyperopia**, or farsightedness, exists when the image is focused behind the retina. **Astigmatism** usually refers to corneal irregularity that requires unequal power in different meridians to place a single image on the fovea. Lenticular astigmatism (due to the lens) is less common than corneal astigmatism. **Presbyopia** is the natural impairment in accommodation often noted around age 40 years. The corrective "add" or bifocal segment to combat presbyopia increases with age.

3. How is myopia related to age?

Myopia is common among premature infants, less common in full-term infants, and uncommon at 6 months of age, when mild hyperopia is the rule. Myopia becomes most prevalent in adolescence (approximately 25%), peaking by 20 years of age and subsequently leveling off. This information is important for determining the appropriate age to consider refractive surgery.

4. What are the goals of refractive surgery?

Goals vary for each patient. Certain patients desire refractive surgery because of professional or lifestyle issues; examples include athletes and police, fire, and military personnel, who may find glasses or contact lenses hindering or even dangerous. Other patients, such as high myopes, may find spectacle correction inadequate because of image minification or may be intolerant of contact lenses. In general, the goals of refractive surgery are to reduce or eliminate the need for glasses or refractive lenses without altering the quality of vision or best corrected vision.

5. What features characterize a good candidate for refractive surgery? Are there any contraindications?

First, patients considering refractive surgery should be at least 18 years of age with a stable refraction. Patients with ocular conditions (severe dry eye syndrome or uveitis) or systemic diseases and patients taking medications that impair wound healing are poor candidates. Keratoconus, a condition in which the cornea is irregularly cone-shaped, remains a contraindication for refractive surgery because results are unpredictable. Analysis of corneal curvature, often using computerized corneal topography, should be performed on all patients before surgery because early keratoconus has a prevalence of up to 13% in this population and may be missed by other diagnostic methods.

Second, patients' motivations and expectations should be explored thoroughly so that unrealistic hopes may be discovered preoperatively. For example, the patient who is constantly cleaning his or her glasses because of "excruciating glare" from dust on the lenses or who desires perfect uncorrected vision is not a good candidate for refractive surgery. A careful discussion of the risks and benefits of surgery is particularly important. Patients may desire a trial of contact lens wear before considering surgery. Also, the concept of presbyopia must be explained; many patients are prepresbyopic and have no understanding that achieving excellent uncorrected vision at distance will require correction for reading at near within a few years.

6. How is corneal topography used in the evaluation of patients undergoing refractive surgery?

Corneal topography typically refers to the use of computer-based videokeratography to evaluate corneal curvature accurately. Most topographic systems use a video camera to detect reflected images of rings projected onto the cornea. A computer generates a topographic "map" of corneal curvature based on the measured distance between the rings reflected from the cornea. Topography is extremely useful for evaluating patients undergoing refractive surgery because it generates precise images of corneal curvature that correspond to a large area of the cornea. Subtle corneal abnormalities, such as early keratoconus or contact lens-induced corneal warpage, may be detected only by this method. In addition, postoperative and preoperative topographic maps may be analyzed to generate "difference" maps that isolate the procedure-induced changes. Computerized corneal topography is also extremely useful for determining the cause of imperfect vision after refractive surgery, which is commonly due to irregular astigmatism.

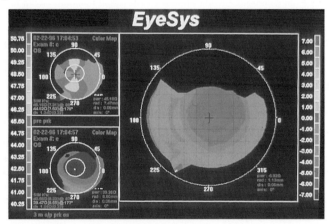

Corneal topography. Upper left shows preoperative myopic astigmatism. Lower left shows central flattening three months after photorefractive keratectomy. On right, the difference map demonstrates treatment effect of excimer laser. (See Fig. 7, Color Plates.)

7. What are the major options for the surgical treatment of myopia?
1. Radial keratotomy (RK)
2. Photorefractive keratectomy (PRK)
3. Laser in-situ keratomileusis (LASIK)

8. How does RK reduce myopia?

Deep radial incisions created with a diamond blade cause steepening of the cornea peripherally, which results in secondary flattening of the central cornea. The number, length, and depth of incisions and the size of the clear, central optical zone determine the refractive effect. Typically, four incisions are used for low myopia and eight incisions for moderate myopia. Optical zones < 3 mm in diameter are associated with greater reduction of myopia but also greater risk of refractive instability and optical aberrations such as glare or starburst.

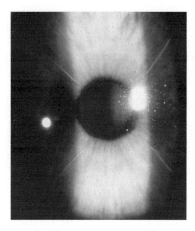

Three weeks after four-incision radial keratotomy.

9. What are the various RK techniques?

1. The American technique involves making centrifugal incisions (from the center toward the limbus) with an angled diamond knife blade.

2. The Russian technique uses centripetal incisions (from the limbus toward the center) with a straight vertical diamond knife blade. The Russian technique gives deeper incisions and more refractive effect; however, there is greater danger of entering the optical zone.

3. A combined bidirectional technique uses an angled blade edge on one side for centrifugal incisions, which are performed first, combined with a vertical blade edge on the other side to perform a second centripetal incision. The vertical blade edge is sharp only at the tip so that the second incision stops at the optical zone. This technique allows the creation of a deep and square rather than a sloped incision near the optical zone.

Based on statistical analysis of previous cases, standardized nomograms are used to determine the number of incisions and optical zone size, depending on the patient's age and desired refractive change. Each ophthalmologist must follow his or her own results to make surgeon-specific modifications in the nomograms.

10. What results have been achieved with RK? What about complications?

Several major investigations have been performed, the most important of which is the Prospective Evaluation of Radial Keratotomy (PERK). This study showed that 60% of treated eyes were within 1 diopter of emmetropia up to 10 years postoperatively. After 10 years, 53% had at least 20/20 uncorrected vision, and 85% had at least 20/40 vision. However, 43% of eyes had a progressive shift toward hyperopia of at least 1 diopter after 10 years. This shift was noted to be worse for eyes with the smaller optical zone of 3.0 mm. Only 3% of patients lost two or more lines of best corrected visual acuity, and all had 20/30 vision or better. Three of more than 400 patients complained of severe glare or starburst that made night driving impossible. Corneal perforations occurred in 2% of cases; none required a suture for closure. Overall, the best results were achieved in the low myopia group (−2.00 to −3.00 diopters).

Waring et al. recently reported similar results in 615 eyes 1 year after RK using the Russian technique. Their data showed that 54% of eyes had 20/20 vision and 93% had 20/40 uncorrected vision 1 year postoperatively. One percent (6 eyes) lost 2–3 lines of best-corrected vision, but all had 20/30 vision or better. Despite a significant increase in glare and fluctuation in vision from baseline, 90% of patients were satisfied with the outcome after RK. As with any invasive procedure, infection is a small but real risk.

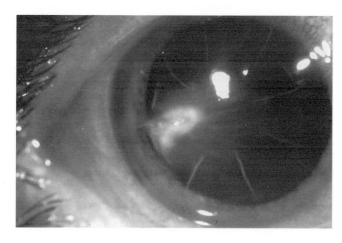

Infection at radial keratotomy incision.

11. How does PRK reduce myopia?

Unlike RK, which causes central corneal flattening indirectly through steepening of the corneal periphery, PRK involves direct laster treatment of the central corneal stroma. Specifically, the **"exci**ted di**mer"** (excimer) 193-nm UV laser causes flattening of the central cornea through a photoablative/photodecomposition process whereby more tissue is removed centrally than peripherally. Under topical anesthesia, the central corneal epithelium is removed either with a spatula or the laser. The laser is then used to ablate a precise quantity of stromal tissue with submicron accuracy to achieve the desired refractive effect.

12. What results have been achieved with PRK? What about complications?

In some respects, the results with excimer laser are comparable to those of RK for the same magnitude of myopia (–1.00 to –6.00 D), as indicated by the Summit and VISX experience at 1 year:

- 68% were within 1 diopter of emmetropia (vs. 60% for RK)
- 60% had at least 20/20 vision (vs. 53% for RK)
- 90% had at least 20/40 vision without correction (vs. 85% for RK)

In the subgroup of patients with low-to-moderate myopia (1.5–2.9 D), 80% had at least 20/20 uncorrected vision. As with RK, a small percentage of patients lost less than 2 lines of best-corrected vision. Postoperative corneal haze was seen in a minority of patients at 3 months and by 1 year was no longer severe in any patient. The refraction was generally stable by 6–9 months, depending on the amount of myopia treated.

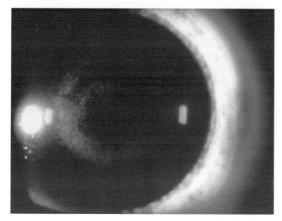

Mild stromal haze, 3 months after photo-refractive keratectomy.

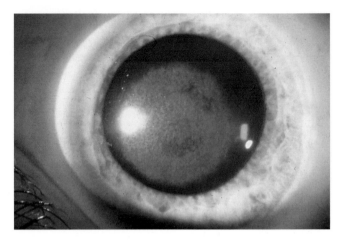

Moderate-to-severe stromal
haze, 6 months after photorefractive keratectomy.

13. Discuss the major advantages and disadvantages of PRK vs. RK.

- The cornea is weakened in RK but not in PRK because RK is an incisional technique. Permanent weakening of the globe may be important in patients who are at risk for blunt trauma (athletes, military personnel).
- Unlike RK, PRK is associated with no diurnal variation in refraction.
- It may be easier to resume soft lens wear after PRK than after RK (for the minority of patients who require contact lenses).
- The "hyperopic shift" associated with RK is much less frequently experienced after PRK. The initial hyperopic phase after PRK, which precedes the return to emmetropia, may be prolonged in patients over the age of 40 because of decreased accommodative reserve.
- A significant advantage of RK is the relative speed of recovery. Patients undergoing RK may have excellent uncorrected vision on postoperative day 1. After PRK, healing of the epithelial defect may delay return of good vision and comfort for several weeks.
- RK currently is less expensive than PRK.

14. What is LASIK?

LASIK, which stands for laser in-situ keratomileusis, is sometimes referred to as the "flap-and-zap" technique. LASIK is currently undergoing a multicenter clinical trial under the supervision of the Food and Drug Administration (FDA). The procedure involves creating a corneal flap to ablate midstromal tissue directly with an excimer laser beam, ultimately flattening the cornea. Whereas earlier techniques of keratomileusis consisted of removing a corneal flap and resecting stromal tissue manually, technologic advancements have revolutionized this procedure into a highly automated process. Contemporary techniques use a suction ring with a blade guide, an automated microkeratome blade, and an excimer laser. After a lid speculum is placed and topical anesthetic is applied, the suction ring is centered on the cornea to apply a constant suction pressure > 65 mmHg on the eye (as measured by any applanation tonometry device). The microkeratome blade is then placed on the guide of the suction ring and advanced to create a hinged flap with a depth approximately 25–30% of the corneal thickness. The blade stops approximately 0.5 mm short of a complete flap resection. The suction on the ring is shut off, and the flap is then lifted and moved to the side on its hinge, exposing a bed of bare stroma. Next, the excimer laser is applied directly to the stromal tissue. Afterward, the corneal flap is replaced to its original position, typically without sutures, and allowed to heal.

15. How have advancements in the LASIK procedure helped to improve results?

The use of a suction ring helps to maintain constant pressure on the eye so that the microkeratome blade makes a smooth and uniform cut through a single plane of corneal tissue.

Automation of the microkeratome with a mechanically operated turbine drive on a blade guide also has contributed to producing a smooth, regular cut with the ability to leave a hinge (so that the corneal flap can be easily realigned to its original position). The excimer laser beam also allows for the controlled and monitored removal of stromal tissue, thereby adding greater precision, predictability, and reproducibility to the results.

16. What is the range of myopia recommended for correction with LASIK?
LASIK is generally recommended for myopia > 5–7 diopters and as high as 30 diopters.

17. What are the advantages and disadvantages of LASIK vs. RK and PRK?
LASIK offers the advantage of minimal postoperative pain as well as earlier recovery of vision because the epithelium is left intact. In addition, patients do not experience the "halos" and "foggy vision" due to wound healing and scarring after RK and PRK. The disadvantages of LASIK include the brief intraoperative period of marked visual loss (due to high intraocular pressures generated by the suction ring), the risk of flap subluxation or dislocation, and the expense of the procedure. Additional problems associated with LASIK include irregular astigmatism and the potential for epithelial ingrowth under the flap.

LASIK offers several advantages to the surgeon. Because the technique involves making a flap in the anterior corneal stroma, the risk of corneal perforation associated with RK is virtually nonexistent. The creation of a uniform smooth flap with preservation of central Bowman's layer also reduces the subepithelial scarring seen with PRK. The overall mechanization of the technique allows little room for surgeon error. However, its automated aspect also poses disadvantages. The surgeon has limited intraoperative control over creation of the flap and ablation of the stroma. The microkeratome also requires extensive care for proper performance. The suction ring device is quite cumbersome and can be difficult to place on a patient with narrow palpebral fissures or deep orbits. If the suction is released during the use of the microkeratome, the corneal flap may be damaged.

18. How do the surgical results of LASIK compare with those of RK and PRK?
Few well-controlled, long-term data about LASIK are available. Salah et al. recently reviewed the results of 88 eyes in 63 patients treated with LASIK. The preoperative refractions ranged from –2.00 to –20.00 D with a mean follow-up of 5.2 months. Thirty-six percent achieved an uncorrected visual acuity of at least 20/20, and 71% achieved an uncorrected visual acuity of at least 20/40. Four percent lost 2 or more lines of best-corrected visual acuity. Similar results were reported in the phase I clinical trials of the Summit study with a 6-month follow-up. When refractive subgroups were analyzed, less predictable results were achieved in the higher myopia groups. Nevertheless, LASIK may be the best technique available for treating higher degrees of myopia. Long-term stability requires further study.

19. Name the potential complications of LASIK.
Complications are uncommon and are not listed in order of frequency:
1. Premature release of suction ring
2. Intraoperative flap amputation
3. Postoperative flap dislocation/subluxation (may require suturing of flap into place)
4. Epithelialization of flap–bed interface (causes regression and light scattering)
5. Irregular astigmatism

20. Are there any other surgical options for the treatment of myopia?
Because the crystalline lens adds about 18 diopters of power to the optical system, clear lens extraction may be used in patients with a comparable level of myopia. However, performing intraocular surgery for a purely refractive goal is controversial. In addition, highly myopic eyes carry a moderate risk of retinal detachment, which is increased after lens extraction.

Another procedure is the intracorneal ring (ICR), which is implanted into the peripheral cornea at approximately $2/3$ stromal depth. The result is a vaulting effect that flattens the central cornea, decreasing myopia. The ICR procedure has the advantage of being reversible.

21. What are the treatment options for astigmatism?

The correction of astigmatism is slightly more forgiving than the correction of myopia. A patient with 3.00 diopters of astigmatism is usually quite pleased with a postoperative residual of 1.25 diopters of cylinder correction because reasonably good vision results. Each of the procedures for myopia has adaptations to address astigmatism alone or simultaneously with myopia. Astigmatic keratotomy (AK) refers to making transverse (straight) or arcuate astigmatic cuts in the mid periphery of the steep corneal meridian. We have learned that crossing of transverse and radial incisions is problematic. Epithelial ingrowth into the stroma, healing difficulties, and significant scarring may result. Excimer laser photo-astigmatic refractive keratotomy (PARK) uses a cylindrical rather than a spherical ablation pattern to remove tissue in a chosen meridian (astigmatic correction). If compound myopic astigmatism is present, an elliptical PRK ablation (a combination of spherical and cylindrical patterns) results in correction of both myopia and astigmatism. Similar astigmatic corrections have been achieved with LASIK. Whichever procedure is employed, the axis of the astigmatism should be marked with the patient seated, because it may shift when the patient reclines.

22. What can be done about astigmatism after a corneal transplant?

There are several options. First, selective removal of sutures in steep meridians may improve astigmatism. A rigid gas-permeable contact lens may be especially effective in alleviating irregular astigmatism. However, many patients do not tolerate or desire contact lenses after corneal transplant surgery. Once all sutures are out and the refraction is stable, arcuate relaxing incisions may be performed in the donor cornea along the steep meridian to reduce astigmatism. An alternative technique involves using a blade to open the wound partially and relax several millimeters of the graft-host junction as opposed to creating incisions in the donor tissue. As described above, the excimer laser also has been used to make cylindrical ablations for the correction of postcorneal transplant astigmatism. Relaxing incisions combined with compression sutures (across the graft-host interface) have been used successfully to correct astigmatism of 5–10 diopters by causing steepening of the cornea in the sutured median. For astigmatism greater than 10 diopters, a wedge resection (of corneal tissue followed by sutured closure of the wound) may be performed in the flat meridian.

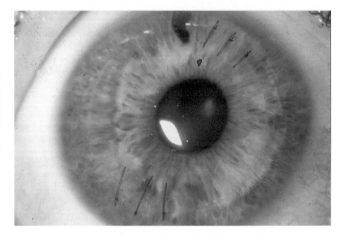

Treatment for postcorneal transplant astigmatism. Compression sutures were placed in the flat meridians (1:00–3:00 o'clock and 6:30–8:00 o'clock) and relaxing incisions were performed in the graft wound 90° away.

23. A 40-year-old Olympic ski coach desires refractive surgery so that he may see distance clearly. His refraction is –3.00 –2.00 × 180 in both eyes. The surgeon performs radial incisions for 3.00 D of myopia and transverse incisions to flatten the steep meridian by 2.00 D at 90°. Is the patient happy?

The patient is unhappy because of residual myopia. He now knows more about the "coupling effect" than his surgeon. When a transverse incision causes corneal flattening in one meridian, there is a compensatory steepening of the unincised corneal meridian 90° away. In the case above, the coupling effect of the incised and unincised meridians (90° apart) should have been anticipated. Radial incisions must be used to correct the 3.00 D of spherical myopia as well as the approximate 1.00 D of steepening induced by the transverse incisions. In general, short incisions tend to cause less steepening of the unincised meridian than longer incisions.

24. What about procedures for hyperopia?

Of the available options, none is as effective or reliable as the procedures for myopia.

1. For low levels of hyperopia, holmium laser thermokeratoplasty has been used in phase II trials with some early success. Eight (or 16) peripheral laser spots are placed in a ring (or two), each spot causing shrinkage of the stromal collagen and resulting in steepening of the central cornea. Problems to be resolved include regression of effect and induced astigmatism.

2. Hyperopic excimer laser PRK is also under investigation. The laser is used to create a large, donut-shaped ablation that requires a generous epithelial defect (often 9 mm or more). A 3.00 D hyperope requires three times as many laser spots as a 3.00 D myope. This may lead to dehydration and decentration during the lengthy procedure and prolonged epithelial healing time postoperatively. Although initial results are encouraging, regression of refractive effect is a problem.

3. Hyperopic LASIK treatments are currently under study. Performing the laser ablation under a corneal flap has the theoretical advantage of decreased haze (ablation performed deep to Bowman's layer) and faster healing response (no large epithelial defect). However, loss of best-corrected visual acuity in a minority of patients remains a problem.

4. Clear lens extraction is a technique already familiar to most surgeons. Phacoemulsification is performed with implantation of one or two intraocular lenses as required by the degree of hyperopia. However, accommodation is completely eliminated by the procedure. Moreover, the risks of intraocular surgery, including endophthalmitis, are difficult to justify in eyes without organic disease.

25. What are the effects of refractive surgical procedures on corneal endothelial cells?

Although endothelial cell loss was an early concern in RK, studies using specular microscopy have demonstrated only a small, nonprogressive loss of endothelial cells. After excimer laser treatment of myopia, studies in animals and humans suggest a small, insignificant loss of endothelial cells that diminishes over time. Nevertheless, ongoing studies are important. As the treated population grows older, patients eventually will require cataract surgery. There are already case reports of a renewed hyperopic shift in post-RK patients undergoing cataract surgery. Is corneal decompensation in Fuchs' endothelial dystrophy accelerated by previous refractive surgery? Many questions remain unanswered. Effects of the laser itself, the inflammatory response, and toxicity of topically applied drugs may contribute to endothelial cell loss and require further study.

26. What is the role of drugs in refractive surgery?

The first issue is pain, which is important in all treatment modalities but most significant for PRK. After PRK, increased levels of prostaglandin E-2 have been found, which sensitize the pain response of nerves. Topical nonsteroidal antiinflammatory drugs (NSAIDs) such as ketorolac and diclofenac sodium have been shown to decrease pain by reducing prostaglandin E-2 levels. However, these agents also increase white blood cell response in the cornea and should be used concomitantly with a topical steroid. One study found increased sterile corneal infiltrates when topical NSAIDs were used alone.

Another issue is corneal haze after PRK. The cornea undergoes a wound-healing response to the excimer laser ablation. Activated keratocytes lay down new collagen and proteoglycan matrix (the haze). This is first apparent at 1 month postoperatively, peaks at 3 months, and then decreases as remodeling ensues. Several experimental and retrospective studies have shown that topical steroids reduce corneal haze after PRK. However, a prospective, double-masked study revealed no benefit from topical steroids vs. placebo. Still, in a subgroup of patients steroids may be beneficial, and they are typically used postoperatively.

Topical steroids also have been studied in the modulation of corneal curvature. Despite controversy in the literature, topical steroids apparently help to prevent regression of myopic effect after PRK. In fact, cessation of steroids has been associated with myopic regression, which may be reversed on reinstituting therapy in certain patients.

BIBLIOGRAPHY

1. Arrowsmith PN, Marks RG: Four-year update on predictability of radial keratotomy. Refract Surg 4:37–45, 1988.
2. Brint SF, Ostrick DM, Fisher C, et al: Six-month results of the multicenter phase I study of excimer laser myopic keratomileusis. J Cataract Refract Surg 20:610–615, 1994.
3. Gartry DS, Kerr Muir KG, Marshall J: Excimer laser photorefractive keratectomy: 18-month follow-up. Ophthalmology 99:1209–1219, 1992.
4. O'Brart DPS, Corbett MC, Lohmann CP, et al: The effects of ablation diameter on the outcome of excimer laser photorefractive keratectomy (PRK): A prospective, randomised, double-blind study. Arch Ophthalmol 113:438–443, 1995.
5. Salah T, Waring GO III, El Maghraby A, et al: Excimer laser in-situ keratomileusis under a corneal flap for myopia of 2 to 20 diopters. Am J Ophthalmol 121:143–155, 1996.
6. Salz JJ (ed): Corneal Laser Surgery. St. Louis, Mosby, 1995.
7. Sanders DR, Dietz MR, Gallagher D: Factors affecting predictability of radial keratotomy. Ophthalmology 92:1237–1243, 1985.
8. Waring GO III (ed): Refractive Keratotomy for Myopia and Astigmatism. St. Louis, Mosby, 1992.
9. Waring GO III, Lynn MJ, Gelender H, et al: Results of the Prospective Evaluation of Radial Keratotomy (PERK) Study one year after surgery. Ophthalmology 92:177–198, 1985.
10. Waring GO III, Lynn MJ, McDonnell PJ, et al: Results of the Prospective Evaluation of Radial Keratotomy (PERK) Study 10 years after surgery. Arch Ophthalmol 112:1298–1308, 1994.
11. Waring GO III, Casebeer C, Dru RM, et al: One year results of a prospective multicenter study of the Casebeer system of refractive keratotomy. Ophthalmology 103:1337–1347, 1996.

III. Glaucoma

16. GLAUCOMA

George L. Spaeth, M.D.

1. What is glaucoma?

Glaucoma is a group of conditions in which tissues of the eye become damaged. Usually the optic nerve is damaged, but in conditions such as acute angle-closure glaucoma, the lens, cornea, and other structures can be affected. Intraocular pressure is one of the factors responsible for the damage. Glaucoma is a highly heterogeneous group of conditions, both from the point of view of pathogenesis and clinical expression. In acute primary closed-angle glaucoma the sole cause for the damage is elevated intraocular pressure; the patient usually has excruciating pain, and blindness may occur in 2 hours. In open-angle, focal, and low-tension glaucoma, the patient has no symptoms until damage is marked. Intraocular pressure plays only a small role in the pathogenesis of the disease, and the pressure may actually be below normal. The condition may need to be present for 15 or more years before the patient becomes symptomatic. All these conditions are called glaucoma, but obviously they are very different.

2. Who gets glaucoma?

Anybody can. Glaucoma affects around 2% of the population and is the first, second, or third leading cause of blindness in every country in the world. Many types of glaucoma are hereditary, such as primary angle-closure glaucoma, which has an autosomal dominant pattern. Some cases are related to constitutional factors; visual loss in glaucoma is far more common in people of black African origin and in people who are overweight. Some glaucomas are related to a specific inciting cause such as trauma to the eye or an intraocular tumor. Newborns may develop glaucoma, related or unrelated to family history. Juveniles who have abnormalities of the 1q chromosome are highly predisposed to developing glaucoma. The most common cause of glaucoma in America and Europe, specifically primary open-angle glaucoma, is strongly related to aging. It is infrequent in people below the age of 50 and relatively common in people 80 years of age and older.

The risk factors for developing open-angle glaucoma are elevated intraocular pressure, genetic predisposition, race, age, hyperopia for angle-closure or myopia for open-angle glaucoma, exfoliation syndrome, pigment dispersion syndrome, and trauma to the eye. Risk factors that make patients with glaucoma more likely to have progressive disease include inabilty to manage one's own life, obesity, and sedentary lifestyle. In addition, any factor that results in inadequate nourishment of the optic nerve predisposes to glaucomatous damage; examples include malnutrition, hypotension, vasospasm, and severe anemia.

Various factors predispose to the development of angle-closure types of glaucoma:

Anatomic features (inherited or congenital)

1. Small anterior segment
   - Hyperopia
   - Nanophthalmos
   - Microcornea
   - Microphthalmos
   - Retinopathy of prematurity
   - Hereditary narrow angle

2. Anterior iris insertion
   - Eskimos
   - Asians
   - Black Africans

3. Shallow anterior chamber
   - Women (as opposed to men)
   - Elderly people, especially with significant nuclear sclerosis
   - Plateau iris syndrome
   - Loose or dislocated lens
   - Large lens

Obstruction of aqueous humor at pupil

1. Contact between iris and pseudophakos, vitreous, or other materials such as silicone
2. Adhesion between iris and other material (lens, pseudophakos, vitreous)
3. Obstruction of aqueous humor posterior to pupil or traumatic angle damage and adhesions secondary to surgery

Anterior rotation of ciliary body

1. Retinal vein occlusion
2. Other obstruction to venous outflow
3. Cyclitis (as follows cyclophotocoagulation)
4. Choroidal effusion
5. Scleral buckling

Anterior displacement of the lens-iris diaphragm

1. Parasympathomimetic agents (miotics)
2. Aqueous misdirection (ciliary block or malignant glaucoma)
3. Pressure from the posterior segment
   - Tumor
   - Expanding gas
4. Loose or dislocated lens

Adherence of iris to trabecular meshwork unrelated to pupillary block

1. Chandler's syndrome
2. Essential iris atrophy
3. Cogan-Reese syndrome
4. Neovascularization of anterior segment
5. Inflammatory adhesions secondary to uveitis or inflammation
6. Adhesion secondary to angle recession or hyphema
7. Adhesion secondary to surgery

Lastly, some optic nerves are more resistant to the damaging effects of intraocular pressure than others. Small nerves with no peripapillary atrophy but small central cups in which it is not possible to see laminar dots are less likely to become damaged than eyes with large optic nerves, large cups, peripapillary atrophy, and prominent laminar dots.

3. Why does intraocular pressure become elevated?

The eye is normally maintained at a level of pressure usually around 15 mmHg. The pressure inside the eye is a consequence of the balance between aqueous humor and blood entering the eye and aqueous humor and blood leaving the eye. When there is little resistance to the outflow of aqueous or the eye makes little fluid, the pressure is low. It is rare that the cause of elevated intraocular pressure is a consequence of excessive production of aqueous humor. Resistance to aqueous outflow may be due to a block in the system at the pupil, in the trabecular meshwork, in the sclera, or in the venous outflow channels into which the aqueous is drained. Clearly, treatment designed to lower intraocular pressure varies depending on the cause of intraocular pressure elevation.

4. The warning flag of glaucoma is loss of peripheral vision. True or false?

False. This is one of the many misunderstandings about glaucoma. For almost everybody, loss of peripheral vision means loss of vision to the side—that is, off to the left side or off to the right side. But, in fact, side vision (that is, temporal vision) is the last to be affected in most types of glaucoma. It is also incorrect to say that central vision is the first part of vision loss in glaucoma, because central vision to most people means vision of the point at which at they are looking. In fact, the first area to be damaged in most people with the most common type of glaucoma is vision just toward the inside, that is, the nasal side of central vision. This fact helps to explain why patients usually do not notice loss of vision until the damage is marked. Both eyes provide vision toward the nasal side, so that a blind spot does not become noted as long as both eyes are open. It is only when nasal loss of vision is marked in both eyes that the person becomes symptomatic.

5. Most people with pressures that are higher than two standard deviations above the norm eventually have glaucoma damage. True or false?

False. Normal intraocular pressure is around 15 mmHg, with a standard deviation of 3 mmHg. Only 5% of people with pressures above 21 mmHg and about 10% of people with pressures above 24 mmHg eventually develop glaucoma. As pressure increases, the likelihood of eventually developing glaucoma increases. Around 50% of people with pressures of 27 mmHg eventually develop glaucoma, and almost everybody who maintains a pressure of 30 mmHg for 10 or 15 years develops some glaucomatous damage.

6. Most people with glaucoma have elevated intraocular pressure. True or false?

True, but "most" does not mean "all." Depending on the study, about five of six people with glaucomatous damage have intraocular pressure above 21 mmHg. Because intraocular pressure fluctuates, any one measurement may show a patient's pressure to be lower than the average reading.

7. The pathogenesis of optic nerve damage in glaucoma is mechanical deformation of the optic nerve caused by pressure higher than the optic nerve can tolerate. True or false?

False.

8. The pathogenesis of glaucoma is ischemia of the optic nerved caused by intraocular pressure higher than the blood vessels can tolerate. True or false?

False.

9. The pathogenesis of glaucoma is either mechanical deformation or ischemia of the optic nerve caused by pressure higher than the eye can tolerate. True or false?

False.

10. So what is the pathogenesis of glaucoma?

The pathogenesis of optic nerve damage in glaucoma has been only partially elucidated. In some cases, mechanical deformation of the optic nerve with posterior bowing of the lamina cribrosa plays an important role in optic nerve damage. This mechanism has been demonstrated in experimental glaucoma in animals and was proved by Shiose's study, in which the intraocular pressure of human eyes was increased by administration of topical corticosteroids, after which the optic nerve became cupped and visual field loss developed. When topical corticosteroids were stopped, the intraocular pressure fell, the cupping disappeared, and visual fields returned to normal. It is possible that other factors, including ischemia, were at work, but mechanical deformation by itself was apparently an adequate explanation of the damage.

In other cases, ischemia appears to be the dominant or perhaps sole cause of damage to the optic nerve. A sudden decrease in blood pressure may cause a sudden decrease in perfusion pressure to the optic nerve. This may be the response to a carotid artery occlusion or treatment of an intracranial aneurysm, in which case sudden progression of cupping is associated with worsening visual field loss from the side with large-vessel hypoperfusion. Cases also have been reported in which sudden lowering of blood pressure in response to bleeding, trauma, or pharmacologic agents has been associated with sudden progression of visual field loss in both eyes.

A different type of ischemia may play a role in some types of low-tension glaucoma associated with focal vasospasm. There is good epidemiologic support for the existence of vasospastic glaucoma as well as corroborating experimental evidence. However, it has not been demonstrated with certainty in humans. Yet another type of ischemic mechanism is secondary to elevation of intraocular pressure. It has been demonstrated repeatedly that increasing intraocular pressure in some people is associated with decreasing blood flow to the optic nerve. However, the exact importance of decreased blood flow to the optic nerve in causing damage in patients with glaucoma has not been demonstrated. Nevertheless, increasing intraocular pressure, even relatively small amounts such as 5 or 10 mmHg, can cause a decrease in blood flow to the optic nerve. When the rise in pressure is sufficiently great that the intraocular pressure exceeds the pressure within the retinal arteries, the glaucoma causes an acute ischemic optic neuropathy, with all of the classic signs and symptoms. The optic nerve becomes pale, the retinal arteries empty, the retina becomes electrophysiologically nonreactive, and vision is lost. In such cases, when the intraocular pressure is again lowered, there is often a surprising recovery of function, although visual field loss and changes in the optic nerve can be documented.

There are probably other pathogenetic mechanisms in addition to mechanical deformation and ischemia. For example, it has been suggested that glutamate toxicity may be involved. What is certain, however, is that multiple different pathogenetic mechanisms are responsible for optic nerve damage in different pateints with glaucoma. In most patients several different pathogenetic mechanisms probably operate simultaneously.

11. Gonioscopy is which of the following: (1) Visualization of the anterior chamber angle? (2) Estimation of the anterior chamber depth? (3) Estimation of the rate of flow of aqueous humor by visualizing the dilution of the eye? (4) Evaluation of the effect of intraocular pressure on the visual field?

Gonioscopy is visualization of the anterior chamber angle. Gonioscopy, ophthalmoscopy, and tonometry constitute the essential triad of evaluating patients with glaucoma. Tonometry, the measurement of intraocular pressure, provides information about the primary risk factor for damage in the future—specifically, the level of intraocular pressure. Ophthalmoscopy, the evaluation of the appearance of the optic nerve head and the interior of the eye, permits the examiner to determine how much damage has already occurred and gives important clues to the pathogenesis of the damage. Gonioscopy allows us to determine the mechanism that controls the intraocular pressure and strongly influences the nature of the recommended treatment. Gonioscopy is important to determine whether the space between the iris and the cornea is adequate for the aqueous to exit; it also determines other abnormalities, such as pigment dispersion syndrome, exfoliation syndrome, adhesions caused by inflammation, and damage caused by trauma. Gonioscopy is an absolutely essential part of the evaluation of every patient with glaucoma.

12. The primary goal of treatment of a patient with glaucoma is to lower intraocular pressure. True or false?

False.

13. The primary goal of treatment of a patient with glaucoma is to preserve vision. True or false?

False.

14. The primary goal of treatment of a patient with glaucoma is preservation or possible enhancement of the patient's health. True or false?

True. One way in which this goal is achieved is to preserve the patient's vision. One way of perserving vision is to lower intraocular pressure. However, sometimes the primary goal is forgotten, especially by patients who are more concerned about the level of intraocular pressure than about their health. The level of intraocular pressure is but one of many factors that relate to the preservation of vision and health. All of the treatments designed to lower intraocular pressure, especially medicinal treatments, have side effects that may be damaging to the patient's health. Unless the primary goal is constantly kept in mind, all too frequently the patient ends up as described in the old medical school saw: "The operation was a success, but the patient died."

15. History is the most important part of the evaluation of a patient with glaucoma. True or false?

True. The aspects that are necessary to determine the type of glaucoma and the appropriate treatment are determination of the stage of glaucoma, the stability of the condition, rhe rate at which the condition is changing, the condition's likely duration of action (that is, the patient's life expectancy), and the mechanism responsible for pressure elevation. If possible, it is also important to understand the damage that is occurring. The mechanism of pressure elevation is determined by gonioscopy. The stage of the glaucoma—that is, how much damage has occurred—is partially determined by ophthalmoscopy, but most importantly by the history: how much functional difficulty, how much pain, does the patient have as a result of the glaucoma? The stability of the glaucoma and the rate of change are determined in part by serial examinations such as repeat evaluation of the optic nerve or visual field. But, most importantly, they are ascertained by careful history. Is the patient getting worse? If so, how quickly? Life expectancy is essential to know, because only by understanding how the long the disease process is likely to operate can the physician develop a rational approach to treatment. Life expectancy is determined largely by history: How long did the patient's parents live? How good is the patient's general health? What is the patient's lifestyle? In addition, the history allows the physician to know who the patient is. The physician must get a sense of the patient's self-management skills, because they are essential in arriving at a rational plan for therapy. For example, patients who show far-advanced glaucomatous optic nerve damage, who become worse, and who know that they have glaucoma but do not take their medications have told the physician that such behavior almost certainly will continue. For such patients, surgery is usually promptly needed. In contrast, patients with moderate glaucomatous damage that occurred asymptomatically and has not progressed since the diagnosis was made and who appear to have their lives well ordered, including knowing how to care for glaucoma, are probably best treated by continuing the medication.

16. Eye drops are hazardous because they are absorbed directly into the blood stream. True or false?

True. It is a misunderstanding to think that eye drops are safer than medications taken by mouth. In fact, one drop of a beta blocker, such as timolol, in a child can produce blood levels in excess of those used for full systemic beta-blocker therapy. Consequently, side effects such as apnea may occur in children in response to a single eye drop.

17. Which of the following is the best treatment of glaucoma?

1. Eye drops	**3. Laser trabeculoplasty**	**5. No therapy at all**
2. Immediate surgery	**4. Removal of the eye**	

There is no "best" treatment for glaucoma. Eye drops are best for some types of glaucoma in certain situations. Immediate surgery is usually appropriate in infants with congenital glaucoma and adults with severe pressure elevation due to angle closure. Argon laser trabeculoplasty is often preferred in patients with glaucoma associated with exfoliation syndrome or pigment dispersion syndrome. Removal of the eye may be the best treatment for glaucoma caused by a tumor or severe neovascularization associated with diabetes mellitus. And in some people with glaucoma, even when they have marked damage, it is best to follow them with no medicinal or surgical therapy.

18. Appropriate treatment of glaucoma results in stabilization of the disease process in what percentage of patients?

The answer is related to the type of glaucoma, the amount of damage, when the glaucoma is first diagnosed, the patient's self-management skills, and various other factors. For example, a 50-year-old woman with almost total excavation of the optic nerve caused by glaucoma in association with aniridia has less than a 10% chance of preserving her vision. Even if the intraocular pressure can be controlled in a range in which the glaucomatous process no longer damages cells (which is almost certainly impossible), the normal death of cells as the person ages will result in continuing loss of neurons and probably in eventual total loss of vision. In contrast, the 70-year-old man with primary open-angle glaucoma that has been present for 30 years, during which the intraocular pressure has averaged around 30 mmHg but the patient has used no medication and has developed the slightest amount of optic nerve damage, will almost certainly maintain good vision until the time of death, even with no treatment. Glaucoma is an extremely heterogeneous group of conditions; appropriate treatment, therefore, is equally heterogeneous.

19. Patients who deserve referral to an ophthalmologist for evaluation for possible glaucoma include patients who:
  1. **Have a family history of glaucomatous visual loss.**
  2. **Have intraocular pressures above 21 mmHg.**
  3. **Are nearsighted.**
  4. **Have a history of smoky vision, often in the evenings, sometimes associated with headaches.**
  5. **Have 20/20 vision in both eyes but sense that their visual function is not as good as it used to be.**

All of the above. The first three are risk factors for the development of glaucoma. The fourth describes the classic symptoms of patients with recurrent angle-closure glaucoma. Patients usually retain normal central vision until the glaucoma is extremely far advanced. Moreover, 20/20 vision does not rule out the probability of severe glaucomatous damage. Infants with tearing and photophobia, especially if the eye appears hazy or large, also should be referred to an ophthalmologist, as should adults with shallow anterior chambers, ocular pain, or reduced vision.

BIBLIOGRAPHY

1. Caprioli J, et al: Primary Open-angle Glaucoma: Preferred Practice Pattern. San Francisco, American Academy of Ophthalmology, 1992.
2. Shields MB, Ritch R, Krupin T: Chronic open-angle glaucoma: Treatment overview. In Ritch R, Shield MB (eds): The Glaucomas, 2nd ed. St. Louis, Mosby, 1996, pp 1507–1521.
3. Ritch R, Low RF: Angle-closure glaucoma: Therapeutic overview. In Ritch R, Shield MB (eds): The Glaucomas, 2nd ed. St. Louis, Mosby, 1996, pp 1521–1535.
4. Liebowitz HM, et al: The Framingham Eye Study monograph. Surv Ophthalmol 24(Suppl):335, 1980.
5. Leske MC: The epidemiology of open-angle glaucoma: A review. Am J Epidemiol 118:166, 1983.
6. Levine RV: Low-tension glaucoma: A critical review and new material. Surv Ophthalmol 24:621, 1980.
7. Hollows FC, Graham PA: Intraocular pressure, glaucoma, and glaucoma suspects in a defined population. Br J Ophthalmol 50:570, 1966.
8. Sommer A, et al: Relationship between intraocular pressure and primary open-angle glaucoma among white and black Americans: The Baltimore Eye Survey. Arch Ophthalmol 109:1090, 1991.
9. Shiose Y, Kanda T: Quantitative analysis of "optic cup" and its clinical application. II: The case study. Jpn J Clin Ophthalmol 28:367–374, 1974.
10. Spaeth GL: The normal development of the human anterior chamber angle: A new system of descriptive grading. Trans Ophthalmol Soc UK 91:709–739, 1971.
11. Spaeth GL: How to suspect, detect, and treat a person with angle-closure glaucoma. In Transactions of the New Orleans Academy of Ophthalmology: A Symposium on Glaucoma. St. Louis, Mosby, 1997.
12. Van Buskirk EM: Adverse reactions from timolol administration. Ophthalmology 87:447, 1980.

17. ANGLE CLOSURE GLAUCOMA

Anup K. Khatana, M.D., and George L. Spaeth, M.D.

1. What landmarks are seen in the anterior chamber (AC) angle?

The structures noted in anterior to posterior sequence are as follows (boldface numbers in parentheses correspond to number labels in the figure):

(1) Schwalbe's line: The peripheral or posterior termination of Descemet's membrane, seen clinically as the apex or termination of the corneal light wedge. It may be visible inferiorly as the most anterior nonwavy pigmented line.

(2) Anterior, nonpigmented, trabecular meshwork (TM): Clear whitish band

(3) Posterior, pigmented, trabecular meshwork (TM): Variably pigmented band of homogeneous width. It is usually most pigmented inferiorly (see figure on next page).

(4) Schlemm's canal: Variably visible light grey band at the level of the posterior TM. Elevated episcleral venous pressure or pressure from the edge of the goniolens will cause blood to reflux, making it appear as a faint red band.

(5) Scleral spur: Narrow white band of sclera invaginating between the TM and ciliary body. It marks the insertion site of the longitudinal muscle fibers of the ciliary body to the sclera.

(6) Ciliary body band (CB band): Pigmented band marking the anterior face of the ciliary body. Variably, iris processes may be seen as lacy projections crossing this band. By definition, iris processes do not cross the scleral spur. Projections that cross the scleral spur to the TM are peripheral anterior synechiae (PAS) and may be focal, pillar-like, or broad sheets.

(7) Iris

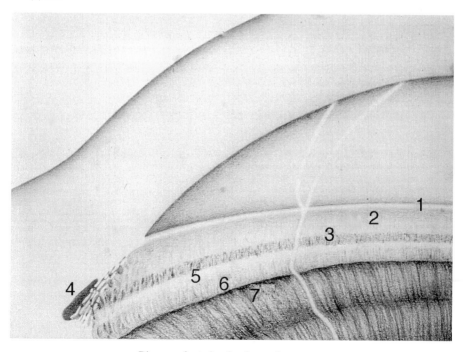

Diagram of anterior chamber angle anatomy.

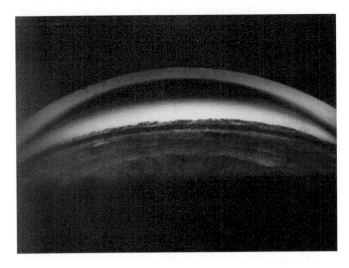

Inferior quadrant of heavily pigmented normal open angle.

2. Why is a goniolens necessary to visualize the AC angle?

Light from the AC angle undergoes total internal reflection at the cornea–air interface, preventing direct visualization. A goniolens changes the refractive index at the interface, enabling visualization.

3. What are the different kinds of goniolenses, and how do they differ?

Direct gonioscopy uses the **Koeppe** contact lens. This technique is cumbersome, requiring a supine patient, a clear viscous liquid coupling medium such as methylcellulose, and a direct viewing system.

Indirect gonioscopy uses a mirrored contact lens, either the **Goldmann** three-mirror lens that also vaults the central cornea and requires a viscous coupling liquid, or the **Zeiss** (see figure), **Posner**, or **Sussman** four-mirror lenses that directly contact the cornea and thus do not require a coupling agent beyond the patient's normal tear film.

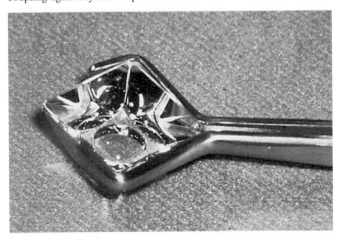

Zeiss goniolens.

4. Which goniolens is preferred by most glaucoma specialists and why?

The Zeiss lens is preferred by a majority of glaucoma specialists for the following reasons:

1. Its speed and ease of use (it does not require a viscous coupling liquid, and, because of its four mirrors, it does not need to be rotated to see all 360 degrees of the angle).

2. The ability to perform indentation gonioscopy (which cannot be performed with the Goldmann lens because of its larger diameter), and its absence of suction effect on the eye (the suction effect of the Goldmann lens can sometimes artificially widen narrow angles). These two qualities can be critically important when evaluating eyes with narrow angles.

3. Elimination of the transient degradation of corneal clarity that is a consequence of the viscous liquid and Goldmann lens manipulation and that can make subsequent fundus examination difficult.

When first mastering gonioscopy, the Zeiss lens can be more difficult than the Goldmann lens.

Warning: In inexperienced hands, excessive indentation can easily occur that will make the angle appear wider than it really is. Zeiss gonioscopy demands a light touch. One way to make sure you are not pressing is for the contact to be so light that you occasionally lose part of the contact meniscus. If you see any corneal striae or if your view is not crystal clear, you are probably indenting.

5. How is gonioscopy performed?
1. Topical anesthesia is essential for patient comfort and cooperation.
2. Rest your elbow on the slit-lamp platform and your ring and/or small fingers on the side bar or on the patient's cheek to help stabilize your hand.
3. Examination can be facilitated by asking the patient to stare straight ahead with the fellow eye without blinking.
4. To facilitate viewing a particular quadrant of the angle with indirect gonioscopy, either tilt the mirror toward the quadrant or have the patient look toward that mirror. For example, when viewing the superior angle, either tilt the inferior mirror upward, toward the superior angle, or have the patient look down slightly, toward the inferior mirror.
5. The superior–inferior relationships in the nasal and temporal mirrors and the nasal–temporal (right–left) relationships in the superior and inferior mirrors are preserved, not inverted as in indirect ophthalmoscopy. For example, when viewing the superior angle through the inferior mirror, an area of PAS seen at five o'clock in the mirror is actually at one o'clock, not eleven o'clock.

6. How can I determine which patients may have narrow angles and need gonioscopy?
The van Herick technique uses a thin slit beam focused at the limbus to approximate angle depth by comparing the peripheral AC depth to corneal thickness. A grade I has a peripheral AC depth less than one-quarter corneal thickness; grade II is one-quarter corneal thickness; a grade III is one-half thickness; and a grade IV is one corneal thickness or more. Patients who are grade I or II certainly have narrow angles and should have gonioscopy. This technique, however, should never replace gonioscopy in eyes with clear media as part of a glaucoma evaluation. It falsely gives the appearance of an open angle in some eyes with plateau iris or anterior rotation of the ciliary body (see classification below).

7. What are the different gonioscopic anterior chamber angle classification systems?

	Grade 0	Grade I	Grade II	Grade III	Grade IV
Scheie		Wide open	Scleral spur visible, CB band not seen	Can only see to anterior TM	Closed
Schaffer	Closed	10°	20°	30°	40°

(Scheie is rarely used. Schaffer is most commonly used, and the angle is graded as a slit when it is between grades 0 and I.)

Spaeth: This system is the most descriptive. The first element is a capital letter (A–E) for the level of iris insertion: **A**—anterior to TM; **B**—behind Schwalbe's line, or at TM; **C**—at scleral spur; **D**—deep angle, CB band visible; **E**—extremely deep. If during indentation gonioscopy, the true iris insertion is noted to be more posterior than originally apparent, the original impression is put in parentheses, followed by the true iris insertion outside parentheses.

(Table continued on following page.)

Spaeth *(cont)*: The second element is a number that denotes the iridocorneal angle width in degrees, usually from **5 to 45°**. The third element is a letter (q, r, or s) describing the peripheral iris configuration: **q**—queer, concave; **r**—regular; **s**—steep.

In addition, the pigmentation of the posterior TM is graded on a scale of 0 (none) to 4 (maximal). *Example:* (A)C10 r, 2+PTM refers to an appositionally closed 10-degree angle that, with indentation, opened to the scleral spur and revealed moderate pigmentation of the posterior TM.

---

8. How do I know if I can dilate a patient safely?

In addition to the angle width in degrees, the apparent and real iris root insertion and peripheral iris configuration can add valuable information when trying to determine if an angle is at risk for closure. Angles that are less than or equal to 15 degrees are at risk for closure and probably should not be dilated. An eye with a 20-degree angle should be watched closely, as it may narrow further with time, and should be reevaluated with tonometry and gonioscopy after dilation. An exception to these general guidelines is plateau iris (discussed later), in which the angle may be wider than 20° and still at risk for closure.

9. How do I know if I can safely dilate a patient if I don't have a slit lamp?

Use a penlight and shine it from the temporal side perpendicular to the central visual axis. The temporal half of the iris will always be illuminated. In an eye with a normal or "safe" anterior chamber depth, the entire nasal half of the iris will be illuminated as well. In an eye with a shallow or questionable anterior chamber depth, none or only part of the nasal half of the iris will be illuminated. This technique does not hold true in eyes with plateau iris.

10. How is angle closure classified?
A. By clinical presentation
   I. Acute
   II. Subacute or intermittent
   III. Chronic
B. By mechanism
   I. Posterior pushing mechanism
     a. Pupillary block (can occur in phakic, pseudophakic, or aphakic eyes)
       1. Relative
       Idiopathic (i.e., primary angle closure)
       Miotic-induced
       Lens-induced
       Plateau iris
       2. Absolute or true: by posterior synechiae from any inflammatory etiology
     b. Lens-induced
       1. Phakomorphic (due to an intumescent cataractous lens or a swollen lens in a diabetic)
       2. Lens subluxation
       Trauma
       Pseudoexfoliation syndrome
       Hereditary/metabolic disorders—Marfan's syndrome, homocystinuria, etc.
       3. Lens pushed forward
       Aqueous misdirection syndrome (malignant or ciliary block glaucoma)
       Mass—tumor, ROP, PHPV, etc.
     c. Plateau iris
       1. True plateau iris
       2. Iris and ciliary body cysts
     d. Swelling/anterior rotation of the ciliary body (there is some overlap within this)
       1. Inflammatory—scleritis, uveitis, after panretinal photocoagulation, etc.
       2. Congestive—after scleral buckling surgery, nanophthalmos, etc.

   3. Choroidal effusion—hypotony after trauma or surgery, uveal effusion, etc.
   4. Suprachoroidal hemorrhage (SCH)—intra- or postoperative
      Risk factors for SCH include previous IOP elevation followed by hypotony, high myopia, advanced age, aphakia, previous vitrectomy, systemic hypertension or atherosclerotic vascular disease, and postoperative Valsalva maneuver.
 II. Anterior pulling mechanism—synechial angle closure
   a. Chronic appositional closure from any of the above
   b. Intraocular inflammation (uveitis)
   c. Neovascular glaucoma
      1. Central retinal vein occlusion (CRVO), accounts for one-third of cases
      2. Diabetes mellitus, accounts for another one-third of cases
      3. Carotid occlusive disease, comprises approximately 13% of cases
      4. Miscellaneous: central retinal artery occlusion (CRAO), tumors, retinal detachment, etc.
   d. Iridocorneal endothelial (ICE) syndrome
      1. Progressive iris atrophy
      2. Chandler's syndrome
      3. Cogan-Reese syndrome

PRIMARY ANGLE CLOSURE (RELATIVE PUPILLARY BLOCK)

11. What is the epidemiology of primary angle closure glaucoma?

For **acute** angle closure, Eskimos (highest incidence) and Asians have a much higher incidence than Caucasians, who in turn have a higher incidence than blacks. It is relatively more common in Northern European Caucasians than in Mediterranean Caucasians. The peak incidence is between the ages of 55 and 65. In Caucasians, women are three to four times more likely to develop angle closure than men. In blacks, the incidence is equal between men and women. There is also a greater incidence in hyperopes. The inheritance appears to be polygenic.

For **chronic** angle closure, blacks have a higher incidence than Asians, who have a higher incidence than Caucasians. In addition, blacks are more likely to develop chronic angle closure than acute angle closure.

12. What are the symptoms of acute angle closure glaucoma?

Patients can complain of ocular pain, redness, blurred or foggy vision, haloes around lights, nausea, and vomiting. The visual symptoms are partly caused by the corneal edema that occurs from the sudden severe rise in intraocular pressure (IOP). This, the most common presentation, is most often induced by stress or low ambient light levels and occasionally by various medications. If the IOP exceeds the pressure in the ophthalmic or central retinal artery, visual loss occurs as a result of ischemia of the optic nerve or retina.

13. Describe the signs or exam findings seen in primary acute angle closure glaucoma.

IOP: Typically greater than 45 mmHg

Conjunctiva and episclera: Dilated vessels

Cornea: Epithelial and stromal edema

Anterior chamber: Shallow; cells or flare variably present

Iris: Dilated vessels (distinguish from neovascularization of the iris), mid-dilated nonreactive or sluggish pupil, and sector atrophy from ischemia (only if previous episodes have occurred)

Lens: Glaukomflecken (not seen acutely, but if present initially may indicate previous episodes of angle closure)

Gonioscopy: With narrow angle or closed angle, one may be unable to view structures owing to corneal edema (glycerin may be used to clear the cornea); superior angle is usually the narrowest and the first to develop peripheral anterior synechia (PAS)

Optic nerve: Occasional swelling and hyperemia from vascular congestion; may mimic papilledema

Retina: May be normal, or may show signs of vascular occlusion

Examination of the fellow eye is very important in making the diagnosis. If the fellow eye has a normal depth AC and a normal angle width, the diagnosis of primary angle closure should be seriously doubted, unless the involved eye is significantly more hyperopic.

14. How does subacute or intermittent angle closure present clinically?

The symptoms are similar to an acute attack but usually less severe, tend to recur over days to weeks, and may be confused for headaches. They resolve on their own, often when the individual goes to sleep or enters a well-lit area (both induce miosis). These episodes can result in chronic angle closure. Between episodes, the IOP is normal and the ocular exam is usually normal, except for the presence of narrow angles and, sometimes, glaukomflecken, cataracts, and PAS on gonioscopy.

15. How does chronic angle closure present clinically?

It is usually asymptomatic, unless marked visual field loss has occurred. Gradual closure of the angle, by simple apposition and/or PAS, leads to a more gradual rise in IOP. The IOP is more variable but tends to be somewhat lower than in acute angle closure. The cornea is usually clear, because the IOP rises gradually, resulting in a lack of pain, redness, decreased vision, or other symptoms. The most frequent exception to this is neovascular glaucoma, which is also caused by PAS but often presents with symptoms and signs similar to acute angle closure.

16. What are the anatomic characteristics of these eyes?

Short axial length, hyperopia, and "anterior segment crowding."

17. What is the pathophysiologic mechanism of relative pupillary block?

The crystalline lens grows throughout life. In eyes that are predisposed, there is a gradually increasing apposition between the posterior iris surface and the anterior lens capsule. As the iridolenticular touch increases, the resistance to aqueous flow from the posterior to the anterior chamber increases, causing a gradual increase in the posterior chamber pressure. Under conditions in which the pupil is in a mid-dilated position (from stress, low ambient light levels, sympathomimetic or anticholinergic medications, etc.), the elevated posterior chamber pressure causes the lax or floppy iris to bow anteriorly and occlude the trabecular meshwork. In thinner or lighter-colored irides, this is more likely to cause an acute rise in IOP. Thicker irides are less likely to flop anteriorly, but rather are gradually pushed anteriorly, especially peripherally, leading to chronic angle closure, with or without PAS, and a more gradual IOP rise.

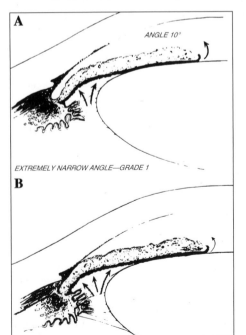

Mechanism of relative pupillary block angle closure. *A,* Extremely narrow (grade I) angle with resistance to aqueous flow between the iris and lens leading to increased posterior chamber pressure. *B,* Closed angle.

18. What nonmedical maneuver may help to lower IOP even before medicating the patient?

Even before starting medical treatment, indentation gonioscopy can sometimes help to lower IOP by pushing aqueous from the central AC peripherally, opening the angle if it is not sealed with PAS. This must be done carefully to avoid abrading the corneal epithelium, which is swollen and may abrade more easily than normal.

19. How would you treat the involved eye medically?

The "kitchen sink" approach is generally preferred, using some combination of the following:

The use of miotics such as pilocarpine in narrow, potentially occludable, angles is a subject of some debate, even among glaucoma specialists. The rationale for miotic use is to pull the peripheral iris away from the TM, which opens the angle and prevents appositional closure. It may, however, make the angle narrower and potentially induce angle closure by causing the lens–iris diaphragm to move anteriorly with contraction of the ciliary muscle, which relaxes zonular tension and makes the pupillary block worse. If pilocarpine is used in such a patient, repeat gonioscopy should be performed 30 to 60 minutes after the initial drop. If the angle is not any wider, some would argue that a laser PI should be performed right away. If this is not feasible, consider adding a beta-blocker to decrease aqueous secretion until the PI is performed.

Topical inhibitors of aqueous secretion—Beta blockers, carbonic anhydrase inhibitors (CAIs), and alpha-2 adrenergic agonists.

Carbonic anhydrase inhibitors—In patients who are not nauseated, an oral CAI is administered. If IV medications are available and the patient is unable to tolerate oral medications, IV acetazolamide is preferred as an adjunct to topical therapy because of its faster onset of action.

Hyperosmotic agents—Hyperosmotic therapy reduces vitreous volume and can be a very powerful weapon in lowering IOP and breaking an attack. Glycerin and isosorbide can be given orally, but glycerin is contraindicated in diabetics because it can cause severe hyperglycemia. Intravenous mannitol is the most potent agent for lowering IOP and is usually used as a last resort owing to the increased risk of systemic cardiovascular side effects.

Topical steroids—Topical steroids (e.g., prednisolone 1% qid) are a useful adjunct to control the usually concurrent intraocular inflammation that may or may not be clinically apparent.

Miotics—Pilocarpine helps to break the attack by pulling the peripheral iris away from the TM and increasing trabecular outflow. However, the pupillary sphincter (but not the ciliary muscle) usually becomes ischemic at IOPs above 40 to 50 mmHg and therefore unresponsive to miotics until the IOP is lowered with other medications. The duration of IOP elevation and sphincter ischemia ultimately determine whether or not the sphincter will respond to miotics even after the IOP is lowered. The usual concentration used is 1 or 2%. Pilocarpine should be used with caution, however, to avoid cholinergic toxicity. Also keep in mind that it may make some cases of angle closure worse. Some believe it should not be used in aphakic or pseudophakic pupillary block.

Topical glycerin—Topical glycerin can be quite helpful to clear the cornea, which facilitates detailed examination of the eye and also laser treatment.

Others—The latest alpha-2 agonist, brimonidine, increases uveoscleral outflow, as does the prostaglandin F-2 alpha agonist, latanaprost. The efficacy of these two agents in angle closure glaucoma has not yet been well studied. It should be noted that the concurrent use of pilocarpine does cause contraction of the ciliary muscle, thereby increasing resistance to uveoscleral outflow.

20. How would you treat the involved eye with laser?

Laser peripheral iridotomy (PI) is the definitive first procedure of choice to relieve pupillary block. Angle closure from any etiology other than pupillary block will not respond to iridotomy. The argon or Q switched YAG lasers may be used. The Nd:YAG laser is used more often because it is faster, easier, requires fewer bursts with less energy (causes less inflammation), and is not dependent on iris color. The argon laser's thermal effect can help prevent bleeding and facilitate penetration of thick irides. There is also some difference of opinion regarding the timing of the laser peripheral iridotomy in acute angle closure. Although the definitive management of

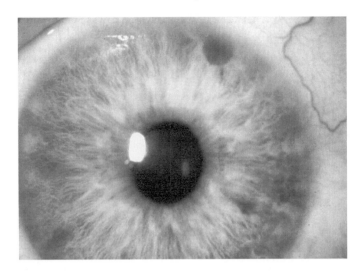

Patent laser peripheral iridotomy.

acute angle closure is laser PI, some glaucoma specialists argue that if an attack has been truly broken, medically, it may be better to defer the iridotomy 1 or 2 days for the following reasons:

1. The corneal edema, from high pressure, and the Descemet's folds, from the abrupt lowering of pressure, can both make visualization and performing the iridotomy more difficult. In addition, because the anterior chamber is shallow, the corneal endothelium is closer to the point of laser energy focus and is more likely to be damaged from the concussion.

2. The iris is usually also somewhat congested, edematous, and inflamed during an attack. This can make the iridotomy more difficult to perform; more power may be required to successfully penetrate the iris, and this can create a situation more uncomfortable for the patient than when the eye is not inflamed.

21. What are the most common complications of laser PI?

The most troublesome problem is a ghost image resulting from light that has entered through the PI.

Argon: Posterior synechiae and localized cataracts. Argon laser PIs are more likely to close than are Nd:YAG PIs.

Nd:YAG: A hemorrhage may occur in up to 50% of eyes. It is usually small and localized to the area of the PI, but sometimes can form a significant hyphema. The bleeding may be controlled by applying gentle pressure on the eye with the contact lens. Even relatively large hyphemas are gone, or almost gone, the next day.

Transient IOP spikes of more than 6 mmHg do occur in up to 40% of patients most often within the first 1 to 2 hours. Perioperative treatment with apraclonidine decreases the incidence and severity of post-laser IOP spikes. Beta blockers and CAIs have been used, but with less success. The incidence and severity of postoperative IOP elevation are similar with argon and Nd:YAG lasers.

22. What are the indications for surgical intervention? What procedure would you perform?

Surgery is indicated in an eye in which the combination of maximal tolerated medical and laser therapy have failed to control the IOP adequately. Evaluation of the disc is essential.

Clear corneal peripheral iridectomy—in an eye with an ongoing or recent acute attack and if unable to successfully perform a laser iridotomy.

Clear corneal peripheral iridectomy combined with goniosynechiolysis—if in the preceding scenario, peripheral anterior synechiae have already formed. This procedure involves breaking the synechiae in the angle to allow it to reopen.

Guarded filtering procedure (GFP), or trabeculectomy—in situations in which the preceding approach has failed or a patent laser PI has failed to resolve the attack.

When operating on these eyes, it is important to remember that they already have shallower chambers and are more likely to develop flat chambers and aqueous misdirection (malignant or ciliary block glaucoma), both of which can complicate intra- and postoperative management. The use of miotics can also increase the chances of aqueous misdirection.

23. When can you consider an attack to be completely "broken"?

When the intraocular pressure in the involved eye is the same or lower than the IOP in the uninvolved eye at initial presentation, and the angle is open.

24. What are the chances of the same thing happening to the fellow eye?

There is a 40 to 80% chance of an acute attack in the fellow eye over the next 5 to 10 years.

25. What would you recommend for the fellow eye?

Prophylactic laser PI, when gonioscopic evaluation reveals a potentially occludable angle. It is sometimes appropriate to treat the fellow eye first (if the angle is occludable), while waiting for the involved eye to quiet down. The use of pilocarpine in the fellow eye to try to prevent angle closure by pulling the peripheral iris away from the TM until PI is performed is not without risk, as discussed in question 19.

26. What are the short- and long-term sequelae to the various structures of the eye after such an attack?

Cornea—Shortly after lowering the IOP, the epithelial microcystic edema will resolve and Descemet's folds may be seen. The stromal edema takes longer to resolve. In all cases, significant endothelial damage does occur. If the attack has caused enough endothelial injury, epithelial and stromal edema may persist. Endothelial pigment may result from the pigment released during iridotomy or from any ischemic atrophic regions of the iris.

Anterior chamber—Even after successful PI, the AC is usually still shallower than normal.

Iris—One may see a mid-dilated, nonreactive, or sluggish pupil, and sector atrophy and stromal necrosis from ischemia. Posterior synechiae may eventually develop long after a PI is performed owing to the alternate route available for aqueous humor flow. The pupil is often vertically oval.

Lens—Glaukomflecken (small whitish anterior subcapsular opacities representing areas of necrotic lens epithelium with adjacent subcapsular cortical degeneration) and development or progression of cataractous changes may be seen.

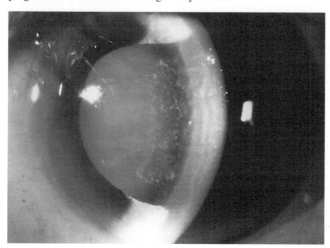

Photograph of an eye after resolution of an acute angle closure attack. Note the corneal Descemet's folds, the PI at 12 o'clock at the upper edge of the photo, and the lacy pattern of glaukomflecken under the anterior lens capsule.

Zonules—Injury from an acute episode may not manifest itself until much later, when zonular weakness is noted during cataract extraction or from spontaneous subluxation or dislocation.

Gonioscopy—PAS.

Optic nerve—The disc congestion and swelling, if present, may take several days to resolve. Acute attacks typically produce more pallor than cupping; chronic angle closure usually produces more cupping than pallor, similar to open-angle glaucoma.

Retina—"Decompression retinopathy" may be seen after rapid lowering of IOP as scattered intraretinal hemorrhages concentrated more around the posterior pole and optic nerve. Peripapillary atrophy can also develop over time, along with focal nerve fiber bundle defects, diffuse thinning of the retina, etc.

27. What types of medications are contraindicated in (narrow angle) glaucoma?

Topical and systemic **sympathomimetic and anticholinergic medications**, such as those found in many over-the-counter antihistamine and cold remedies, should be avoided by people with eyes that have narrow and potentially occludable angles until a prophylactic laser iridotomy is performed. These two classes of medications are not contraindicated in patients with eyes that have narrow but not occludable angles, or eyes with a patent iridotomy or iridectomy, or in patients with open-angle glaucoma.

Topical **miotics** should be used with caution in patients with narrow angles, regardless of whether they ar potentially occludable, because of the potential for causing further narrowing by anterior displacement of the lens–iris diaphragm. At the very least, these patients should have repeat gonioscopy after commencing miotic therapy to rule out this possibility. If the angles do become significantly narrower, then one must consider discontinuation of miotic therapy or a prophylactic PI if there is a compelling reason for continuing miotic therapy.

28. What are some possible causes for a persistent or recurrent IOP elevation after a successful PI?

1. Peripheral anterior synechiae formation and/or undetected injury to the TM during the period of angle closure

2. Nonpupillary block angle closure (see question 10, classification, Ib-d)

3. Incomplete iridotomy will result in persistent IOP elevation. Occlusion of the iridotomy with debris or a membrane may cause a recurrent episode of pupillary block angle closure.

4. Underlying or residual open angle glaucoma component

PLATEAU IRIS

29. Describe the epidemiology of plateau iris.

These patients are usually younger (typically fourth and fifth decades) and less hyperopic than patients with primary angle closure; they may even be myopic.

30. How does it present clinically?

It may be noted on routine examination or present as an acute or chronic angle closure glaucoma.

31. What is plateau iris configuration (PIC)?

Anteriorly positioned ciliary processes force the peripheral iris more anterior than normal. The central AC is usually near normal depth. The iris has a relatively flat contour, with a sharp peripheral drop-off at the angle approach. A component of pupillary block is frequently present. With dilation, the peripheral iris folds into the angle and occludes the TM.

32. How can plateau iris be distinguished from relative pupillary block (primary) angle closure on slit-lamp examination?

Primary angle closure normally presents with a shallow central AC and moderate to significant iris convexity, which is in contrast to the appearance of PIC noted above. With indentation gonioscopy, the angle is much harder to open and does not open as widely as a typical narrow angle. Persistence of the plateau iris appearance despite a patent iridotomy would help to confirm the diagnosis clinically. High-resolution ultrasound biomicroscopy can also confirm the diagnosis.

33. What is plateau iris syndrome?

Acute or chronic angle closure that develops with dilation, or even spontaneously, in an eye with plateau iris configuration and a patent PI.

34. How is plateau iris treated?

The primary procedure of choice in an eye with (or at risk for) angle closure is **laser peripheral iridotomy** to eliminate any component of pupillary block that may be present. In general, the older the patient, the more the pupillary block contributes, as a percentage, to the mechanism of angle closure.

Laser peripheral iridoplasty may be necessary in patients whose angle approach remains very narrow despite a patent PI. This technique uses the argon laser to apply burns circumferentially to the peripheral iris, which cause it to contract and pull away from the angle.

Chronic miotic therapy can also be a useful alternative or adjunct to iridoplasty in eyes with a narrow approach despite a patent PI. However, the angle should be examined with gonioscopy after instillation of pilocarpine, and at regular 6- to 12-month intervals afterwards, to document the effect on angle configuration.

AQUEOUS MISDIRECTION SYNDROME (MALIGNANT/CILIARY BLOCK GLAUCOMA)

35. What is aqueous misdirection syndrome?

Posterior misdirection of aqueous into the vitreous cavity causes an anterior displacement of the lens–iris diaphragm. It most commonly occurs after ocular (typically glaucoma filtering) surgery, but can occur after laser procedures or, rarely, spontaneously. Miotic use and previous angle closure glaucoma increase the risk of occurrence. It typically presents within the first postoperative week with a shallow to flat anterior chamber and a high IOP, but the IOP may be normal in an eye with a functioning filter. Serous choroidal effusion/detachment, pupillary block, and suprachoroidal hemorrhage should be ruled out.

36. How is aqueous misdirection treated medically?

Cycloplegics relax the ciliary muscle, which increases zonular tension and pulls the lens–iris diaphragm posteriorly. Cycloplegics are also essential in the management of angle closure due to anterior rotation of the ciliary body. They may be required indefinitely.

Aqueous suppressants
Hyperosmotic agents
Miotics are contraindicated.

37. How can aqueous misdirection be treated with laser if it is unresponsive to medication?

The goal of therapy is to reestablish aqueous flow from the posterior chamber to the anterior chamber, and to try to create a channel for aqueous flow from the posterior segment to the anterior segment.

Nd:YAG laser hyaloidotomy: In pseudophakes and aphakes, using the Nd:YAG laser to disrupt the anterior vitreous face can be successful in resolving aqueous misdirection.

Argon laser treatment of ciliary processes: Regardless of the lens status, this procedure can only be done if a surgical iridectomy or a relatively large laser iridotomy is present.

38. How can aqueous misdirection be treated surgically if refractory to medical therapy and/or laser?

The timing and mode of intervention depend on the following factors:
1. Duration of misdirection without resolution

2. Presence and duration of flat anterior chamber

3. Lens status: IOL–corneal touch is more harmful to the corneal endothelium than crystalline lens–corneal touch.

4. IOP and optic nerve status.

Anterior chamber reformation: Can be performed at the slit lamp by injecting a small amount of air followed by viscoelastic through a peripheral corneal paracentesis wound. The initial air helps to confirm complete penetration of the needle through the cornea into the AC before injecting any viscoelastic.

Pars plana vitrectomy (PPV): Aqueous misdirection can occasionally persist or recur even after PPV, especially in phakic eyes.

Lens extraction: May be combined with vitrectomy. The posterior capsule and anterior hyaloid are usually incised to allow aqueous passage to the anterior chamber.

NEOVASCULAR GLAUCOMA

39. What typically causes neovascular glaucoma (NVG)?

Posterior segment (retinal) ischemia results in the production of angiogenic factors that stimulate the formation of a fibrovascular membrane on the iris (NVI). As the membrane first grows into the angle and across the scleral spur to the TM, the angle appears anatomically open. Later, the membrane contracts, pulling the peripheral iris up to the TM and peripheral cornea, creating PAS. This latter process can occur over significant areas of the angle very quickly (often in a few days) producing an acute angle closure glaucoma. Common causes of NVG are CRVO (1/3), proliferative diabetic retinopathy (1/3), and carotid occlusive disease (approximately 13%).

40. How is neovascular glaucoma treated?

1. The underlying etiology of the neovascularization must be diagnosed and treated, usually with panretinal photocoagulation (PRP) or, if the lack of clear visualization of the retina precludes PRP, peripheral retinal cryotherapy for posterior segment ischemic processes.

2. **Medical:** The percent of angle that is closed with PAS as well as the outflow resistance of the TM still open will determine the potential for successfully treating the glaucoma medically. Even if the angle is completely closed, maximal tolerated aqueous suppressant and, if necessary, hyperosmotic therapy, should be used in an attempt to temporize until surgery is performed. Miotics should not be used, because they decrease uveoscleral outflow.

3. **Surgical:** One of the most important principles to remember when operating on these eyes, especially eyes with florid NVI, is to try to avoid rapid decompression of the eye; the fragile new vessels may rupture, creating a spontaneous hyphema that can significantly complicate subsequent management.

   - The **guarded filtering procedure (trabeculectomy)** has been used to control IOP in these eyes with poor results. The success rate is somewhat better if an adjunctive antimetabolite such as mitomycin C is used. The risk of filtration failure due to fibrosis is higher, presumably owing to the presence of angiogenic factors in the aqueous.
   - **Aqueous tube shunts** have become the procedure of choice for many glaucoma surgeons, but still have success rates of only approximately 70% owing to the often poor prognosis of the underlying pathologic process.

4. **Laser/cryo cyclodestruction:** This may be a viable option in eyes with minimal visual potential, as an attempt to control IOP for long-term comfort, and to prevent the need for enucleation for pain due to high IOP.

MISCELLANEOUS

41. What are the different mechanisms of producing angle closure secondary to inflammation?

1. PAS formation from any etiology
2. Complete pupillary block (secluded pupil) from posterior synechiae resulting in iris bombe

3. Uveal effusion causing anterior rotation of the ciliary body (uncommon)
4. Exudative retinal detachment pushing lens–iris diaphragm forward (rare)

42. What is nanophthalmos?

A bilateral condition in which the globes are significantly shorter than normal, with an axial length defined as less than 20 mm (mean 18.8 mm), with a corresponding hyperopia. In addition, the corneal diameter is smaller (mean 10.5 mm vs. 12 mm for a normal adult) and the sclera is much thicker (often at least twice as thick) than normal. This impediment to uveoscleral outflow predisposes to choroidal effusions, either spontaneously or after surgery, and angle closure. Angle closure glaucoma can also occur as a result of anterior segment crowding without uveal effusions.

BIBLIOGRAPHY

1. Albert D, Jakobiec F: Principles and Practice of Ophthalmology. Philadelphia, W.B. Saunders, 1994.
2. American Academy of Ophthalmology Basic and Clinical Science Course: Section 10, Glaucoma. 1997.
3. American Academy of Ophthalmology Preferred Practice Pattern: Primary Angle Closure Glaucoma. 1996.
4. Davidorf J, Baker N, Derick R: Treatment of the fellow eye in acute angle-closure glaucoma: A case report and survey of members of the American Glaucoma Society. J Glaucoma 5:228–232, 1996.
5. Ritch R: The pilocarpine paradox [editorial]. J Glaucoma 5:225–227, 1996.
6. Ritch R, Shields B, Krupin T: The Glaucomas, 2nd ed. St. Louis, Mosby, 1996.

18. SECONDARY OPEN-ANGLE GLAUCOMA

Janice A. Gault, M.D.

1. A 72-year-old man presents for a routine exam. He states that his vision in the left eye is getting bad. On exam, he has vision of 20/30 in the right and counts fingers at 3 feet in the left. The intraocular pressure in the right eye is 25 mmHg; in the left eye, 42 mmHg. The optic nerve appears somewhat cupped on the right, severely so on the left. Visual fields reveal a significant nasal step in the right eye and a temporal island on the left. He does not have pseudoexfoliation syndrome or a Krukenberg spindle in either eye. His angles are deep. What do you suspect?

A history of trauma. The patient's prior occupation was boxing, and he was often hit in his left eye. Angle-recession glaucoma can be asymptomatic until many years later when visual loss occurs. On gonioscopy, the angle recession is determined by torn iris processes and posteriorly recessed iris, revealing a widened ciliary body band. Comparison with the other eye may help to identify this condition. Any patient with traumatic iritis or hyphema needs to be warned of this complication, which may occur many years later. Treatment is the same as with open-angle glaucoma except that miotic agents are ineffective and may even increase the intraocular pressure.

2. What should you look for to make a diagnosis of pseudoexfoliation glaucoma?

Fibrillar, "dandruff-like" material is deposited on the anterior lens capsule in a characteristic bull's eye pattern, most easily seen after pupillary dilation (figure *A*). This material is also seen clinically in the angle and on the iris. Gonioscopy reveals a heavily pigmented trabecular meshwork and a Sampolesi's line, which is pigment deposited anteriorly to Schwalbe's line (figure *B*). Pseudoexfoliation syndrome is thought to be part of generalized basement membrane disorder, because it can be found histologically in other parts of the body. It may be unilateral or bilateral with asymmetry. Although pseudoexfoliation is infrequent in the United States, it accounts for more than 50% of open-angle glaucoma in Scandinavia. The condition is often more resistant to medical therapy than primary open-angle glaucoma and may require argon laser trabeculoplasty (ALT) or surgical therapy.

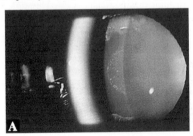 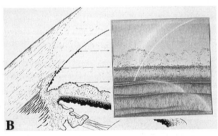

A, Patients with pseudoexfoliation may have deposits in a bull's eye pattern. Look for these deposits on the iris edge. (From Tasman W, Jaeger EA: Wills Eye Hospital Atlas of Clinical Ophthalmology. Philadelphia, Lippincott-Raven, 1995, with permission.) (See Fig. 8, Color Plates.) *B,* Sampaolesi's line is a scalloped band of pigmentation anterior to Schwalbe's line. (From Alward WLM: Color Atlas of Gonioscopy. St. Louis, Mosby, 1994, with permission.)

3. Is the condition cured after cataract extraction?

No. The deposits continue, and cataract surgery has a higher risk in such patients. The zonules are weak, and synechiae are often present between the iris and anterior lens capsule. The risk of posterior capsular rupture is increased.

4. A 24-year-old man with sarcoidosis presents with an intraocular pressure of 35 mmHg in the right eye and 32 mmHg in the left eye. He notes mild pain and some decreased vision but is otherwise asymptomatic. On examination, you notice 2+ cell and flare in both eyes as well as significant posterior synechiae and mutton-fat keratic precipitates. Gonioscopy reveals an open angle with no peripheral anterior synechiae. A dilated exam reveals no significant cupping of either optic nerve. What do you do?

Most likely, the inflammatory cells have clogged the trabecular meshwork. Intensive topical steroids and a cycloplegic should decrease the inflammatory load and break the synechiae to prevent angle closure from becoming an issue in the future. Antiglaucoma medications are also appropriate until the pressure decreases. However, miotics are contraindicated because they may cause further synechiae and precipitate angle closure. The aggressiveness with which you lower the pressure depends a great deal on optic nerve cupping.

5. The same patient returns 14 days later with pressures of 40 mmHg and 45 mmHg in the right and left eye, respectively. Exam reveals minimal cell and flare in each eye as well as a significant decrease in the keratic precipitates. He has been using prednisolone acetate 1% every hour and atropine 1% 3 times/day. What should you do?

Gonioscopy. Provided the angle is open and without neovascularization, the most likely cause is response to steroids. The increased intraocular pressure may occur anywhere from a few days to years after initiating therapy. The response has been noted in or around the eye after oral and intravenous administration of steroids and even with inhalers. Patients with Cushing's syndrome with excessive levels of endogenous steroids are also at risk. Optic nerve evaluation is crucial to determine the risks of damage. Decrease the steroid concentration or dosage, and start antiglaucoma therapy. A topical nonsteroidal agent is appropriate in certain situations, such as uncomplicated cataract surgery. Fluorometholone is also less likely to increase intraocular pressure than other formulations of steroids; however, it has less potency in decreasing inflammation.

6. What does a Krukenberg spindle look like? What does it mean?

A Krukenberg spindle is a vertical pigment band on the corneal endothelium. It is typically found in patients with pigmentary dispersion syndrome. The iris is often bowed posteriorly and rubs against the lens zonules. This process causes midperipheral spokelike iris transillumination defects. Gonioscopy reveals a densely pigmented trabecular meshwork for 360°. The patient is often asymptomatic but may notice blurred vision, eye pain, and halos around lights after exercise or pupillary dilation. Pigmentary dispersion syndrome is more common in young adults and white, myopic males. It is usually bilateral.

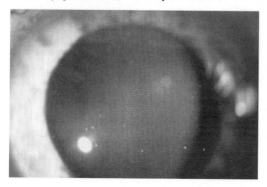

A Krukenberg spindle is made of pigment deposited on the endothelium in pigmentary dispersion syndrome (From Alward WLM: Color Atlas of Gonioscopy. St. Louis, Mosby, 1994, with permission.) (See Fig. 9, Color Plates.)

7. How is pigmentary dispersion treated?

If no optic disc damage is noted and the visual fields are normal, the patient may be observed. Treatment for intraocular pressure over 28 mmHg is usually indicated, although this point is controversial. Once damage is noted, miotics may be the first line of therapy because they minimize contact between the zonules and iris. However, miotics also cause myopic fluctuation and may not be practical in young patients. Laser peripheral iridectomies (PI) have been recommended; they treat the posterior bowing of the iris and may theoretically cure the disorder. Patients also respond well to argon laser trabeculoplasty because of the increased pigment of the trabecular meshwork.

8. A 95-year-old woman presents with a markedly red, painful right eye of two days' duration. Her vision is hand motions at one foot and 20/400 in the right and left eye, respectively. Exam of the right eye reveals a steamy cornea with a pressure of 60 mmHg and no view of the anterior chamber. The left eye has a brunescent cataract but appears to be deep and quiet with a pressure of 18 mmHg. With topical glycerin, the cornea clears in the right eye to reveal iridescent particles floating in the anterior chamber with a Morgagnian cataract. Gonioscopy reveals bilateral open angles. No view is obtained of either posterior chamber. What do you do now?

The patient denies a history of uveitis. A B-scan of both eyes reveals only significant cataract without retinal detachment or intraocular tumor. The leakage of lens material through an intact lens capsule is obstructing the trabecular meshwork. If the diagnosis is in question, paracentesis may be done to examine the anterior chamber reaction microscopically. Macrophages are filled with cortical material (phacolytic glaucoma). Typically, the lens is hypermature, as in this patient. The intraocular pressure must be reduced and the inflammation controlled before surgical therapy is attempted. A steroid such as prednisolone acetate 1% every hour, a cycloplegic such as scopolamine 0.25%, 3 times/day, and antiglaucoma medications are started immediately. Cataract extraction is performed in the next day or two once the eye is in better condition.

9. A 64-year-old woman who had cataract surgery in the left eye 1 week ago presents to the emergency department complaining that the eye is red and painful with decreasing vision. What is your concern?

First, you must think of endophthalmitis. Any patient presenting after surgery with a red, painful eye with decreased vision must be presumed to have endophthalmitis until it is ruled out. The exam reveals vision of hand motions at two feet, a severely injected eye with corneal edema, 4+ cell and flare, and an intraocular pressure of 47 mmHg. The anterior chamber is filled with lens cortical material, and a rupture in the posterior capsule is seen. A large chunk of nuclear material is in the vitreous. The optic nerve is mildly cupped.

Because the lens material is seen in the anterior chamber, treatment with steroids and antiglaucoma medications is appropriate, along with close observation. The diagnosis is most likely lens-particle glaucoma. The patient is started on prednisolone acetate 1% every 2 hours, scopolamine 0.25%, 3 times/day, latanoprost once daily, a beta blocker twice daily, apraclonidine twice daily, and acetazolamide sequels twice daily. In addition, because her pressure is so high, mannitol is given. When the pressure improves to 25 mmHg, she is sent home. The next day, she counts fingers at five feet, her intraocular inflammation is subsiding, and the pressure is 23 mmHg. Once her eye is less inflamed and the pressure well controlled, she is scheduled for removal of the remaining lens material. If the retained lens material is minimal, patients sometimes can be maintained on medical therapy until the eye clears without surgery.

10. What other type of open-angle glaucoma can be caused by the lens?

Phacoanaphylactic glaucoma, which occurs after penetrating trauma or surgery. The patient is sensitized to the lens protein during a latent period and develops a granulomatous uveitis. This feature distinguishes it from lens particle glaucoma. Patients are treated medically and may need surgery to remove the lens if they do not respond adequately.

11. What is Posner-Schlossman syndrome? Who gets it?

Patients are young to middle-aged. They notice unilateral attacks of mild pain, decreased vision, and halos around lights. Episodes tend to recur. Also known as glaucomatocyclitic crisis, this disorder is idiopathic. On exam, intraocular pressure is high, usually between 40–60 mmHg. The angle is open on gonioscopy without synechiae, and the eye is minimally injected. Anterior chamber reaction is minimal. The corneal epithelium may be edematous because of the acute rise in pressure. A few fine keratic precipitates may be present on the corneal endothelium, often inferiorly. Treatment includes steroids and antiglaucoma medications to reduce aqueous production. A cycloplegic agent is necessary only if the patient is symptomatic. The attacks usually resolve in a few hours to a few weeks. No therapy is needed between attacks. However, the risk of chronic open-angle glaucoma is increased in both eyes.

12. What is the classic triad of Fuchs' heterochromic iridocyclitis?

Heterochromia, cataract, and low-grade iritis. The iritis is mild and does not cause synechiae. Characteristic stellate, colorless keratic precipitates are seen over the inferior endothelium. Fine new vessels may be seen in the angle but do not cause closure. The glaucoma is difficult to control and often does not correspond to the degree of inflammation. Steroids are not often helpful.

13. A patient reports for postoperative check-up 1 day after cataract surgery. The pressure in the operated eye is 40 mmHg, and the patient complains of nausea. What is the most likely cause?

Retained viscoelastic from surgery, which usually begins 6 or 7 hours after surgery and normalizes within 24–48 hours, depending on the type of viscoelastic. Most eyes tolerate short-term pressures up to 30 mmHg; of course, tolerance depends on preexisting optic nerve status. Medical treatment and paracentesis to remove the viscoelastic are indicated to decrease pressure quickly and relieve nausea. Paracentesis is somewhat controversial because of the increased risk of endophthalmitis.

14. What else can cause postoperative glaucoma?

Hyphema, pigment dispersion, generalized inflammation, aphakic or pseudophakic pupillary block, malignant glaucoma (aqueous misdirection syndrome), and steroid-response glaucoma. In patients who have undergone an intracapsular cataract extraction, alpha-chymotrypsin is injected into the anterior chamber to dissolve the zonules. The zonular debris may block the trabecular meshwork postoperatively. Epithelial ingrowth may occur many months to years after surgery or trauma and block outflow.

15. A patient had cataract surgery 1 year ago but continues to have episodes of anterior chamber cell and flare with increased intraocular pressure. Some of the cells are red blood cells. What is the diagnosis?

Uveitis-glaucoma-hyphema (UGH) syndrome. The cells may actually layer out to produce a hyphema, usually as a result of irritation from an anterior chamber intraocular lens, although a posterior chamber lens may be involved. Gonioscopy may reveal where the irritation is occurring. Treatment consists of atropine, topical steroids, and antiglaucoma medications until the pressure is reduced. Argon laser of the bleeding site, if it can be identified, may be curative. However, removal of the intraocular lens may be necessary.

16. How can raised episcleral venous pressure cause glaucoma?

Aqueous drains from the anterior chamber through the trabecular meshwork, Schlemm's canal, and intrascleral channels to the episcleral and conjunctival veins. Normal drainage depends on an episcleral venous pressure that is lower than the pressure of the eye. Usually, it ranges from 8–12 mmHg. However, if it is higher than intraocular pressure, drainage does not occur. Drugs that reduce aqueous humor formation are obviously the most effective medical treatment.

17. What are causes of raised episcleral venous pressure?

Thyroid ophthalmolopathy, carotid and dural fistulas, superior vena cava syndrome, retrobulbar tumors, orbital varices, and Sturge-Weber syndrome.

18. A patient with long-standing diabetes has had recurrent vitreous hemorrhage. While you are observing him waiting for the condition to clear, intraocular pressure increases to 35 mmHg. What should you suspect?

When intraocular hemorrhages clear, hemolytic or ghost cell glaucoma may develop. Hemolytic glaucoma occurs because macrophages full of hemoglobin block the trabecular meshwork. Reddish cells can be seen in the anterior chamber. In ghost cell glaucoma, degenerating red blood cells block the aqueous outflow. Khaki cells in the anterior chamber may layer out to form a pseudohypopyon. Both conditions can be treated medically until the hemorrhage clears. However, because the intraocular pressure may become markedly raised, washout of the anterior chamber and/or vitrectomy often becomes necessary. In addition, the patient may be developing neovascular glaucoma; thus it is important to check the angles for new vessels and angle narrowing.

19. What other conditions may cause open-angle glaucoma?

1. Intraocular tumor may cause secondary open-angle glaucoma by invasion of the chamber angle or blockage of the trabecular meshwork by tumor debris.

2. Siderosis or chalcosis from a retained metallic foreign body.

3. Chemical injuries from acid or alkali can shrink the scleral collagen or cause direct damage to the trabecular meshwork.

4. Iridocorneal endothelial syndrome (ICE) is a spectrum of three entities that overlap considerably:

    (1) Essential iris atrophy—iris thinning leads to iris holes and pupillary distortion

    (2) Chandler's syndrome—mild iris thinning and distortion with hammered metal appearance of corneal endothelium

    (3) Cogan-Reese syndrome—pigmented nodules on the iris surface with variable iris atrophy

Such patients are generally asymptomatic, middle-aged adults. Usually findings are unilateral with increased intraocular pressure and corneal edema. No treatment is necessary unless corneal edema and glaucoma are present.

5. Posterior polymorphous dystrophy is a bilateral and autosomal dominant disease. Vesicles are seen at Descemet's membrane. Corneal edema occurs in severe cases. Iridocorneal adhesions may occur. Glaucoma is associated in 15%.

20. What types of secondary open-angle glaucoma occur in children?

1. Glaucoma associated with mesenchymal dysgenesis is a spectrum of disease, but two main categories are recognized:

    (1) Axenfeld's anomaly consists of a prominent Schwalbe's ring with attached iris strands. Axenfeld's syndrome is the anomaly with coincident glaucoma and occurs in 50% of cases. It is autosomal dominant or sporadic.

    (2) Rieger's anomaly is Axenfeld's anomaly plus iris thinning and distorted pupils. Sixty percent of patients develop glaucoma; it is also autosomal dominant or sporadic. Rieger's syndrome is the anomaly associated with dental, craniofacial, and skeletal abnormalities.

2. Aniridia is a bilateral, near-total absence of the iris. The strands may be seen only by gonioscopy. Glaucoma, foveal hypoplasia, and nystagmus may occur. The disorder may be autosomal dominant or sporadic. Patients with sporadic inheritance need to be evaluated for Wilms' tumor, which is associated in 25% of cases.

3. Oculocerebrorenal syndrome (Lowe) is an X-linked recessive disease. Patients have aminoaciduria, hypotonia, acidemia, cataracts, and glaucoma.

4. Congenital rubella may be associated with cataracts and pigmented retinal lesions. Cardiac, auditory, and central nervous abnormalities are often coexistent.

5. Sturge-Weber syndrome

6. Neurofibromatosis

7. Glaucoma after cataract removal is a long-term risk for such patients

BIBLIOGRAPHY

1. American Academy of Ophthalmology Basic and Clinical Science Course, Section 10. San Francisco, American Academy of Ophthalmology, 1992.
2. Cullom RD, Chang B: The Wills Eye Manual: Office and Emergency Room Diagnosis and Treatment of Eye Disease, 3rd ed. Philadelphia, J.B. Lippincott, 1994.
3. Danyluk AW, Paton D: Diagnosis and management of glaucoma. Clin Symp 43:2–32, 1991.
4. Shields MB: Textbook of Glaucoma, 4th ed. Baltimore, Williams & Wilkins, 1998.

. THE MEDICAL TREATMENT OF GLAUCOMA

Richard P. Wilson, M.D.

1. What classes of medications are used to treat glaucoma?

Commonly Used Agents for Glaucoma Management

CHEMICAL NAME	STRENGTH	USUAL DOSAGE	SIZE
Miotics			
(Mechanism of action—constrict longitudinal muscle of ciliary body and open spaces in trabecular meshwork, thereby mechanically increasing aqueous outflow)			
Pilocarpine hydrochloride	0.25, 0.5, 1, 2, 4, 6, 8, 10%	2–4 times/day	15, 30 ml
Ocusert-Pilo	20, 40%	Weekly	Box of 8
Pilopine-HS gel	4% gel	At bedtime	4-gm tube
Pilocarpine nitrate	1, 2, 4%	2–4 times/day	15 ml
Carbachol	0.75, 1.5, 2.25, 3%	2–3 times/day	15, 30 ml
Echothiophate iodide	0.03, 0.06, 0.125, 0.25%	1–2 times/day	5 ml
Adrenergics			
(Mechanism of action—epinephrine and dipivefrin increase aqueous outflow; apraclonidine and brimonidine decrease aqueous inflow)			
Dipivefrin hydrochloride	0.1%	1–2 times/day	5, 10, 15 ml
Epinephrine hydrochloride	0.5, 1, 2%	1–2 times/day	5, 10, 15 ml
Apraclonidine hydrochloride	0.5%	2–3 times/day	5 ml
Brimonidine tartrate	0.2%	2 times/day	5 ml
Prostaglandins			
(Mechanism of action—increase uveoscleral outflow)			
Latanoprost	0.005%	Daily	5 ml
Beta blockers			
(Mechanism of action—decrease aqueous inflow)			
Betaxolol hydrochloride suspension	0.25%	2 times/daily	2.5, 5, 15, ml
Carteolol hydrochloride	1.0%	1–2 times/day	5, 10 ml
Levobunolol hydrochloride	0.25, 0.5%	1–2 times/day	2, 5, 10 ml
Metapranolol	0.3%	1–2 times/day	5, 10 ml
Timolol maleate	0.25, 0.5%	1–2 times/day	2.5, 5, 10, 15 ml
Timolol XE gel-forming solution	0.25, 0.5%	Daily	2.5, 5 ml
Carbonic anhydrase inhibitors			
(Mechanism of action—decrease aqueous inflow)			
Acetazolamide sodium	125, 250 mg	3–4 times/day	NA
Acetazolamide sequels	500 mg	2 times/day	NA
Dichlorphenamide	50 mg	2–4 times/day	NA
Methazolamide	50 mg	2–4 times/day	NA
Dorzolamide	2%	2–3 times/day	5, 10 ml
Hyperosmotic agents			
(Mechanism of action—increase osmolality of blood to draw aqueous from posterior chamber)			
Glycerin	50%	1–1.5 gm/kg (orally)	NA
Isosorbide	45%	1.5 gm/kg (orally)	NA
Mannitol	5–20%	0.5–2 gm/kg (IV)	NA

2. How do these medications work?

Miotics constrict the longitudinal muscle of the ciliary body, which is attached to the scleral spur anteriorly and to the choroid posteriorly. When the longitudinal muscle constricts, it pulls the scleral spur posteriorly, pulling open the spaces between the trabecular beams and mechanically increasing the capacity for aqueous outflow.

Adrenergic agonists: Epinephrine and dipivefrin initially decrease aqueous production slightly, but their major action is to increase outflow through the trabecular meshwork. Iopidine and brimonidine decrease aqueous production.

Beta blockers and **carbonic anhydrase inhibitors** decrease aqueous production.

Prostaglandins increase outflow through the uveoscleral outflow channels. Aqueous is absorbed from the anterior chamber into the face of the ciliary body or into the trabecular meshwork and then flows posteriorly around the longitudinal muscle fibers of the ciliary body posteriorly. It is absorbed into the choroid or passes out through the sclera.

Hyperosmotic agents increase the osmolality of the blood, which in turns draws fluid from the posterior chamber into the blood vessels of the ciliary body.

3. For patients in good health with primary open-angle glaucoma, what is the first drug to try?

Most ophthalmologists start with a beta blocker. The cardioselective beta blocker, betaxolol, has far fewer systemic side effects than the nonselective beta blockers. In patients in whom adequate control can be obtained with a 20% drop in intraocular pressure, betaxolol is often effective. If a greater effect is required and the patient is healthy, one of the nonselective beta blockers may be chosen. For the most part, they can be used in the ¼% dosage once daily for patients with light irides and the ½% dosage once daily for patients with dark irides. Beta blockers block intrinsic beta$_1$ and beta$_2$ receptor tone; thus, when patients are asleep, beta blockers are ineffective because there is little tone. However, because aqueous production also declines at night, this fact is usually considered inconsequential. Thus, many ophthalmologists prescribe beta blockers once daily when patients awake in the morning. Brubaker's study, however, suggested that a nighttime dose may be the most effective. For patients with more advanced disease, a twice-daily regimen of ¼% for lighter irides and ½% for darker irides is common. This regimen guards against going for a day without medication in patients who miss one prescribed drop.

4. How does one choose among the five nonselective beta blockers?

In terms of effectiveness, there is little difference. However, each medication offers a slight advantage compared with the others. Carteolol raises triglycerides and lowers high-density lipoproteins the least. Thus, in patients with hyperlipidemias or atherosclerotic cardiovascular disease, it is the best choice. Levobunolol lasts the longest of the compounds that have been tested as once-daily drugs. Metapranolol is the least expensive and in once-daily dosage can fit many budgets when other beta blockers may not. Timolol was the first beta blocker and still enjoys the largest market share. It has more recently been formulated as a drop that becomes viscous on contact with the eye. This new formation, named Timoptic XE, remains in the tear film longer; consequently, intraocular absorption is greater. This drug provides the best diurnal curve for pressure control with once-daily dosing.

5. Under what conditions should a drug other than a beta blocker be used as the first treatment?

In patients who are in poor health, especially if they have a pulmonary or cardiac condition or suffer from serious depression, dorzolamide is the first choice if a beta blocker cannot be used.

6. Since both dorzolamide and pilocarpine, like beta blockers, decrease aqueous production, which should be added to the treatment regimen in patients in whom beta blockers have a significant but inadequate effect?

Both pilocarpine, the most commonly used miotic, and dorzolamide, a carbonic anhydrase inhibitor, have similar additive effects when combined with a beta blocker. Because dorzolamide avoids the miosis and blurred vision associated with pilocarpine and because it can be used 2–3 times/day instead of 3–4 times/day like pilocarpine, dorzolamide has replaced pilocarpine as the second-line drug.

7. Can pilocarpine be added to the combination of a beta blocker and dorzolamide if additional control is needed?

Yes. In patients who are old enough to have little remaining accommodation but still retain clear lenses (late 50s and 60s), pilocarpine is often excellently tolerated. It provides a pinhole effect that gives an increased depth of field for most patients. Many patients can read without reading glasses when taking pilocarpine, and no one needs trifocals if the pupils are adequately miotic.

8. If the patient is uncontrolled on beta blockers, dorzolamide, and miotics, are adrenergic agonists then used?

Adrenergic agonists may be broken down into two groups. Epinephrine and dipivefrin, which is converted into epinephrine by the eye, make up the first group; they increase trabecular meshwork outflow. Iopidine and brimonidine make up the second; they are alpha$_2$ agonists that reduce aqueous production rather than increase trabecular meshwork outflow.

The epinephrine compounds are characterized by a high allergic reaction rate. Epinephrine is said to have a 50% allergic rate by 5 years, and iodipine has an approximately 20% allergic rate by 1 year. The main complaint about epinephrine and dipivefrin is that they add only 1–2 mmHg effect in combination with a nonselective beta blocker. If combined with a selective beta blocker, the added effect is greater, but the effectiveness of the selective blocker is less than that of the nonselective beta blocker to begin with. Therefore, betaxolol plus dipivefrin gives the same effect as any of the nonselective beta blockers plus dipivefrin. In addition, Lavin has pointed out that topical epinephrine is a strong risk factor for filter failure in patients who have taken it for a long time. For these reasons, epinephrine compounds are no longer commonly used.

However, one or two circumstances may be well treated by dipivefrin or epinephrine. The first is glaucoma in a pregnant woman. Because the fetal effects of most glaucoma drops have not been adequately tested, the use of an endogenous compound like epinephrine is reassuring. The same comfort level with the systemic side effects of dipivefrin leads many glaucoma specialists to use it in patients who have elevated intraocular pressure and enough risk factors to suggest that an elevated intraocular pressure will cause damage with time. This approach seems prudent compared with use of a strong medication with marked side effects in a patient who does not have definite disease.

Iopidine and brimonidine are relegated to the last-resort category of topical antiglaucoma medications. Although both are quite powerful, the increased allergic rate and a tachyphylaxis rate reported to be 30–65% at 1 year restrict iodipine to short-term use for the most part. Tachyphylaxis and allergy are less with brimonidine.

9. What prevents most practitioners from using oral carbonic anhydrase inhibitors until just before surgery—if at all?

Acetazolamide and methazolamide cause myriad side effects. The most common complaints are lack of energy and lethargy, lack of appetite and weight loss, nausea and/or an upset stomach, and a metallic taste to foods. The most dangerous side effect is hypokalemia, especially when a carbonic anhydrase inhibitor is combined with a potassium-losing diuretic. This combination is dangerous in patients taking digitalis. Depression and anemia, which in rare cases is aplastic and deadly, are other serious side effects. Because complaints are frequent with oral carbonic anhydrase inhibitors, most ophthalmic surgeons offer them as an alternative to surgical intervention.

10. Latanaprost is a new medication that recently received regulatory approval. Where does it fit in the above therapeutic outline?

Latanaprost is an extremely powerful medication. In a 0.005% concentration it is 100 times more powerful than timolol or levobunolol. Because it works by an altogether different mechanism from any of the other glaucoma drugs, it is additive to all of them, even the miotics. Because miotics tighten the ciliary body, reducing the space between the muscle bundles through which the uveoscleral outflow travels, it seems that miotics would cancel the effects of latanaprost. However, at this point it seems that pilocarpine plus latanaprost is more effective than either drug alone. Although it is marketed as an adjunctive medication to beta blockers, its slightly greater strength than the nonselective beta blockers, combined with negligible systemic side effects and once-daily dosing, may quickly move it to the drug of choice in almost all glaucomas. The two most common side effects of latanaprost are conjunctival injection and increased pigmentation of the iris. Increased pigmentation seems to occur only in patients with light irides and darker nevi.

11. What are the general rules for prescribing eye drops?

1. Allow at least 10 minutes between applying any two topical eye medications.

2. A medication used 4 times/day, such as pilocarpine, is usually taken every 4 hours. This schedule compresses the drops into two 12-hour periods. Because pilocarpine has a maximal effect for only 6 hours, the last 6 hours of the second 12-hour period are untreated.

3. Topical medications that have serious systemic side effects if absorbed should be taken with punctal occlusion. The patient puts a clean finger over the nose where the two lids come together and pushes down on the bone. The drop is then instilled in the eye and the lids are gently closed; this position is held for 3 minutes. This procedure dramatically reduces the amount of drug entering the system. Because a drug coming into contact with the nasal mucosa is absorbed rapidly and almost completely, it attains serum levels quite similar to those achieved by intravenous administration. Absorption through the nasal mucosa avoids a first pass by hepatic enzymes, which gives the liver a chance to metabolize or detoxify the medication.

4. The most important rule to remember (except for pilocarpine, which seems to have a much more consistent effect) is that topical medications should be prescribed with a one-eye therapeutic trial. For example, only 90% of the population responds to a topical, nonselective beta blocker. Of the 90% that responds, only 90% would also respond to a selective beta blocker. Therefore, a selective beta blocker will work in only 81% of the population and a nonselective beta blocker in 90% of the population. If one adds a topical beta blocker to both eyes and sees the patient in 2 weeks to check the results, a lower intraocular pressure may signal an effective response to the beta blocker or a decrease secondary to the patient's diurnal curve. If the beta blocker is prescribed in only one eye, the therapeutic effect will be clear. There is, however, an approximately 2-mmHg contralateral effect in the untreated eye with most nonselective beta blockers. This contralateral effect needs to be factored into determining the results of the therapeutic trial. A therapeutic trial is essential; continuation of a dangerous and expensive medication is unjustified unless one is sure that it effectively lowers intraocular pressure.

12. What are the dos and don'ts of initiating therapy with pilocarpine?

Because pilocarpine produces a strong contraction of the longitudinal and circular muscle of the ciliary body, it may cause miotic spasm as well as fatigue ache around the eye, extending into the brow. The effect of pilocarpine on the circular muscle of the ciliary body is to constrict the anular ring of muscle, relaxing the zonules and allowing the lens to become more round and globular—in effect, more powerful. This effect increases myopia if patients are young enough to have much accommodation. A severe brow ache and blurred vision may completely turn off a patient who otherwise would be helped by pilocarpine. Therefore, it is essential to start the patient at a low enough dose that the ache and change in vision are tolerable. This is usually ½% for light irides and 1% for dark irides. This percentage is increased as tolerated to a maximum of 2% for gray irides, 4% for light brown irides, and 6% for dark brown irides.

In younger patients with a healthy amount of accommodation, pilocarpine Ocuserts are handy. Ocuserts are permeable wafers that allow slow but steady leakage of pilocarpine solution across the membrane into the tear film. Compared with a large bolus of medication, as with drop therapy, the small but constant amount of medication is more comfortable and does not blur vision nearly as much. The myopic shift in vision is fairly constant and often may be corrected with a change in glasses.

For older patients, an alternative to therapy 4 times/day is the Pilopine HS ophthalmic gel, which is placed in the inferior cul-de-sac at bedtime and remains in the tear film in contact with the cornea overnight. A large amount of pilocarpine is absorbed into the eye. During the day, the retained pilocarpine is gradually washed out but provides a 4% pilocarpine effect until early evening. A substantial effect is still apparent at bedtime. This form of pilocarpine is especially useful in patients for whom noncompliance is a problem. Often a more responsible person in the household can administer a drop of nonselective beta blocker, followed 10 minutes later by pilopine gel at bedtime, and obtain substantial 24-hour intraocular pressure control. However, because a massive amount of pilocarpine is absorbed into the eye overnight, the tone of the ciliary body must be increased with lower percentage drops before the pilopine gel can be tried.

13. Pilocarpine is often used in the treatment of angle closure glaucoma. What is its effect on the anterior chamber?

As mentioned above, pilocarpine contracts the longitudinal muscle of the ciliary body, pulling on the scleral spur and mechanically opening the interstices in the trabecular meshwork. However, it also pulls the lens-iris diaphragm forward, shallowing the anterior chamber. The contraction of the circular muscle of the ciliary body relaxes the stress on the zonules, allowing the lens to become more round, to float forward on a longer tether, and to act more like a natural cork in the pupil. This effect increases pupillary block and blows the peripheral iris closer to the trabecular meshwork. All of these effects tend to shallow the anterior chamber and narrow the anterior chamber angle. Luckily, these effects are balanced by the miosis caused by the contraction of the sphincter muscle of the iris. Miosis pulls the peripheral iris away from the trabecular meshwork. Therefore, in most patients, although the anterior chamber depth is decreased by pilocarpine, the peripheral angle is slightly widened. In some patients, however, angle crowding is more of a problem than pupillary block. In such patients, pilocarpine may cause angle closure. Therefore, one should gonioscope all patients with a narrow angle for whom a miotic is prescribed.

14. If a patient does not show an expected response to a topical glaucoma medication, what should the ophthalmologist consider?

1. Ineffective medication. Make sure that any medication except pilocarpine is used in a one-eye therapeutic trial.

2. Noncompliance. The most common cause for an ineffective medication is failure to take it. Kass performed a study in which a microchip placed in the bottom of pilocarpine bottles recorded when the bottle was tipped upside down. The chip was camouflaged, and patients did not know that Kass was able to monitor when they took the drops. He found that 76% of the prescribed doses were taken and that 6% of patients took less than 25% of the drops, whereas 15% took only 50%. However, 97% of his patients reported that they were taking all of their medication. Kass found that compliance was best on the day before the office visit. This effect has been popularized by Heuer as the dental floss syndrome, because most people floss their teeth on the morning that they visit the dentist. This syndrome explains why many patients have completely controlled intraocular pressures in the ophthalmologist's office but have a worsening disc appearance and declining fields. Kass also found that 30% of his patients compressed their 4/times/day schedule to every 4 hours. It is essential, therefore, to tell patients on a 4 times/day schedule to take pilocarpine on awakening and then at lunch, dinner, and bedtime. This approach not only yields an optimal spread but also provides a daily event to remind patients that another drop is due. Many of Kass's patients allowed no interval between drops. At least a 10-minute interval optimizes the effect of multiple topical medications.

15. The *Physicians' Desk Reference* relates that pilocarpine should be used 4 times/day, whereas iopidine and dorzolamide should be used 3 times/day. Because using a medicine 3 times/day requires one to take a drop in the mid-afternoon when few activities act as a reminder, can these recommendations be stretched?

If patients put a drop in their eye, cover their punctum, and close their eye gently for 3 minutes, the contact time of the drug with the cornea is increased markedly. With this technique all three medications can be used twice daily. Even without this technique, iopidine can be used twice a day with no noticeable drop-off compared with 3 times/day. Dorzolamide is slightly less effective at twice daily dosing. However, often twice-daily usage gives an adequate response.

16. If a patient needs oral carbonic anhydrase inhibitors, how do you start? What is the maximal dose?

Methazolamide has a 12-hour duration of action and fewer side effects than acetazolamide pills. Therefore, it is prudent to start with methazolamide, 25 mg 2–3 times/day after meals in elderly patients and 50 mg 2–3 times/day after meals in younger patients. If the maximal dose is needed, acetazolamide, 500-mg sequels 2 times/day after meal, gives the greatest effect with the least number of side effects. If acetazolamide is prescribed, one should write to the patient's medical doctor explaining its side effects. If the patient is on a potassium-losing medication, the ophthalmologist should make it clear that it is the personal physician's responsibility to monitor the electrolyte balance. If the physician cannot do so, he or she should notify the treating ophthalmologist.

17. Many patients taking topical medications complain of dry or irritated eyes. What should the treating ophthalmologist include as a routine part of the examination of all patients taking topical medication?

The treating ophthalmologist should flip the lower lid and observe the conjunctiva. If only papillae are present, the patient does not have a chronic allergy. If, however, there are 3–4 plus follicles, the patient is more likely allergic to the topical drops.

18. In a patient with an ocular allergy secondary to topical medication, what is the most likely offender?

Among the medications now in use, apraclonidine has the highest incidence of allergic reaction, followed (in order) by epinephrine, dipivefrin, and beta blockers and pilocarpine.

19. In a patient who takes apraclonidine, timolol, and pilocarpine to control intraocular pressure but shows a topical allergic reaction, how should the medication be changed?

1. Stop the apraclonidine.
2. Change the beta blocker to carteolol, which seems to be the best tolerated of all beta blockers.
3. Change the pilocarpine to carbachol.

Pilocarpine 4–10% should be changed to carbachol 1.5% 3 times/day, whereas pilocarpine 1–2% should be changed to carbachol ¾% or ⅜% 3 times/day.

In patients who take their medications bilaterally, change the beta blocker in one eye and the pilocarpine in the other. On the patient's return, one should be able to tell whether the offending medication was apraclonidine or one of the other two medications. It is important to avoid a chronic allergic conjunctival reaction, which may reduce the success of filtering surgery later or lead to dry eyes or worse.

BIBLIOGRAPHY

1. Retty ES, Larsson LT, Brubaker RF: The effect of topical timolol on epinephrine stimulated aqueous humor flow in sleeping humans. Invest Ophthalmol Vis Sci 35:554–559, 1994.
2. Lavin MJ, Wormald RPL, Migdal CS, Hitchings RA: The influence of prior therapy on the success of trabeculectomy. Arch Ophthalmol 108:1543–1548, 1990.
3. Kass MA, Meltzer DW, Gordon M, et al: Compliance with topical pilocarpine treatment. Am J Ophthalmol 101:515–523, 1986.

20. TRABECULECTOMY SURGERY

Marlene R. Moster, M.D.

1. What are the indications for trabeculectomy surgery?

Traditionally, after both topical medication and argon laser trabeculoplasty have failed to control intraocular pressure, the next step is to perform a trabeculectomy or guarded filtration procedure. Indications include anticipated or documented optic nerve damage and visual field loss despite maximal tolerated medical therapy. If the surgeon believes that the deterioration is progressing at such a rate that it can diminish the patient's visual potential or quality of life, surgical intervention is suggested. Indications for surgery usually include change in the appearance of the optic disc or visual field and an intraocular pressure that is too high for the long-term health of the optic nerve.

2. What is the goal of glaucoma surgery?

The goal of glaucoma surgery is to lower intraocular pressure sufficiently to stabilize the optic nerve and visual field. The postoperative pressure goal should be 30% lower than the average intraocular pressure before trabeculectomy surgery. This goal has been associated with stabilization and even improvement of optic nerve cupping by photographic analysis, and one-third of patients show improvement in computerized visual fields. Because one-third to one-half of patients with glaucoma do not initially appear to have elevated intraocular pressure, the goal of glaucoma surgery is not to reduce pressure to less than 21 mmHg but to reduce intraocular pressure by a percentage. We must set a target pressure to maximize the likelihood of arresting the glaucomatous process.

3. How do we inform patients about the risks of trabeculectomy surgery?

The risks and benefits of glaucoma surgery must be carefully outlined to all patients in language that is easily understood. It is imperative to explain clearly the remote possibility of blindness or loss of the eye due to hemorrhage or infection. In addition, the possibility of sudden or permanent visual loss, late infection, serious bleeding, failure to control intraocular pressure (which may be too high or too low), need for second surgery, droopy lid, and significant blurring for at least 2 weeks should be elaborated. Later risks include endophthalmitis, progression of glaucoma, or worsening of cataract.

4. What factors are related to success of glaucoma filtering surgery?

Favorable factors include a normal quiet eye, operative success in the other eye, Caucasian race, early-to-moderate stage of disease, and no history of steroid response or prior ocular surgery.

5. What factors are related to failure of glaucoma filtering surgery?

Unfavorable factors include previous surgical failure; pigmented skin (non-Caucasian); a history of keloid formation; neovascular changes; youth; intraocular inflammation; shallow anterior chamber; extreme hyperopia; dislocated lens with vitreous; thick, thin, or otherwise abnormal sclera; inability to use corticosteroids; scarred or abnormal conjunctiva; and an inexperienced surgeon.

6. Does a fornix vs. a limbal conjunctival approach affect outcome?

Fornix-based and limbal-based approaches produce similar results after trabeculectomy surgery. We prefer a limbal-based approach when using antimetabolites because the risk of a wound leak is much smaller. However, as long as a fornix-based flap is closed tightly at the limbus, excellent filtration can result. Often in the presence of scarred conjunctiva, a fornix-based flap is favored because the chance of creating a conjunctival buttonhole is reduced. If a limbal-based flap is chosen, it should be made sufficiently posterior so that the closure is at least 10 mm or more from the limbus. This technique decreases the likelihood of leakage and scarring because the conjunctival wound can heal far from the scleral flap.

7. What medications should be stopped before filtration surgery?

We generally ask that patients stop aspirin 2 or more weeks before surgery. If possible, patients should discontinue Coumadin 1–4 days before surgery by arrangement with the internist. Oral carbonic anhydrase inhibitors, pilocarpine, carbachol, and echothiophate are stopped the night before surgery.

8. What are the choices of anesthesia?

We recommend a facial nerve block of 7 ml of mepivacaine with a short, 25-gauge needle, using a Nadbath technique. The facial nerve block is followed by a peribulbar block on a 25-gauge, tapered 1½-inch needle with a 50–50 mixture of mepivacaine and bupivacaine with hyaluronidase. Another alternative to the traditional method is a standard facial nerve block followed by a temporal sub-Tenon's injection of 1.0 cc mixture of bupivacaine/mepivacaine and wydase with a short, 30-gauge needle. The conjunctiva and Tenon's capsule are ballooned for 360°, and the trabeculectomy can be performed without difficulty. With the subconjunctival/sub-Tenon's approach, a superior rectus suture cannot be placed because of patient sensation. Instead, an 8-0 vicryl suture is passed through clear cornea at the superior limbus and used as a traction suture.

9. Does a triangular vs. a rectangular flap affect outcome?

The shape of the scleral flap is surgeon-dependent; there is no difference in clinical outcome with a triangular or rectangular flap. Although the shape of the flap is not important, its thickness is. A ⅓–½-thickness flap has been shown to afford better long-term filtration. Regardless of the shape of the scleral flap, sufficient sutures are necessary to prevent overfiltration.

10. Does the size of the internal block affect outcome?

In removing the trabeculectomy specimen, it is usually recommended that the size should be ½–⅔ of the scleral flap. Assuming the average-sized flap is approximately 4 × 2 mm, a 2–3 × 1 mm block is usually sufficient. More filtration results when one edge of the internal block coincides with one edge of the scleral flap. The more aggressive the surgery, the closer the internal block comes to one edge of the flap. The flap can be closed tightly and released by laser suture lysis in the postoperative period. The internal block can be removed with Vanass scissors and 0.12 forceps or a Gass punch if the surgeon prefers.

11. Are iridectomy and paracentesis always necessary during filtration surgery?

Yes. An iridectomy is always performed to ensure that pupillary block does not occur. In addition, if the chamber shallows, the iris is less likely to occlude the ostium. Iridectomies should be basal and large enough so that the iris does not occlude the trabeculectomy opening. A paracentesis can be made with either a sharp blade temporally or a TB syringe with a 27-gauge needle. Paracentesis is essential with each procedure because it allows reformation of the anterior chamber toward the end of surgery. By refilling the anterior chamber via the paracentesis, the surgeon has an appreciation of how much flow is present under the scleral flap.

12. How tight should I make the scleral flap? Are releasable sutures necessary?

The number of sutures and their tightness depend on the depth of the anterior chamber, the preoperative intraocular pressure, and how much leak is desired at the time of surgery. If the intraocular pressure is inordinately high, it makes sense to use more and tighter sutures so that the postoperative pressure does not fall too dramatically. The sutures can be lysed with an argon laser anywhere from day 1 through the first 3 weeks or even longer if antimetabolites are used. If the anterior chamber is shallow, as in chronic angle closure, tighter sutures are recommended initially to avoid a flat chamber postoperatively. Again, sutures can be selectively lysed. We tend to use additional releasable sutures tied into clear cornea because of the ease with which they can removed at the slit lamp. The flap can be closed moderately tight with permanent sutures, and the releasable sutures decrease the flow further. Selective removal between the first postoperative day and 1 month can easily be done at the slit lamp. If more filtration is desired, argon suture lysis may follow. With low-tension glaucoma, looser sutures with more flow may be indicated to ensure a lower initial postoperative intraocular pressure. Such sutures may be combined with releasable sutures that are cut early in the postoperative period to ensure a high flow around the edge of the scleral flap. Although releasable sutures are convenient, they are not necessary to achieve a good result.

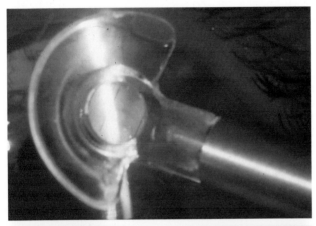

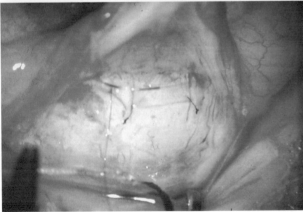

Top, Argon laser suture lysis with a Hoskins lens. *Bottom,* Two 10-0 nylon sutures closing the scleral flap with releasable suture to control aqueous flow.

13. What are the best suture and technique to close a limbal-based flap?

Different suture types as well as varied needles may be used to close a limbal-based flap successfully. We prefer one continuous-running, 8-0 vicryl suture and close Tenon's capsule and the conjunctiva separately. Tenon's capsule is closed with a locking technique, whereas the conjunctiva is closed in a nonlocking, water-tight layer. Other techniques include use of of 9-0 vicryl suture, 10-0 nylon suture, or 9-0 polydioxanone suture (PDS) in a single or double layer. More important than the type of suture is the meticulous nature of the closure, which should be water-tight and checked at the end of the procedure. Otherwise, the trabeculectomy is doomed to failure.

14. Does it matter if the limbal-based conjunctival flap is not carried out anteriorly?

Yes. The conjunctiva and Tenon's capsule should be dissected with either Wescott scissors or a Weck-cell sponge until no fibers are crossing the corneoscleral sulcus. A 67-Beaver blade held at 45° from the direction of the incision can remove these fibers easily. The dissection is continued anteriorly until the lumbus cannot be cleaned further. The corneoscleral sulcus should be visualized easily for the width of 5 mm or more. If the conjunctiva is not cleaned from the corneoscleral limbus, it will be difficult to make an anteriorly placed scleral flap.

15. Does it matter if the scleral flap is made through episcleral tissue?

Yes. The episcleral tissue should be actively removed from the bare sclera before making the scleral flap. This step is essential because the episcleral tissue may grow over and occlude the radial portions of the scleral flap and cause the surgery to fail. The true limbus must be visualized, with the episcleral tissue reflected from it, before the scleral flap is made. The limbus is probably the single most important landmark with regard to filtration surgery. Dissection of the flap can then be carried out with relative ease into clear cornea. Because the trabecular meshwork usually lies in close proximity, its removal is then facilitated.

16. Does it matter how far I dissect the scleral flap anteriorly?

In large myopic eyes, a perpendicular incision just anterior to the corneoscleral sulcus carries the flap well anterior to the iris root. In contrast, in small hyperopic eyes, an incision at the same point terminates just in front of the iris root. In removing the internal block in a myope, a satisfactory corneoscleral removal results. In a high hyperope, a slightly anterior incision is necessary to ensure that the ciliary processes are not unroofed. It is imperative to enter the anterior chamber anteriorly in patients with peripheral anterior synechiae to ensure success of the procedure.

17. Should Tenon's capsule be excised at the time of trabeculectomy surgery?

Some surgeons remove Tenon's capsule, especially when it appears to be redundant or diffuse. Removal may result in a thinner, more cystic conjunctival filtration bleb. With the advent of antimetabolites, removal of Tenon's capsule has the disadvantage of predisposition to a thinner, more fragile bleb with a greater incidence of postoperative complications; it is therefore discouraged.

Thin cystic bleb that may result after Tenon's capsule has been removed.

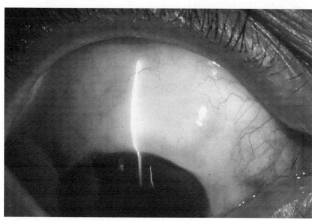

18. Should atropine be used during the procedure?

A small, sterile vial of 1% atropine is used to dilate the pupil maximally and to move the lens iris diaphragm posteriorly. This technique decreases the likelihood of a flat anterior chamber in the early postoperative period. Atropine 1%, 2–4 times/day, may be used at the surgeon's discretion postoperatively in patients who are prone to a flat chamber (e.g., chronic angle closure).

19. How often are steroids used in the postoperative period?

Prednisolone acetate 1%, every 2 hours while awake, is used for the first week, then changed to 4 times/day for 1 month and tapered quickly 2 weeks later. A broad-spectrum topical antibiotic is used 4 times/day for 1 week and then stopped.

20. How can you avoid a flat anterior chamber after trabeculectomy?

The amount of leakage around the scleral flap ultimately determines the postoperative pressure. To minimize the chance of a flat anterior chamber, more 10-0 nylon sutures, with or without releasable sutures, should be used to minimize the flow at the end of the procedure. Laser suture lysis may then be used to increase selectively the flow under the scleral flap and improve control. If the sutures are cut too aggressively, a flat anterior chamber may result.

21. What do you do when you have a wound leak in the immediate postoperative period?

If the leak is near the limbus, either a collagen shield or a bandage contact lens with patching often results in healing of the wound leak within the first few days. If antimetabolites have been used, healing may take longer. When the wound leak is found along the closure of a limbal-based flap, either patching or cyanoacrylate glue may help. If in the early postoperative period a button-hole at the dome of the bleb is noted, surgical closure is necessary to allow the bleb to fill adequately. When a fornix-based conjunctival suture breaks and a wound leak is present at the limbus, a simple restitching of the wound is indicated.

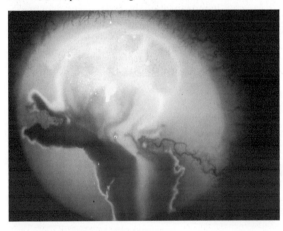

Buttonhole at dome of bleb with marked leakage, as noted with fluorescein. (See Fig. 10, Color Plates.)

22. What do you do if there is vitreous in the wound at the time of the trabeculectomy?

When faced with the appearance of vitreous through a wound that is either inappropriately posterior or at the site of a disturbed zonular face, it is best to close the wound promptly and move to a different location. Sometimes a limited cellulose sponge and scissors vitrectomy is all that is necessary to eliminate the vitreous from under the flap, and the surgery can continue. If possible, an alternate trabeculectomy may be fashioned where vitreous is not present. If an inordinate amount of vitreous is present, it is probably best to proceed with a full anterior vitrectomy, using contemporary surgical technique. Vitreous loss is rare in phakic eyes that have no history of trauma, prior iridectomy, or other predilection toward lens dislocation. Vitreous loss is more frequent in eyes that are aphakic or pseudophakic in the presence of zonular weakening (e.g., pseudoexfoliation).

23. Which ocular conditions may predispose to vitreous loss during trabeculectomy surgery?

Preoperative conditions such as ocular syphilis, Marfan's syndrome, pseudoexfoliation, homocystinuria, and high myopia may predispose to vitreous loss during trabeculectomy surgery.

24. When are antimetabolites indicated in trabeculectomy surgery?

The most important innovation in glaucoma filtering surgery in the past decade is undoubtedly the introduction of 5-fluorouracil and mitomycin C, which impair normal wound healing and facilitate the formation of highly functioning filtering blebs. Although current antifibrotic agents have improved surgical outcomes, their associated complications, ocular toxicity, and lack of standardization in terms of concentration and duration may limit their use. Continued search for wound-healing inhibitors that are safer is paramount. The indications for antimetabolite use with trabeculectomy include cases with scarring of the superior conjunctiva, previously failed filters, age younger than 50 years, pseudophakia, aphakia, or advanced optic nerve and visual field injury with desired postoperative pressure less than 14 mmHg.

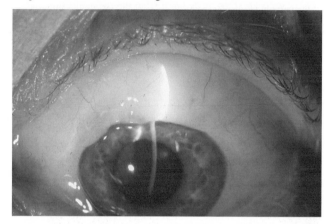

Appearance of bleb 2 months after administration of mitomycin C, 0.4 mg/cc, for 2 minutes.

25. Does 5-fluorouracil differ from mitomycin C?

Mitomycin C (MMC) is 100 times more potent than 5-fluorouracil (5-FU). Whereas 5-FU affects primarily the S-phase of the cell cycle, MMC inhibits fibroblastic proliferation regardless of the phase of the cell cycle. Intraoperative 5-FU (50 mg/ml) may be placed on a Weck-cell sponge on the sclera under the conjunctiva and Tenon's capsule and left in place for 5 minutes. The sclera is irrigated copiously with 30 cc of balanced salt solution. MMC may be used at a concentration of 0.2–0.4 mg/ml. Optimal concentration and optimal timing of the length of exposure with MMC are not known. I generally use 0.4 mg/cc MCC on a cut Weck-cell sponge (1 mm × 4 mm) and apply it to the sclera (draping Tenon's capsule and the conjunctiva over it) before making the scleral flap. Depending on the amount of scarring and risk factors, the sponge is left in place from 1.5 to 3.5 minutes.

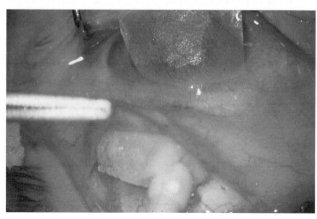

Application of mitomycin C to sclera with a cut Weck-cell sponge.

26. Are antimetabolites indicated in primary trabeculectomies?

Although MMC and intraoperative 5-FU may increase the success rate of trabeculectomy to 86–93%, the postoperative complications of suprachoroidal hemorrhage, choroidal detachment, late endophthalmitis, flat anterior chambers, and wound leaks are much more common. Therefore, a prospective, randomized, multicenter trial is under way to address the issue of antifibrotic agents in primary surgeries.

27. What do you do when the iris blocks the trabeculectomy site in the immediate postoperative period?

One option is to place miochol via the paracentesis into the anterior chamber in an attempt to constrict the pupil and dislodge it from the trabeculectomy site. A viscoelastic agent is then injected, and either a cannula or 30-gauge needle can be used to remove the iris carefully from the trabeculectomy site. On occasion, the iris does not occlude the ostium completely, and good filtration may occur around it.

28. What if the ciliary processes roll anteriorly and block the trabeculectomy site during surgery?

Ciliary processes commonly block the trabeculectomy site in small hyperopic eyes, chronic angle closure, and nanophthalmos. After the trabeculectomy specimen is removed, the ciliary processes may roll into the filtering site. In upward of 90% of cases, closure of the scleral flap, reforming the anterior chamber, and reestablishing normal anatomy allow the ciliary processes to revert to their normal positions. If, after deepening the anterior chamber, the ciliary processes continue to block the trabeculectomy opening, they can be cauterized and cut away. Care must be taken not to disturb the vitreous face. Surprisingly, this technique is not associated with great discomfort and may improve the outcome of the surgery.

29. What is the best way to remove a cataract with a preexisting filter?

The most successful way to ensure the long-term function of the preexisting trabeculectomy is to do either a temporal clear corneal or limbal temporal phacoemulsification, placing a foldable intraocular lens within the capsular bag. The least manipulation possible is recommended to ensure that the filter continues to function in the postoperative period.

30. When intraoperative 5-FU is used, it is necessary to give postoperative 5-FU injections?

Supplementary 5-FU injections, 0.1 mg (5 mg), may be given in the postoperative period if the bleb is thickened, red, and vascularized. This option is left to the surgeon's discretion. Usually supplementary 5-FU injections are not needed.

31. What do you do if the bleb starts to fail?

If the eye is red and injected, an intensified steroid regimen with the addition of a nonsteroidal antiinflammatory agent is indicated. Digital massage in the early postoperative period increases the flow, and aggressive suture lysis may be considered. Sometimes, regardless of all efforts, the bleb fails and may have to be repeated in another location. At that time, an antifibrotic agent is indicated. We occasionally use digital compression in the early postoperative period; however, we do not believe in long-term use of this modality, because the pressure traumatizes the eye and rarely improves long-term results.

32. What is the differential diagnosis for a flat anterior chamber?

The most common cause of a flat chamber after glaucoma surgery is excessive filtration. Other possibilities include a serous choroidal detachment, hemorrhagic choroidal detachment, pupillary block, and malignant glaucoma. With excessive filtration, the intraocular pressure is low as with a serous choroidal detachment. With a hemorrhagic choroidal detachment, the intraocular pressure may be low, normal, or high and usually is associated with pain. With both pupillary block and malignant glaucoma, the intraocular pressure is elevated, the chamber flat, and the cornea often edematous.

33. How serious is a flat anterior chamber?

Grade I flat anterior chambers (contact between the peripheral iris and the cornea) commonly occur in the presence of excessive filtration. Treatment includes vigorous use of cycloplegics and mydriatics and careful observation. Improvement is usually spontaneous. In some cases, a grade I flat anterior chamber becomes a grade II flat anterior chamber (contact between the peripheral iris and cornea up to the pupil). This progression may be a poor prognostic sign, especially if the pressure is falling and the bleb is flattening. Grade II flat anterior chambers may recover spontaneously or progress to grade III (contact between the corneal endothelium and lens). Grade III flat anterior chambers are a surgical emergency and must be corrected promptly or the cornea will decompensate.

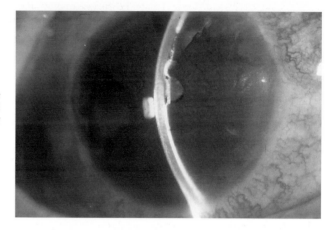

Grade III flat anterior chamber with contact between lens and cornea. (See Fig. 11, Color Plates.)

34. What options are available to treat a grade II flat anterior chamber?

1. Observe the patient without performing further surgery and see whether the chamber spontaneously reforms.

2. Reform the anterior chamber with air, viscoelastic material, or saline either at the slit lamp or in a surgical suite.

3. Drain the choroidal detachment, reform the anterior chamber, and reestablish the normal anatomic relationship of the anterior chamber.

35. What are the indications to drain a choroidal detachment?

Whenever the pressure consistently falls, the bleb flattens, and the chamber shallows despite reformation with viscoelastic material, drainage of the associated choroidal detachment is indicated. Reformation of the anterior chamber is done simultaneously through the paracentesis tract.

36. What do I do if the intraocular pressure rises immediately after surgery? Why not use a beta blocker?

If in the immediate postoperative period the intraocular pressure is elevated, either digital decompression or selective suture lysis may be used to lower the intraocular pressure. We discourage the use of beta blockers or alpha agonists at this point because we do not want to decrease aqueous flow. Aqueous flow is needed to maintain a patent fistula and successful bleb. If within 6 weeks encapsulation of the bleb or Tenon's cyst occurs, suture lysis may not help. At this point, medical therapy, including beta blockers, may be instituted for 4–5 weeks until the Tenon's cyst softens and the intraocular pressure falls. If medical therapy is not possible or not successful, needling of the bleb at the slit lamp may lower the intraocular pressure and maintain its function.

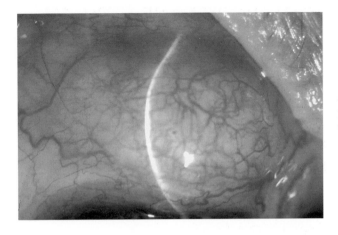

Tenon's cyst with vascularized localized bleb and elevated intraocular pressure.

37. What do you do if the intraocular pressure is zero after a trabeculectomy?

If the anterior chamber is deep and formed, dilating drops and a less aggressive steroid regimen may be used. One must meticulously check for a postoperative wound leak and make sure that the patient wears a plastic shield when sleeping. Often self-induced trauma lowers the intraocular pressure dramatically in the postoperative period. If the chamber is formed, close observation is indicated because the intraocular pressure usually rises spontaneously over the next several days to weeks.

BIBLIOGRAPHY

1. Albert DM, Jakobiec JA: Principles and Practice of Ophthalmology, vol 3. Philadelphia, W.B. Saunders, 1994.
2. Costa VP, Spaeth GL, Eiferman RA, Nania SO: Wound healing modulation in glaucoma filtering surgery. Ophthal Surg 24:152–170, 1993.
3. Feldman RM, Dietze PJ, Gross RL, Oram O: Intraoperative 5-fluorouracil administration in trabeculectomy. J Glaucoma 3:302–307, 1994.
4. Fluorouracil Filtering Surgery Study Group: Three-year follow-up of the Fluorouracil Filtering Surgery Study. Am J Ophthalmol 115:82–92, 1993.
5. Lieberman MF: Complications of glaucoma surgery. In Charlton JF, Weinstein GW (eds): Ophthalmic Surgery: Complications, Prevention and Management. Philadelphia, J.B. Lippincott, 1995.
6. Prata JA, Minckler DS, Baerveldt G, et al: Site of mitomycin-C application during trabeculectomy. J Glaucoma 3:296–301, 1994.
7. Salmon JF: The role of trabeculectomy in the treatment of advanced chronic angle-closure glaucoma. J Glaucoma 2:285–290, 1993.
8. Sastry SM, Street DA, Javitt JC: National outcomes of glaucoma surgery: Complications following partial and full-thickness filtering procedures. J Glaucoma 1:137–140, 1992.
9. Skuta GL, Beeson CC, Higgenbotham EJ, et al: Intraoperative mitomycin versus postoperative 5-fluorouracil in high risk glaucoma filtering surgery. Ophthalmology 99:438–444, 1992.
10. Spaeth GH, Katz LJ, Terebuh A: Glaucoma surgery. In Tasman W, Jaeger E (eds): Clinical Ophthalmology. Philadelphia, J.B. Lippincott, 1994.

21. TRAUMATIC GLAUCOMA AND HYPHEMA

Annette K. Terebuh, M.D., and Martha Motuz Leen, M.D.

1. What is a hyphema?

A hyphema is blood in the anterior chamber. The appearance of a hyphema may range from microscopic, seen only at the slit lamp as erythrocytes circulating in the aqueous, to a total hyphema that fills the entire anterior chamber.

2. List the etiologies of a hyphema.

There are three major causes: trauma to the globe, intraocular surgery, or spontaneous anterior segment hemorrhage in association with ocular or systemic conditions, such as neovascularization of the iris, intraocular tumors, or clotting disorders.

Hyphema Classification by Etiology

I. Trauma
   A. Blunt—rupture of iris or ciliary body blood vessels
   B. Penetrating—direct severing of blood vessels

II. Intraocular surgery
   A. Intraoperative bleeding
      1. Ciliary body or iris injury—most common when performing cyclodialysis, peripheral iridectomy, guarded filtration procedure, and cataract extraction
      2. Laser peripheral iridectomy—bleeding is more common with the YAG laser than with the argon laser
      3. Argon laser trabeculoplasty—rarely
   B. Early postoperative bleeding
      1. Dilation of a traumatized uveal vessel that was previously in spasm
      2. Conjunctival bleeding that enters the anterior chamber through a corneoscleral wound or a sclerostomy
   C. Late postoperative bleeding
      1. Disruption of new vessels growing across the corneoscleral wound
      2. Reopening of a uveal wound
      3. Chronic iris erosion from an intraocular lens

III. Spontaneous
   A. Neovascularization of the iris
      1. Retinal detachment
      2. Central retinal vein occlusion, central retinal artery occlusion, carotid occlusive disease
      3. Proliferative diabetic retinopathy
      4. Chronic uveitis
      5. Fuchs' heterochromic iridocyclitis
   B. Intraocular tumors
      1. Malignant melanoma
      2. Juvenile xanthogranuloma
      3. Retinoblastoma
      4. Metastatic tumors
   C. Iris microhemangiomas—may be associated with diabetes mellitus and myotonic dystrophy
   D. Clotting disorders
      1. Leukemia
      2. Hemophilia
      3. Anemias
      4. Aspirin
      5. Coumadin
      6. Ethanol
      7. NSAIDs

Modified from Gottsch JD: Hyphema: Diagnosis and management. Retina 10:566, 1990.

3. What is the most common cause of a traumatic hyphema?
Blunt anterior segment trauma.

4. Describe the pathophysiology of a traumatic hyphema.
Blunt ocular trauma results in ocular indentation, which causes a sudden expansion of ocular tissues and an immediate rise in the intraocular pressure. The sudden forceful displacement of the cornea and limbus posteriorly and peripherally may result in splitting or tearing of these tissues. As the tissues tear, blood vessels in the vicinity may rupture, resulting in a hyphema.

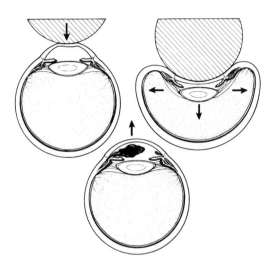

Compressive force results in vascular disruption and bleeding into the globe. (From Shingleton BJ, Hersh PS, Kenyon KR: Eye Trauma. St. Louis, C.V. Mosby, 1991, p 105, with permission.)

5. List the anterior segment structures that may split or tear in response to blunt ocular injury.
1. Central iris—sphincter tear
2. Peripheral iris—iridodialysis
3. Anterior ciliary body—angle recession
4. Separation of ciliary body from the scleral spur—cyclodialysis
5. Trabecular meshwork—trabecular meshwork tear
6. Zonules/lens—zonular tears with possible lens subluxation
7. Separation of the retina from the ora serrata—retinal dialysis

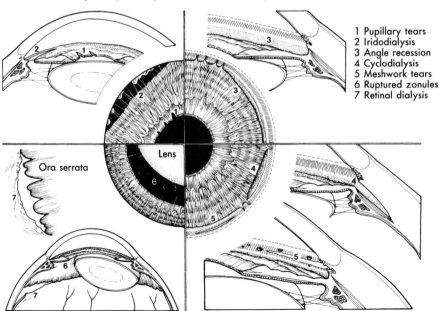

1 Pupillary tears
2 Iridodialysis
3 Angle recession
4 Cyclodialysis
5 Meshwork tears
6 Ruptured zonules
7 Retinal dialysis

The seven typical anterior tears that occur following blunt trauma to the eye. (From Shingleton BJ, Hersh PS, Kenyon KR: Eye Trauma. St. Louis, C.V. Mosby, 1991, p 118, with permission.)

6. When a patient presents with a hyphema due to blunt ocular trauma, which anterior segment structure is the most likely source of the hemorrhage?

Hyphema as a result of blunt ocular trauma most commonly occurs as a result of angle recession, a tear in the anterior face of the ciliary body between the longitudinal and circular ciliary body muscles. Rupture of the blood vessels in the vicinity of the tear results in a hyphema. The most frequently ruptured blood vessels include the major arterial circle of the iris, arterial branches to the ciliary body, and the recurrent choroidal arteries and vein crossing between the ciliary body and episcleral venus plexus.

7. What are the ocular injuries that may be associated with a traumatic hyphema?

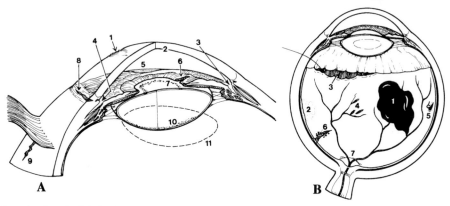

Associated ocular injuries in eyes with traumatic hyphema. *A,* 1, Corneal abrasion; 2, corneal endothelial injury with or without bloodstaining; 3, angle recession; 4, cyclodialysis; 5, iridodialysis; 6, iris sphincter tears; 7, Vossius ring; 8, corneoscleral rupture; 9, scleral rupture; 10, cataract; 11, lens subluxation. *B,* 1, Vitreous hemorrhage; 2, retinal edema; 3, retinal dialysis; 4, retinal hemorrhages; 5, horseshoe tear; 6, choroidal rupture; 7, optic nerve injury. (From Shingleton BJ, Hersh PS, Kenyon KR: Eye Trauma. St. Louis, C.V. Mosby, 1991, p 106, with permission.)

8. Describe an appropriate approach toward the workup of a patient with a hyphema.

Past medical and ocular history may identify risk factors for the bleeding episode and the chance of future complications. Sickle cell test and Hgb electrophoresis are suggested for all black and hispanic patients and anyone with a positive family history. Establishing the exact nature of the trauma helps to estimate the likelihood of a possible ocular or orbital foreign body and/or ruptured globe. The exact timing of the injury is crucial in enabling one to predict when a patient will be at greatest risk for a rebleed, and to help determine the expected time of clearing and the length of necessary treatment.

A search for a ruptured globe and ocular foreign body is suggested in all patients who present with a traumatic hyphema. The color, character, extent of the hyphema, and associated ocular injuries including corneal blood staining status should be documented. Gonioscopy is usually best deferred, but if necessary it may be performed gently, taking care to avoid a rebleed. Before a possible rebleed obscures the view, a dilated lens and fundus examination should be performed without scleral depression.

Four to six weeks after the injury, careful gonioscopy of the recovered eye may reveal an angle recession. At this time, one may also perform a dilated fundus examination with scleral depression to rule out peripheral retinal injury, such as described in the figure.

9. What are pertinent questions to ask a patient who presents with a traumatic hyphema and why?

1. **When did your injury occur?** Establishing the exact time of the injury is important because there is an increased rate of rebleed in patients who present more than 24 hours after trauma, and it will help to determine how soon a patient will be at greatest risk for a rebleed.

2. **What type of injury did you sustain?** The type and severity of an injury is important to help assess the likelihood of associated systemic injuries, an ocular or intraorbital foreign body, and the possibility of a ruptured globe.

3. **Do you or any of your family members have a medical history of bleeding disorders or sickle cell disease?** The answer to this question may help to establish a possible etiology for the hyphema and to determine what type and how aggressive the treatment should be.

4. **What types of medications do you take (including alcohol intake)?** Antiplatelet or anticoagulant effects of aspirin, NSAIDs, coumadin, and alcohol may predispose a patient to developing a hyphema or a rebleed after trauma and should be discontinued if possible.

10. How are hyphemas managed?

There is no consensus regarding the appropriate treatment for hyphema. Traditionally, most patients with a hyphema were admitted to the hospital for bed rest and sedation, and were given a monocular or binocular patch for approximately 5 days. Today, compliant patients with a microhyphema and a low risk for rebleed are often followed as outpatients. It still appears prudent to hospitalize those patients who have a layered hyphema, who are at increased risk for rebleed, who have sickle cell disease, or who are not compliant.

Patients are given a protective shield over the affected eye to decrease any inadvertent trauma. The head is elevated, and systemic blood pressure is controlled in an attempt to decrease the hydrostatic pressure in the traumatized blood vessels to minimize the risk of recurrent hemorrhage. Patients should be examined gently once or twice a day.

The medical management of hyphema includes the following:
1. Discontinuation of antiplatelet and anticoagulant medications
2. Treatment with cycloplegic drops, oral or topical steroids, antiemetics, and antifibrinolytics
3. Intraocular pressure control as necessary
   - Beta blockers
   - Alpha agonists
   - Carbonic anhydrase inhibitors, and hyperosmotics (except in sickle cell disease or trait) because of the risk of increased sickling with these medications
   - Avoid miotics, as they may increase inflammation

11. Explain the rationale for the use of antifibrinolytic agents in the treatment of hyphema.

Antifibrinolytic agents are used in an effort to reduce the chance of recurrent hemorrhage. Their use is controversial, especially in populations with a low risk of rebleeding. Fibrinolysis of a clot that seals a recently ruptured blood vessel may result in a repeat hemorrhage from that site. Tranexamic acid and aminocaproic acid decrease the rate of clot hemolysis by initiating the conversion of plasminogen to plasmin, which results in stabilization of the clot that seals the ruptured blood vessel. The injured vessel now has more time to heal permanently prior to fibrinolysis of the clot, thus reducing the risk of recurrent hemorrhage.

12. Name the most common adverse effects associated with aminocaproic acid treatment.

Nausea, vomiting, and postural hypotension are frequently encountered side effects of aminocaproic acid. It is therefore recommended that patients who receive aminocaproic acid be transported via wheelchair, particularly during the first 24 hours, to prevent possible complications from postural hypotension. Antiemetics may be used as necessary.

13. In what setting is aminocaproic acid contraindicated?

Aminocaproic acid use is contraindicated in the presence of the following:
1. Active intravascular clotting disorders, including cancer
2. Hepatic disease
3. Renal disease
4. Pregnancy

Cautious use is recommended in patients at risk for myocardial infarction, pulmonary embolus, and cerebrovascular disease.

14. Why are patients with sickle cell disease or sickle cell trait at a particularly high risk for developing complications from a hyphema?

Once pliable biconcave erythrocytes transform into elongated ridged sickle cells, they are unable to pass through the trabecular meshwork easily. The trabecular meshwork becomes obstructed with these cells, leading to a marked rise in intraocular pressure, even in the setting of a relatively small hyphema. Factors that encourage sickling include acidosis, hypoxia, and hemoconcentration. Patients with sickle cell are also predisposed to infarction of the optic nerve, retina, and anterior segment at minimally elevated intraocular pressures. This predisposition is thought to occur because of vascular sludging by sickled cells, which leads to ischemia and microvascular infarction. Therefore, vigorous and aggressive therapy for intraocular pressure control is suggested for patients with sickle cell disease.

All glaucoma medications except beta blockers are generally avoided because they may increase sickling:

1. Carbonic anhydrase inhibitors, particularly acetazolamide, may increase the concentration of ascorbic acid in the aqueous, which decreases the pH and leads to increased sickling in the anterior chamber.

2. Epinephrine compounds and alpha agonists may cause vasoconstriction with subsequent deoxygenation and increased intravascular and intracameral sickling.

3. Hyperosmotics may cause hemoconcentration, which may lead to vascular sludging and sickling, which increases the risk of infarction in the eye as well as other organs.

15. What level of intraocular pressure is considered medically "uncontrolled"?

An intraocular pressure that is considered uncontrolled depends upon the patient in question. Surgery is generally not indicated in a patient with a healthy optic nerve unless, despite medical therapy, the intraocular pressure is around 50 mmHg for 5 days, or greater than 35 mmHg for a more prolonged period of time. In the patient with previous glaucomatous optic nerve damage, however, the threshold for surgical intervention is lower and depends upon the level at which the intraocular pressure is considered to be likely to cause further optic nerve damage. In such patients, surgery may be appropriate within hours or days of the initial trauma. As previously discussed, aggressive therapy is required for patients with sickle cell disease, as these patients are predisposed to optic nerve damage and central retinal artery occlusion at minimally elevated intraocular pressures. Surgery is generally indicated in a patient with sickle cell disease if the intraocular pressure exceeds 24 mmHg for more than 24 hours despite medical therapy.

16. List the indications for surgical intervention in the management of a hyphema.

As a rule, patients with true eight-ball hyphemas require prompt surgical intervention (see question 26); in contrast, approximately 5% of all traumatic hyphemas demand surgical management. Indications for surgical intervention include the following:

1. A large hyphema that persists for more than 10 days

2. A total hyphema that persists for more than 5 days (after which time peripheral anterior synechiae are more likely to develop)

3. Early corneal blood staining

4. An intraocular pressure that cannot be controlled medically and threatens to damage the optic nerve or cornea or result in retinal vascular occlusion.

17. Name the major complications associated with a hyphema.

1. Corneal blood staining
2. Recurrent hemorrhage
3. Secondary glaucoma

In addition to the preceding complications, patients with sickle cell anemia or sickle cell trait have a predisposition to central retinal artery occlusion and optic nerve damage at only minimally elevated intraocular pressure owing to vascular sludging of the sickled cells, which leads to ischemia and vasoocclusion. Antiglaucoma medications may be used more aggressively in these patients.

18. What is corneal blood staining?
Endothelial cell decompensation results in passage of erythrocyte breakdown products into the stroma, creating a yellowish-brown discoloration of the posterior stroma. Corneal blood staining may resolve over months or years, first peripherally and then posteriorly.

19. What percent of patients with a hyphema develop corneal blood staining?
Five percent.

20. In which setting is corneal blood staining most likely to occur?
1. Recurrent hemorrhage
2. Compromised endothelial cell function
3. Larger hyphemas that are prolonged in duration
4. Usually, but not always, in association with an elevated intraocular pressure

21. What is the differential diagnosis of the appearance of bright red blood in the anterior chamber within the first 5 days after a patient has suffered a traumatic hyphema?
1. Recurrent hemorrhage
2. Fibrinolysis and hemolysis of a clotted hyphema
Recurrent hemorrhage must be differentiated from hemolysis that occurs as a clotted hyphema resorbs, particularly if the patient has been treated with aminocaproic acid. A rise in intraocular pressure associated with accelerated hemolysis can mimic a rebleed and may occur 24 to 96 hours after use of aminocaproic acid has been discontinued.

A patient who has been treated with aminocaproic acid should continue to have his or her intraocular pressure monitored several days after discontinuation of therapy in the event that there is a spike in intraocular pressure associated with accelerated hemolysis.

22. In the setting of a traumatic hyphema, when is a patient at greatest risk for developing a recurrent hemorrhage?
Two to five days following blunt ocular trauma, perhaps due to clot fibrinolysis and retraction.

23. How common is a recurrent hemorrhage?
A recurrent hemorrhage generally occurs in 4 to 35% of patients who suffer a traumatic hyphema.

24. What is the significance of a recurrent hemorrhage, and why is it important to try to prevent this event?
A recurrent hemorrhage carries a poorer prognosis than the initial hyphema. Most rebleeds are larger than the initial hyphema and carry an increased risk of developing a secondary glaucoma and corneal blood staining; visual outcome is worse, and there is a more frequent need for surgical intervention.

25. List the risk factors that may be associated with an increased risk of developing a recurrent hemorrhage.
1. Antiplatelet or anticoagulant ingestion
2. Black and hispanic race
3. Hypotony
4. Younger age
5. Larger initial hyphema

26. What is an eight-ball hyphema?
An eight-ball or black-ball hyphema is a hyphema that has clotted and taken on a black or purple color. The black or purple appearance of an eight-ball hyphema is due to impaired aqueous circulation, which leads to a subsequent decrease in the oxygenation of the intracameral blood and results in the characteristic black- or purple-colored clot. It is believed that impaired aqueous circulation occurs as a result of either pupillary block from the clot or direct tamponade effect by the

clot at the level of the trabecular meshwork. The impairment in aqueous circulation prevents the clotted black-ball hyphema from being reabsorbed. These hyphemas carry a graver prognosis with respect to developing secondary glaucoma.

27. How is an eight-ball hyphema different from a total or 100% hyphema?

An eight-ball hyphema describes blood in the anterior chamber that has clotted and taken on a black or purple appearance. A total, or 100%, hyphema is one in which the blood filling the anterior chamber appears bright red. A hyphema that consists of bright red blood indicates that there is continuous aqueous circulation within the anterior chamber, which results in a significantly more favorable prognosis than an eight-ball hyphema.

28. What is the prognosis for an eight-ball hyphema?

Patients who develop an eight-ball hyphema carry a poor prognosis with respect to developing secondary glaucoma. Most, if not all, patients develop an elevated intraocular pressure that is usually severe and frequently difficult to control with medical therapy. Surgical intervention to evacuate the clot and/or decrease the intraocular pressure is generally required for most patients with an eight-ball hyphema.

29. When is the optimal time to remove a clotted or eight-ball hyphema and why?

It is thought that the optimal time for evacuation of a clotted hyphema is 4 to 7 days after the hemorrhage, because it is at this time that there is maximal consolidation and retraction of a clot from adjacent structures and thus a decreased risk of causing new bleeding.

30. What types of surgical techniques can be used to evacuate a hyphema?

Surgical techniques in managing a hyphema include (1) paracentesis and anterior chamber washout alone or in association with a guarded filtration procedure, (2) clot expression with limbal delivery, (3) automated clot removal with a vitrectomy instrument, and (4) peripheral iridectomy with or without a guarded filtration procedure to relieve pupillary block, which may be associated with an eight-ball hyphema.

The algorithm at the top of the following page is helpful for the workup and management of a patient who presents with a hyphema.

31. List the types of secondary glaucoma associated with a traumatic hyphema.

An acute rise of intraocular pressure is generally due to obstruction of the trabecular meshwork by erythrocytes or their breakdown products. The intraocular pressure at which medical or surgical therapy is initiated should be individualized and depends upon the presence of previous glaucomatous optic nerve damage, corneal endothelial dysfunction, or sickle cell disease.

Late secondary glaucoma may develop weeks to years after a hyphema. Causes of late secondary glaucoma are listed in the table below.

Secondary Glaucomas Associated with Traumatic Hyphema

A. Early
    1. Trabecular meshwork obstruction with fresh red blood cells and fibrin, resulting in secondary open-angle glaucoma
    2. Pupillary block by the blood clot, resulting in secondary angle-closure glaucoma
    3. Hemolytic glaucoma
    4. Steroid-induced glaucoma from treatment

B. Late
    1. Angle recession glaucoma
    2. Ghost-cell glaucoma
    3. Peripheral anterior synechiae formation, resulting in secondary angle-closure glaucoma
    4. Posterior synechiae formation with iris bombé, resulting in secondary angle-closure glaucoma
    5. Hemosiderotic or hemolytic glaucoma

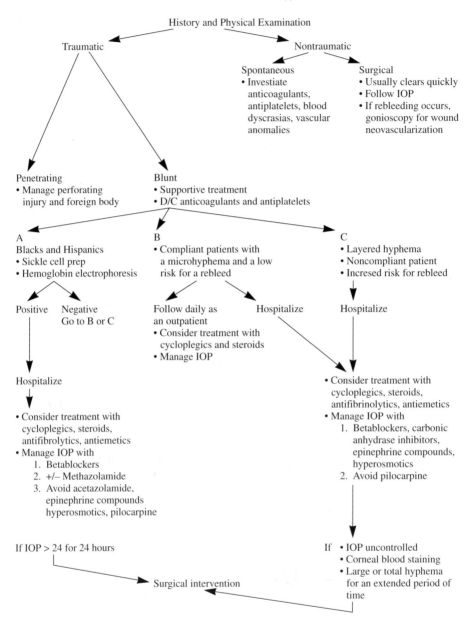

Treatment algorithm for hyphema. (Modified from Gottach JD: Hyphema: Diagnosis and management. Retina 10:566, 1990.)

32. Is the chance of developing secondary glaucoma related to the size of the hyphema?

Although there are conflicting reports, the chance of developing a secondary glaucoma may be related to the size of the hyphema. Secondary glaucoma occurred in 13.5% of those eyes in which blood filled half of the anterior chamber, in 27% of those eyes in which blood filled greater than half of the anterior chamber, and in 52% of those eyes in which there was a total hyphema.

Recurrent hemorrhages are often larger than the initial hyphema and carry a greater risk for developing secondary glaucoma.

Patients with eight-ball hyphemas develop glaucoma virtually 100% of the time.

33. Why and when is it important to perform gonioscopy on patients who have suffered a hyphema?

The gonioscopic appearance of angle recession may change with time. Immediately following blunt eye trauma, a hyphema may obscure adequate visualization of the angle. Thorough gonioscopic evaluation with indentation is recommended approximately 6 weeks after trauma, at which time the eye has recovered, the hyphema has resolved, and the risk of further injury has been minimized. Clues that may help the ophthalmologist diagnose an old angle recession include the presence of torn iris processes, depression or tears of the trabecular meshwork, and increased whitening of the scleral spur.

Up to 10% of patients with greater than 180° of angle recession will eventually develop a chronic traumatic glaucoma. The term **angle recession glaucoma** may also be used to describe the chronic traumatic glaucoma that occurs in association with an angle recession.

34. Given a history of ocular trauma, how can one make the diagnosis of angle recession on gonioscopic examination?

Angle recession can be diagnosed by careful gonioscopic examination of the injured eye and by comparing it with the fellow, nontraumatized eye. Gonioscopy may reveal an irregular widening of the ciliary body, indicating a tear between the longitudinal and circular muscles of the ciliary body. A normal, nonrecessed ciliary body band is usually not as wide as the trabecular meshwork and should be roughly even in width throughout its entire circumference. Angle recession is found in 60 to 90% of patients with a traumatic hyphema.

35. Explain the difference between a cyclodialysis and an angle recession.

Although not as common as angle recession, cyclodialysis can occur secondary to blunt compressive trauma. Traumatic cyclodialysis occurs when the ciliary body is torn from its attachment at the scleral spur. A cyclodialysis differs from an angle recession in the following manner: an angle recession is a tear within the ciliary body itself, whereas a cyclodialysis is a tear between the ciliary body and the scleral spur. Disinsertion of the uvea from the sclera allows free passage of the anterior chamber aqueous fluid to the suprachoroidal space, therefore permitting direct

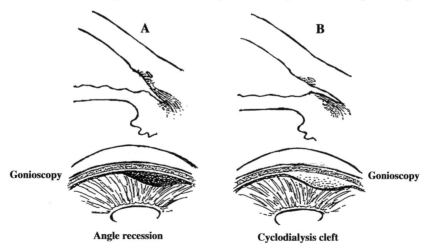

Cross-sectional and corresponding gonioscopic appearance of angle recession and cyclodialysis. (From Shields MB: Textbook of Glaucoma, 3rd ed. Baltimore, Williams & Wilkins, 1992.

access to the uveoscleral outflow pathway. Temporary or permanent hypotony is usual. A cyclo-dialysis cleft should be suspected and carefully searched for when the intraocular pressure remains low after ocular trauma.

36. Once a cyclodialysis cleft is suspected, how can it be diagnosed?

A traumatic cyclodialysis cleft can be diagnosed by careful gonioscopic examination (see figure on previous page). Although the wall of the cyclodialysis cleft is white (i.e., sclera), it appears shaded owing to the fact that one is looking down into a hole. This is opposed to the gonio-scopic appearance of angle recession, which appears simply as an enlarged ciliary body band secondary to a tear in the ciliary body itself. Treatment for a cyclodialysis cleft includes atropine, laser, and surgical repair.

37. How long after a traumatic hyphema is a patient at risk for developing angle recession glaucoma?

Angle recession glaucoma may develop weeks to many years following blunt ocular trauma.

Patients who develop angle recession glaucoma may have an underlying predisposition to primary open-angle glaucoma (POAG). It is believed that the infliction of trauma to a meshwork that is already predisposed to reduced aqueous outflow (POAG) may be just enough to push an already compromised trabecular meshwork over the edge, resulting in an angle recession glaucoma. Evidence to support this underlying predisposition to reduced aqueous outflow (POAG) includes the unusually high incidence of POAG in the nontraumatized fellow eye and an increased tendency for the intraocular pressure to be increased by topical corticosteroids.[19] Therefore, management of patients with angle recession includes long-term follow up of both the injured and uninjured eyes.

38. Explain the pathophysiology of angle recession glaucoma. Is it a direct result of injury to the ciliary body?

No. Angle recession is merely a marker for anterior segment contusion injury, specifically injury to the trabecular meshwork. Angle recession glaucoma is thought not to be due to the angle recession itself (i.e., a tear in the ciliary body) but rather due to (1) direct trabecular meshwork damage from the blunt trauma or (2) an extension of a Descemet's-like membrane covering the trabecular meshwork.

39. Describe treatment for angle recession glaucoma.

Angle recession glaucoma often does not respond well to conventional therapy. Eyes with secondary traumatic glaucoma have reduced conventional outflow owing to trabecular meshwork injury, and may therefore shift over to primarily uveoscleral outflow. Miotics may actually para-doxically increase the intraocular pressure, possibly by decreasing uveoscleral outflow. Laser tra-beculoplasty does not have a high rate of success in this setting. Beta blockers, carbonic anhydrase inhibitors, cycloplegics, and filtration surgery are the most effective treatments for angle recession glaucoma.

BIBLIOGRAPHY

1. Berrios RR, Dreyer EB: Traumatic hyphema. Ophthalmol Clin 35(1):93–103, 1995.
2. Caprioli J, Sears ML: The histopathology of black-ball hyphema: A report of two cases. Ophthalmic Surg 15(6):491–495, 1984.
3. Chi TS, Netland PA: Angle recession of glaucoma. Int Ophthalmol Clin 35(1):117–126, 1995.
4. Coles WH: Traumatic hyphema: An analysis of 235 cases. South Med J 61:813, 1968.
5. Crouch ER, Frenkel M: Aminocaproic acid in the treatment of traumatic hyphema. Am J Ophthalmol 81:355–360, 1976.
6. Dietse MC, Hersh PS, Kylstra JA, et al: Intraocular pressure increase associated with epsilon aminocaproic acid therapy or traumatic hyphema. Am J Ophthalmol 106:383–390, 1988.
7. Goldberg MF: Antifibrinolytic agents in the management of traumatic hyphema. Arch Ophthalmol 101:1029–1030, 1983.

8. Gottsch JD: Hyphema: Diagnosis and management. Retina 10:S65–S71, 1990.
9. Herschler J: Trabecular damage due to blunt anterior segment injury and its relationship to traumatic glaucoma. Trans Am Ophthalmol Otolaryngol 83:239–248, 1977.
10. Kennedy RH, Brubaker RF: Traumatic hyphema in a defined population. Am J Ophthalmol 106:123–130, 1988.
11. Kutner B, Fourman S, et al: Aminocaproic acid reduces the risk of secondary hemorrhage in patients with traumatic hyphema. Arch Ophthalmol 105:206–208, 1987.
12. McGetrick JJ, Jampol LM, Goldberg MF, et al: Aminocaproic acid decreases secondary hemorrhage after traumatic hyphema. Arch Ophthalmol 101:1031–1033, 1983.
13. Parrish R, Bernardino V: Iridectomy in the surgical management of eight-ball hyphema. Arch Ophthalmol 100:435–437, 1982.
14. Ritch R, Shields MB, Krupin T: The Glaucomas, 2nd ed. St. Louis, C.V. Mosby, 1996.
15. Sears ML: Surgical management of black-ball hyphema. Trans Am Acad Ophthalmol Otolaryngol 74:820–827, 1970.
16. Shields MB: Textbook of Glaucoma, 4th ed. Baltimore, Williams & Wilkins, 1998.
17. Shingleton BJ, Hersh PS, Kenyon KR: Eye Trauma. St. Louis, C.V. Mosby, 1991, pp 95–125, 135–142.
18. Spaeth GL, Levy PM: Traumatic hyphema: Its clinical characteristics and failure of estrogens to alter its course. A double-blind study. Am J Ophthalmol 62:1098, 1966.
19. Tesluk GC, Spaeth GL: The occurrence of primary open-angle glaucoma in the fellow eye of patients with unilateral angle-cleavage glaucoma. Ophthalmology 92(7):904–912, 1985.
20. Volpe NJ, Larrison WI, Hersh PS, et al: Secondary hemorrhage in traumatic hyphema. Am J Ophthalmol 112:507–513, 1991.
21. Wilson FM: Traumatic hyphema pathogenesis and management. Ophthalmology 87(9):910–919, 1980.
22. Wilson TW, Jeffers JB, Nelson LB: Aminocaproic acid prophylaxis in traumatic hyphema. Ophthalmic Surg 21:807–809, 1990.
23. Wolff SM, Zimmerman LE: Chronic secondary glaucoma. Am J Ophthalmol 54:547–562, 1962.

IV. Cataracts

22. CATARACTS

Richard Tipperman, M.D.

1. Where does the term *cataract* come from?

Cataract comes from the Greek word *cataractos*, which describes rapidly running water. Rapidly running water turns white, as do mature cataracts.

2. What is a nuclear sclerotic cataract?

A nuclear sclerotic cataract describes the sclerosis or darkening that is seen in the central portion of the lens nucleus. This type of cataract is typically seen in older patients. As the equatorial epithelial cells of the lens continue to divide, they produce compaction of the more central fibers and sclerosis.

3. What produces the brown color seen in cataracts?

The brown color comes from urochrome pigment.

4. What is "second sight"? How is it associated with nuclear sclerotic cataracts?

As patients develop nuclear sclerotic cataracts, the increased density of the lens causes the patient to become increasingly nearsighted. As a result of their nearsightedness, many patients who required spectacles to help them read find that they are able to read small print up close without glasses. In the past, this phenomenon was termed "second sight." Of interest, patients erroneously believe that their eyes are getting stronger or better, whereas the opposite is the case. Second sight indicates progression of the cataract.

5. What are the typical symptoms of nuclear sclerotic cataracts?

In general, all types of cataracts cause decreased vision. Nuclear sclerotic cataracts tend to cause problems with distance vision but preserve reading vision because of the above-mentioned nearsightedness.

6. What are posterior subcapsular cataracts?

Posterior subcapsular cataracts are granular opacities seen mainly in the central posterior cortex just under the posterior capsule. They have a hyaline type of appearance.

7. What are the symptoms of posterior subcapsular cataracts?

Unlike patients with nuclear sclerotic cataracts, patients with posterior subcapsular cataracts often have good distance vision but typically have blurred near vision. In addition, patients with posterior subcapsular cataracts often have extreme difficulty with glare so that in dim illumination they function well, whereas with bright illumination their vision decreases significantly.

8. What are the associated systemic findings in patients with cataracts?

In general, **nuclear sclerotic cataracts** are seen in elderly patients, although they may occur in younger patients as well. In younger patients, they are often associated with high myopia.

Posterior subcapsular cataracts are common in patients with diabetes, patients who have taken steroids, and patients with a history of intraocular inflammation, such as uveitis.

9. What are the major potential causes of cataracts in infants?

Common causes of congenital cataracts include familial inheritance, intrauterine infection (e.g., rubella), metabolic diseases (e.g., galactosemia), and chromosomal abnormalities. Complete evaluation by a pediatrician is mandatory for any infant with a congenital cataract.

10. What is a Morganian cataract?

A Morganian cataract is a mature cataract in which the cortex liquefies and the mature central nucleus can be seen within the liquefied cortex.

11. What is phacolytic glaucoma?

Phacolytic glaucoma may occur with Morganian and mature cataracts. Liquefied cortex traverses the capsular membrane and enters the anterior chamber, producing an inflammatory response that clogs the trabecular meshwork and results in elevated intraocular pressure.

12. What is phacomorphic glaucoma?

As the cataract matures, the lens becomes enlarged (intumescent). As the lens enlarges, it pushes the iris root and ciliary body forward, narrowing the angle between the iris and peripheral cornea in the region of the trabecular meshwork. If the angle becomes narrow enough, the pressure may become elevated because of angle closure. Treatment involves removal of the cataract.

13. What is pseudoexfoliation? What is its relationship to cataracts?

Pseudoexfoliation is a condition in which basement membrane material from the zonules and lens capsule is liberated onto the anterior lens capsule and anterior chamber. Patients with pseudoexfoliation have a predisposition for the development of glaucoma, presumably because of clogging of the trabecular meshwork by the exfoliated material. Patients with pseudoexfoliation often present a challenge for the cataract surgeon because their pupils tend to dilate poorly and they often have weak or loose zonules that can cause intraoperative complications with disinsertion of the zonules. Because of their propensity for developing glaucoma, patients often have postoperative pressure elevations.

14. What is true exfoliation syndrome as opposed to pseudoexfoliation syndrome?

True exfoliation was seen in glassblowers who stood in front of hot furnaces throughout the day. They often developed large sheets of material that came off the anterior lens capsule. Such cataracts are termed **glassblower's cataracts**. With modern techniques of processing glass, they are no longer seen. Because the type of material produced in pseudoexfoliation seemed similar to the material produced in a glassblower's cataract, it was termed pseudoexfoliation to distinguish it from the exfoliative material produced by heat exposure.

15. What systemic syndrome should be considered in a patient with a spontaneously dislocated lens?

Spontaneous dislocation of the lens is most common in Marfan's syndrome and homocystinuria. Typical patients with Marfan's syndrome are tall, thin, and lanky and exhibit arachnodactyly. The lenses in Marfan's syndrome tend to dislocate superiorly. In homocystinuria, the lenses tend to dislocate inferiorly. Trauma should be considered in all patients with a dislocated lens.

16. What other clinical findings are common in patients with a traumatic cataract?

Blunt trauma may produce a cataract. Patients often have associated sphincter tears and may even have iridodialysis or angle recession. If the trauma has been severe, some or all of the zonules may be broken, causing the lens to be mobile within the eye. This phenomenon is termed **phacodenesis**. Retinal detachment and optic neuropathy also may be present and cause decreased vision.

17. What is the indication for cataract surgery?

The indication for cataract surgery is reduced visual function that interferes with activities of daily living. This indication obviously varies, depending on the patient's age and degree of activity. For instance, a 40-year-old accountant with an early posterior subcapsular cataract may be much more symptomatic than an 85-year-old who no longer reads or drives. Cases in which cataract surgery is medically necessary (e.g., phacomorphic and phacolytic glaucoma) are extremely uncommon. Patients with cataracts should be informed that cataract surgery is almost always an elective procedure and that leaving the cataract alone will not hurt or damage the eye.

BIBLIOGRAPHY

1. Datilles M: Clinical evaluation of cataracts. In Tasman W, Jaeger E (eds): Duane's Clinical Ophthalmology, vol 1, 73B [looseleaf]. Philadelphia, Lippincott-Raven, pp 1–15.
2. Datilles M, Kinoshita J: Pathogenesis of cataract. In Tasman W, Jaeger E (eds): Duane's Clinical Ophthalmology, vol 1, 72B [looseleaf]. Philadelphia, Lippincott-Raven, pp 1–9.
3. Datilles M, Magno B: Cataract: Clinical types. In Tasman W, Jaeger E (eds): Duane's Clinical Ophthalmology, vol 1, 73 [looseleaf]. Philadelphia, Lippincott-Raven, pp 1–25.

23. TECHNIQUES OF CATARACT SURGERY

Sydney Tyson, M.D., M.P.H.

1. What are the indications for cataract surgery?

In general, the decision to have cataract surgery is elective. It is based on a patient's personal needs and the physician's judgment as to the probability of visual improvement. For some people, even a slight loss of vision is unacceptable. Others may choose to delay surgery because their cataracts do not seriously interfere with their lives. They key question is whether the patient perceives the cataract to interfere with his or her quality of life.

2. What are two nonsurgical methods of managing a cataract?

1. Refraction. Patients with cataract may experience a myopic (near-sighted) shift or so-called second sight. Occasionally, glasses can compensate for such shifts. However, if the shift is large and unilateral, binocular vision may be compromised by image size differences between the two eyes.

2. Pupillary dilation. An expanded pupil allows light rays to enter around a central cataract (such as a posterior subcapsular [PSC] cataract) rather than be blocked by light rays that attempt to pass through a hazy cataract.

3. What preoperative tests are used to gauge visual impairment?

No single test adequately describes the effect of cataracts on a patient's visual functioning, but the most widely used are:

1. Snellen visual acuity (i.e., 20/20)

2. Potential acuity testing. This test estimates postoperative visual acuity by projecting a Snellen acuity chart through the patient's cataract. It is most often used to determine whether a patient's visual symptoms are due more to cataract or retinal disease.

3. Glare/contrast sensitivity testing. This test simulates lighting conditions outdoors and determines a patient's vision when functioning in more normal conditions. The high-contrast situation in a Snellen test can overestimate a patient's abilities. A patient may have 20/40 acuity in a dark room but may have 20/100 with glare testing, which could significantly impair driving.

4. What are the basic steps in removing a cataract?

1. The pupil is dilated.
2. The skin around the eyelids is disinfected with an antiseptic, usually iodine-based.
3. The eye and lids are anesthetized and a speculum is placed to open the lids.
4. An incision is made into the anterior chamber (AC).
5. A viscoelastic (viscous, protective gel) is injected into the AC.
6. The anterior capsule is opened to gain access to the lens mass with a capsulotomy or capsulorhexis.
7. The nucleus is removed manually or by phacoemulsification.
9. The residual cortex is removed.
9. An intraocular lens (IOL) is inserted.
10. The wound is sutured closed (optional with self-sealing wounds).

5. How is the eye anesthetized for surgery?

Most surgeons prefer local rather than general anesthesia for adult cataract surgery. Facial akinesia with a short-acting agent such as lidocaine and hyaluronidase (a diffusion enhancer) is often desired to prevent squeezing of the eyelids during surgery. There are three types of local anesthesia:

1. Retrobulbar. Anesthetic (usually a combination of a short- and long-acting agent with hyaluronidase) is injected inside the muscle cone to achieve akinesia and anesthesia of the globe.

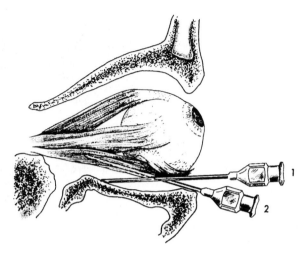

Retrobulbar injection. If tip of needle strikes floor of orbit as it is inserted (1), it is withdrawn slightly and directed more superiorly (2). (From Jaffe NS, Jaffe MS, Jaffe GF: Cataract Surgery and Its Complications. St. Louis, Mosby, 1990, with permission.)

2. Peribulbar. Anesthetic is injected outside the muscle cone. Although this block takes longer to take effect (12–25 min), there are fewer potential complications because a shorter needle is used.

3. Topical. Advances in technology have allowed skilled surgeons to perform the cataract procedure in 10–15 min. With such short operative times, prolonged anesthesia and akinesia become less critical. Topical drops of short-acting agents such as lidocaine or tetracaine may be used to anesthetize the eye sufficiently to complete the procedure. The advantage to the patient is instant, binocular vision postoperatively without the risk of injection-related, potentially sight-threatening complications.

6. What are the disadvantages of topical anesthesia for cataract surgery?
1. Because there is no akinesia, the eye can move during surgery.
2. Patient selection is crucial. Patients need to follow the commands of the surgeon.

7. What is couching?
Couching is one of the most ancient surgical procedures. It was the first known technique of cataract removal and was first described by the Indian physician Susruta circa 800 B.C. It remained popular in the United States until the 1850s. Couching involves piercing the eye with a needle, then dislocating the entire lens backward and downward into the posterior chamber. Although it may seem crude by modern surgical standards and prone to myriad complications, it is still commonly performed in the Third World, where advanced technology is not available.

8. What are the two most common ways to remove a cataract?
1. Intracapsular surgery was the procedure of choice from its discovery by Jacques Daviel in 1752 until the early 1970s. It is accomplished with a cryo (freezing) probe. Intracapsular surgery is rarely performed in the United States today except in cases of dislocated lenses.

2. Extracapsular surgery (ECCE) is the most popular technique. There are two types: manual extraction and phacoemulsification. Both methods require the use of an operating microscope that permits magnification. In extracapsular surgery, the anterior capsule of the lens is removed, the hard nucleus is expressed, and the remaining soft cortical fragments are removed with either an automated or manual device. The advantage of extracapsular surgery is preservation of the posterior capsule, which permits a pocket for an intraocular lens. This method also minimizes the complications associated with vitreous loss.

Extracapsular extraction. *A*, Multiple small cuts are made in the anterior capsule. *B*, Full-thickness incision is completed with scissors. *C*, Nucleus removed. *D*, Cortex aspiration. *E*, Inferior haptic insertion through incision and passed under the iris. *F*, The tip of the superior haptic is grasped with a forceps and advanced into the anterior chamber; as the superior pole is clearing the edge of the pupil, the arm is pronated to ensure that when the haptic is released it will spring open under the iris and not out of the incision. (From Kanski JJ: Clinical Ophthalmology: A systematic Approach, 2nd ed. Boston, Butterworth Heinemann, 1989, with permission.)

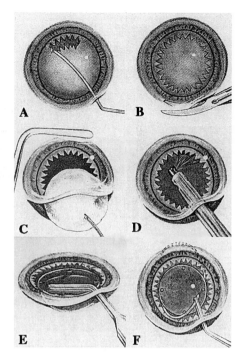

9. What is phacoemulsification?

"Phaco" was invented by Dr. Charles Kellman in 1967 and is probably one of the most significant advances in cataract surgery. It is a sophisticated form of extracapsular surgery that permits mechanical removal of a cataract through a 3.0-mm incision. This reduction in incision size results in faster visual recovery and fewer complications. Conventional extracapsular surgery requires a wound size of 150° (about 10 mm).

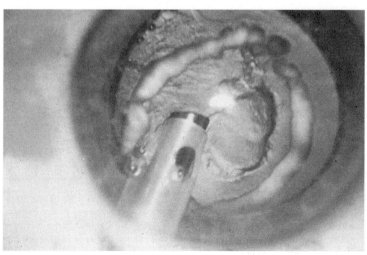

The removal of nuclear material by phacoemulsification. (From Koch PS, Davidson JA: Textbook of Advanced Phacoemulsification Techniques. Thorofare, NJ, Slack, 1991, with permission.)

10. How does the machine work?

Although the machine is complex, its functions are simple: irrigation, aspiration, and ultrasonic vibration via a handpiece. The phacoemulsification handpiece consists of a hollow 1-mm titanium needle that fragments a cataract by vibrating at 40,000 times per second. The fragmented pieces are then aspirated through the tip of the needle and into a drainage bag. An irrigation solution flows from a bottle suspended above the machine and into the eye through the needle. This fluid serves to cool the needle and to maintain proper anterior chamber depth.

11. What are the advantages and disadvantages of phaco?

Phacoemulsification

ADVANTAGES	DISADVANTAGES
Small incision	Machine-dependent
Fewer wound problems	Longer learning period
Less astigmatism	Complications while learning
More rapid physical rehabilitation	Expensive equipment
Less risk of expulsive hemorrhage	Difficult with hard nucleus
	Need good pupil dilation

12. How is a capsulotomy performed?

There are two types of capsulotomies: Can-opener capsulotomy and continuous-curve capsulorhexis (CCC). The can-opener capsulotomy is a series of jagged punctures performed with a bent needle. Although it is simple to perform, it is prone to peripheral extension of its jagged edges. The CCC is made by tearing the capsule so that the edges remain sharp, well-demarcated, and strong. This approach permits safe utilization of phaco techniques that employ shearing or rotational forces. Implants are held more securely and center better.

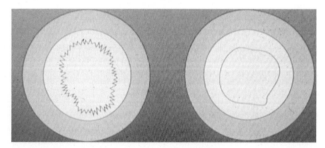

Left, Can opener capsulotomy. *Right*, Continuous curve capsulorhexis. (From Koch PS, Davidson JA: Textbook of Advanced Phacoemulsification Techniques. Thorofare, NJ, Slack, 1991, with permission).

Location. The nucleus can be disassembled in the anterior chamber or in the capsular bag. Anterior chamber removal is less popular because of the higher risk of corneal endothelial damage. However, in cases with capsular rupture, this method of removal can prevent nuclear pieces from moving posteriorly into the vitreous.

Nucleus handling. The nucleus can be disassembled as a whole (sculpting) or by first splitting it (nucleofractis) into quadrants. Harder nuclei are more readily and safely removed with a splitting technique within the capsular bag. However, a capsulorhexis is mandatory because the forces exerted during splitting may cause peripheral extension of a can-opener capsulotomy with possible posterior capsular rupture.

The type of capsulotomy and anticipated method of cataract extraction are closely interrelated. The planned location and technique of nucleus emulsification is affected by variables such as nucleus consistency (hard or soft lens), pupil size, zonular (lens ligament) integrity, and the presence of intraoperative complications.

13. Are lasers used to remove cataracts?

Not yet, although promising developments are in the pipeline. Currently, lasers are used to open cloudy capsular membranes that develop after surgery.

14. Once a cataract is removed (aphakia), what are the options to restore vision?

1. Glasses. Thick aphakic glasses are rarely used today because they create visually annoying magnification (about 25%) and distortion.

2. Contact lenses are a better alternative to visual restoration (magnify only 7%), but many elderly patients do not possess the manual dexterity necessary to handle them. Long-term extended wear lenses can help in this regard.

3. Intraocular lenses (IOLs) are the best and most common alternative to restoration of normal vision after cataract surgery. IOLs almost duplicate the phakic eye. Magnification is minimal, and peripheral vision is normal.

15. Who invented intraocular lenses?

Ridley was the first to insert an implant into the posterior chamber in 1949. Most authorities agree that this was one of the most significant advances in cataract surgery.

16. Of what are implants made?

During World War I it was noted that British Spitfire fighter pilots who had plexiglass (PMMA) embedded in their eyes from shattered canopies tolerated the material well. PMMA lenses then became the gold standard. Advances in technology led to the creation of soft or foldable materials made from silicone and acrylic material. These materials have come into favor mainly because they can be inserted through much smaller, unenlarged incisions.

17. Describe the most common design and shape of IOLs.

Implants are composed of an optical portion called the "optic" and a nonoptical portion called the "haptic," which is used for fixating the IOL.

Most optic designs are unifocal (distance only). Multifocal designs, which eliminate the need for reading glasses, are on the horizon. Optics can be round or oval, with or without positioning holes, and range in size from 5–7 mm. Lens haptics can be looped or plate style (mostly seen in foldable implants) and made of the same or different material as its optic. Anterior chamber lenses are designed with special haptics that allow proper fixation in the delicate anterior chamber angle.

18. What are the most common positions of IOLs?

Capsular bag, ciliary sulcus, and anterior chamber. Capsular bag fixation is preferred because it affords excellent lens stability far away from the corneal endothelium.

19. Is an implant indicated in every aphakic patient?

No. Implants are generally not used in children or in eyes with severe anterior segment disease or inflammation.

20. How is the power of an IOL determined?

The most common method of determining IOL power (P) uses a regression formula called SRK. The formula is $P = A - 2.5 L - 0.9 K$. The components of this formula include axial length (length of the eye) measurement (A), which is determined by A-scan ultrasonography; average corneal curvature (K), which is determined by keratometry; and an A constant (A), which is specific for each lens type. The closer the implant to the retina, the greater the A constant. Therefore, the A constant is greater in posterior chamber implants than in anterior chamber implants.

21. How is the surgical wound closed?

The need for wound closure is directly related to wound size and construction. Larger ECCE incisions can be reapproximated with 10-0 nylon sutures, in a radial, running, or combination technique. The major consideration with these closure techniques is postoperative astigmatism. The more tightly sutures are tied, the greater the astigmatism and the more distorted the early postoperative vision. Phaco incisions are smaller and valvelike in construction. This makes them essentially self-sealing and astigmatism-free, although some surgeons sleep better at night if at least one suture is placed.

22. How should patients be managed postoperatively?

The postoperative patient is seen within the first 48 hours of surgery—preferably within 24 hours. Intraocular pressure, wound integrity, anterior chamber inflammation, and IOL positioning are assessed. Typical postoperative medications include (1) antibiotic solutions for infection control and (2) steroids and/or nonsteroidal antiinflammatory drugs for control of inflammation. Patients are then seen at 1-week, 1-month, and 3–6-month intervals. In advanced small-incision surgeries, refractions are usually stable by 1 month. Glasses may be given at this visit.

23. What are the most significant trends in cataract surgery?

1. Topical vs. retrobulbar anesthesia for cataract surgery
2. Clear corneal vs. scleral incisions
3. Conversion to phacoemulsification from ECCE
4. Foldable IOLs vs. rigid PMMA lenses
5. Sutureless wound closure

BIBLIOGRAPHY

1. American Academy of Ophthalmology: Cataract in the Otherwise Healthy Adult Eye (Preferred Practice Patterns). San Francisco, American Academy of Ophthalmology, 1989.
2. Jaffe N, Horowitz J: Lens and cataract. In Podos S, et al (eds): Textbook of Ophthalmology, vol 3. New York, Gower Medical Publishing, 1992.
3. Johnson S: Phacoemulsification. In Focal Points (Clinical Modules for Ophthalmologists), vol XII. San Francisco, American Academy of Ophthalmology, 1994.
4. Kratz R, Shammas H: Cataracts. In Wright K (ed): Color Atlas of Ophthalmology. Philadelphia, J.B. Lippincott, 1991.
5. Maloney W, Grindle L: Textbook of Phacoemulsification. Fallbrook, CA, Lasenda Publishers, 1988.
6. Stein H, Slatt B, Stein R: The Ophthalmic Assistant, 6th ed. St. Louis, Mosby, 1994.
7. Steinert R: Cataract Surgery: Technique, Complications, and Management. Philadelphia, W.B. Saunders, 1995.

24. COMPLICATIONS OF CATARACT SURGERY

Robert S. Bailey, Jr., M.D.

1. What complications may result from local anesthesia for cataract surgery?

1. Retrobulbar hemorrhage is the most common complication from retrobulbar injection. Blood collects in the retrobulbar space, often causing proptosis of the involved eye and a tense orbit. If not treated, it may lead to severe, irreversible optic nerve ischemia.

2. Ocular perforation may occur if the needle perforates the globe. The risk of this complication is greatest in highly myopic eyes with long axial lengths.

3. Optic nerve sheath hemorrhage may occur if the needle penetrates the optic nerve. It may result in a secondary central retinal vein and/or central retinal artery occlusion.

Peribulbar injections given with a shorter needle have become more popular recently, as has topical anesthesia for cataract surgery.

2. How do you treat a retrobulbar hemorrhage?

Blood collecting in the retrobulbar space may cause a secondary increase in intraocular pressure from the pressure of the blood on the globe. When a retrobulbar hemorrhage occurs intermittent pressure is applied initially to the globe to tamponade the bleeding. The intraocular pressure should be measured. If it is significantly elevated, a lateral canthotomy should be performed. This technique is often successful in relieving the pressure on the globe. Surgery is usually cancelled when a retrobulbar hemorrhage occurs.

3. What are the common complications related to the cataract wound?

1. **Wound leak or dehiscence** occurs when apposition of the cataract wound is inadequate. Aqueous humor can be seen leaking from the involved area of the wound.

2. **Hypotony.** If a wound leak is present a low intraocular pressure is usually found.

3. **Flat anterior chamber.** If the wound leak is large enough, the anterior chamber becomes shallow and may become flat with iris contacting the cornea.

Most wound leaks require repair in the operating room with additional sutures to achieve a water-tight closure.

4. What is iris prolapse? How is it treated?

If a wound leak is present, iris often becomes incarcerated in the wound and may prolapse through the wound, leading to increased inflammation and increased risk of infection (see figure). Prolapse requires repair in the operating room . If the iris is viable, it can be reposited in the eye; if not, it can be excised. Additional sutures are then applied to the area of the wound dehiscence.

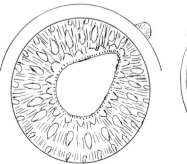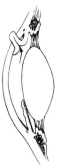

Iris prolapse (front and side views). (From Jaeger E, Tasman W (eds): Clinical Ophthalmology. Philadelphia, J.B. Lippincott, 1995, with permission.)

5. What types of intraocular hemorrhage may occur during or after cataract surgery?

1. **Hyphema or blood in the anterior chamber** can be seen as a layering or meniscus of blood in the anterior chamber. Blood vessels in the base of the cataract wound or possibly from the iris are usually the source of the blood. Most often the blood clears spontaneously, and no treatment is required. The intraocular pressure needs to be monitored closely because secondary elevation may occur.

2. **Expulsive choroidal hemorrhage** is the most feared complication of cataract surgery. It is caused by rupture of choroidal vessels, most often during surgery. The rupture causes a rapid rise in intraocular pressure with loss of the anterior chamber, iris prolapse, and possible prolapse of the entire intraocular contents if not recognized and treated promptly. Fortunately, it has a recurrence rate of 0.2 percent.

6. What are some of the risk factors for expulsive choroidal hemorrhage? How are they treated?

Patients with advanced age, systemic hypertension, arteriosclerosis, glaucoma, and long axial length eyes are at greater risk. The most important factor in treatment is time. The wound must be closed as quickly as possible; the surgeon may tamponade the wound with his or her thumb until a suture is ready. Sutures should be rapidly placed and the eye closed. Some surgeons advocate performing posterior sclerotomies to release accumulated blood. The prognosis for visual outcome is usually quite poor.

7. What are the causes of postoperative inflammation?

1. **Operative trauma.** All eyes show some postoperative uveitis seen as cell and flare reaction in the anterior chamber. Despite individual variation, the degree of inflammation is usually proportionate to the degree of trauma induced by the surgical procedure. Procedures with longer surgical times and/or additional procedures (i.e., vitrectomy or iris manipulation) show greater amounts of inflammation.

2. **Retained lens material.** Fragments of lens material—either nucleus or cortical remnants—may cause inflammation. In almost all cases cortical remnants resorb and require no additional treatment. Nuclear fragments may become a source of chronic inflammation that leads to macular edema. Most nuclear remnants require surgical removal.

3. **Bacteria/fungi.** Microorganisms introduced at the time of surgery also may be a source of inflammation. Intraocular infection may lead to rapid loss of visual function; therefore, prompt recognition and treatment are important.

8. How does infectious endophthalmitis present? When does it usually occur? How is it treated?

The classic presentation includes severe ocular pain, decreased vision, lid swelling, conjunctival chemosis, and hypopyon. Corneal edema and diminution or loss of the red reflex often occur. This condition must be suspected in any patient who presents with more inflammation than expected postoperatively.

The prospective Endophthalmitis Vitrectomy Study was performed to evaluate the treatment and course of endophthalmitis. On average patients developed signs and symptoms 6 days after surgery. More than three-fourths of patients developed signs and symptoms within 2 weeks. In the EVS study the most common causative pathogens were gram-positive, coagulase-negative organisms (e.g., *Staphylococcus epidermidis*), followed by other gram-positive organisms such as *Streptococci* and *Staphylococcus aureus*.

Treatment includes immediate culture of aqueous and vitreous, intravitreal and topical antibiotics. The EVS study showed that intravenous antibiotics are of no benefit. The role of systemic steroids is still controversial. The study also showed that immediate vitrectomy had significant benefit to patients presenting with vision of light perception or worse. It is essential that patients be treated promptly.

9. What are the causes of corneal edema after cataract surgery?

Corneal edema frequently occurs adjacent to the cataract wound and usually resolves spontaneously. Surgical trauma, preexisting endothelial corneal dystrophy, and elevated intraocular pressure may cause central corneal edema. Treatment of elevated intraocular pressure and topical steroids as necessary for inflammation are important. Most often central edema resolves. Corneal transplant can be performed for patients when corneal edema persists.

10. What are the causes of vitreous loss during cataract surgery? Why is vitreous loss important?

Vitreous loss may result from (1) rupture of the posterior lens capsule or (2) weakness or dehiscence of lens zonular apparatus. Vitreous loss increases risk of retinal detachment, cystoid macular edema, and endophthalmitis. The additional surgical trauma also may lead to an increase in corneal trauma and secondary central corneal edema.

11. What is the incidence of retinal detachment following cataract surgery? What patients are at greater risk?

Retinal detachment occurs in 1–2% of patients in most reported series. Patients predisposed to retinal detachment by high myopia, lattice degeneration, and a history of retinal detachment in the fellow eye are at greater risk. Vitreous loss at the time of surgery also raises the risk of retinal detachment. The risk of retinal detachments after cataract surgery has decreased with the advent of extracapsular cataract extraction, which has replaced intracapsular extraction.

12. What is cystoid macular edema?

Cystoid macular edema (CME) occurs when fluid accumulates in the cells in and around the center of the macula known as the fovea. Fluid may leak from the capillaries surrounding the fovea. CME typically presents 4–8 weeks after cataract surgery with a decrease in central visual acuity.

13. What patients get CME? How is it treated?

CME is more common after intracapsular than extracapsular cataract extraction. It is also more common when vitreous loss occurs, especially if vitreous or iris becomes incarcerated in the wound. It may occur in uncomplicated cases.

Treatment of CME is controversial because a significant percentage of cases resolve spontaneously. Initial treatment often includes topical steroids or nonsteroidal antiinflammatory medications. Acetazolamide has been shown to reduce edema in some cases and is often used as an oral medication. When vitreous or iris is adherent to the wound, lysis of vitreous strands with surgery, Nd:YAG laser, or wound revision may be beneficial.

14. What is a secondary membrane?

A secondary or "after-cataract" membrane develops after extracapsular cataract surgery. The posterior capsule opacifies when persistent lens fibers adhere to the capsule, or the remaining lens fibers undergo metaplasia. Patients typically present with progressive decrease in vision or problems with glare after surgery.

15. When does a secondary membrane develop? How frequently does it occur?

Usually secondary membrane begins to develop several months after surgery, although in many cases the membrane may take 1 year or more to become visually significant. The opacification rate varies from 8–50% in various series.

16. How is a secondary membrane treated? What complications may occur?

A capsulotomy can be performed as a primary or secondary surgical procedure by cutting open the posterior capsule with a needle knife. This technique has been largely replaced by use of the Nd:YAG laser (see figure). Complications of laser capsulotomy include transient intraocular pressure rise, retinal detachment, and CME.

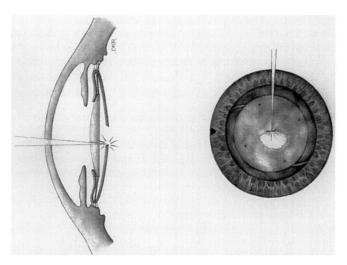

Nd:YAG laser posterior capsulotomy. (From Jaeger E, Tasman W (eds): Clinical Ophthalmology. Philadelphia, J.B. Lippincott, 1995, with permission.)

17. What are the most common complications related to intraocular lenses (IOLs)?

1. **Implantation of the wrong power IOL** may result in unacceptable refraction.

2. **Decentration or dislocation of the IOL** may produce unwanted optical images, including monocular double vision.

3. **Chronic inflammation** may be caused by mechanical chafing of the IOL against the iris or ciliary body. Chronic uveitis and secondary glaucoma, CME, or corneal decompensation may develop.

Patients with these complications may require IOL repositioning or exchange.

18. Why are patients with diabetes at greater risk when undergoing cataract surgery?

Diabetic retinopathy may accelerate dramatically after cataract surgery. This risk is greatest if the posterior capsule ruptures.

19. What are the major problems in managing patients with preexisting glaucoma and cataracts?

1. Many patients have been on glaucoma therapy, including miotics that constrict the pupil. Such therapy may make cataract surgery more difficult and often requires surgical maneuvers to enlarge the pupil.

2. Postoperative pressure may rise because of retained viscoelastic material, and inflammation. This elevation in pressure is often more severe and prolonged in patients with glaucoma. Elevation of pressure may cause additional optic nerve damage and visual field loss and result in loss of central vision in patients with advanced glaucoma. A glaucoma procedure may be combined with cataract surgery in patients with advanced or poorly controlled glaucoma.

3. Patients with glaucoma who have had previous filtration surgery and develop cataracts may require a different approach to cataract surgery. A shift in the location of the incision to avoid damage to the filtration site is often necessary. Inflammation from the surgical procedure may cause failure of a previously functioning filter postoperatively.

BIBLIOGRAPHY

1. Endophthalmitis Vitrectomy Study Group: Results of the Endophthalmitis Vitrectomy Study: A randomized trial of immediate vitrectomy and of intravenous antibiotics for the treatment of postoperative bacterial endophthalmitis. Arch Ophthalmol 113:1479–1496, 1995.

2. Jaeger E, Tasman W (eds): Clinical Ophthalmology. Philadelphia, J.B. Lippincott, 1995.
3. Jaffe GJ, Burton TC, Kuhn E, et al: Progression of nonproliferative diabetic retinopathy and visual outcome after extracapsular cataract extraction and intraocular lens implantation. Am J Ophthalmol 114:448–459, 1992.
4. Jaffe NS: Cataract Surgery and Its Complications, 5th ed. St. Louis, Mosby, 1990.
5. Maloney WF, Grindle L: Textbook of Phacoemulsification. Fallbrook, CA, Lasenda, 1988.
6. Smith SG, Lindstrom RL: Intraocular Lens Complications and their Management. Thorofare, NJ, Slack, 1988.
7. Spaeth GL (ed): Ophthalmic Surgery Principles and Practice, 2nd ed. Philadelphia, W.B. Saunders, 1990.
8. Steinert RF, Fine IH, Gimbel HV, et al (eds): Cataract Surgery: Techniques, Complications, and Management. Philadelphia, W.B. Saunders, 1995.
9. Tipperman R, Lichtenstein SB: LEO Clinical Topic Update: Cataract. San Francisco, American Academy of Ophthalmology, 1996.

V. Ocular Deviations

25. AMBLYOPIA

Steven E. Brooks, M.D.

1. What is amblyopia?

A loss of visual acuity, in one or both eyes, without an identifiable organic lesion of the visual pathways, occurring during the critical period of early visual development.

Because amblyopia is the functional consequence of abnormal visual experience during a sensitive period of development of the visual system, it may be more appropriate to think of amblyopia in a broader sense. For example, amblyopes typically have reduced stereoacuity and binocular visual function and may have altered contrast sensitivity and motion perception. Patients with strabismus develop a profound loss of binocular visual function even though monocular visual acuities may remain intact.

2. Explain the concept of the "critical" or "sensitive" period.

This period is central to amblyopia and describes the time frame early in life during which there is plasticity within the visual system, particularly the visual cortex. This process is not complete at birth but continues until approximately 6 to 9 years of age. In fact, there are probably different critical periods within the visual system for each specific visual function. During this time, normal development depends on normal visual experience. Problems can lead to significant developmental abnormalities at both the structural and functional levels. After the critical period, the visual system is no longer vulnerable to amblyopia. Similarly, it is difficult, if not impossible, to treat amblyopia successfully after the critical period has passed.

3. How is amblyopia classified?

Amblyopia is classified according to the underlying problem that caused it: (1) strabismic, (2) optical defocus, (3) pattern or form deprivation, and (4) congenital or organic.

Optical defocus encompasses anisometropia (asymmetry of refractive error) as well as bilateral severe ametropia (any refractive error). Pattern or form deprivation refers to amblyopia that results from lesions that obstruct the visual axis, such as congenital cataract, corneal opacity, vitreous hemorrhage, or ptosis. Congenital or organic amblyopia refers to the loss of vision that occurs secondary to a congenital organic lesion of the visual pathways such as a macular scar or coloboma. This type of visual loss does not really meet our definition of amblyopia, however, since the causative lesion is identifiable and not treatable. In spite of the fact that there may also be some secondary visual developmental abnormalities present, this cannot be proved.

4. How does strabismus lead to amblyopia?

Strabismus may lead to a loss of vision in one eye if the child develops a preference for the use of one eye over the other. Because of the strabismus, both eyes cannot be used simultaneously without visual confusion or diplopia. Therefore, the image from one or the other eye must be suppressed at all times. If one eye is preferentially used for fixation and the vision from the other eye is chronically suppressed, the nonpreferred eye can become amblyopic. Although suppression is an adaptive and compensatory mechanism for alleviating double vision, amblyopia may be a serious consequence.

5. How prevalent is amblyopia?

In the United States it is estimated to be 2–5%.

6. **What medical or family history factors place children at increased risk for amblyopia?**
Developmental delay
Positive family history
Prematurity
These factors lead to a two- to six-fold increase in a child's chance of developing amblyopia.

7. **What anatomic changes have been shown to occur in amblyopia?**
Although few human data are available, extensive animal studies have shown several neuroanatomic alterations in amblyopia. The primary abnormality appears to be a loss or atrophy of cells in the lateral geniculate nucleus and visual cortex serving the amblyopic eye. These changes can be partially or wholly reversed if the amblyopia is successfully treated.

8. **How early should children be screened for amblyopia?**
The American Academy of Ophthalmology recommends the following time points for routine screening of vision in children:
Newborn to 3 months
6 months to 1 year
3 years
5 years
The optimal time to diagnose and treat amblyopia is as soon as it occurs, but it is critical to do so before the close of the critical period (prior to 5 years of age).

9. **What are some of the ways to check for amblyopia in nonverbal children?**
A unilateral decrease in visual acuity can often be inferred by documenting a significant difference in visual function between the two eyes without ever actually measuring the vision quantitatively. Fixation preference testing is especially useful in this regard (see figure on facing page). In children with manifest strabismus, a lack of spontaneous alternation in visual fixation between the two eyes suggests amblyopia in the nonpreferred eye. In children without strabismus, a vertical tropia can be induced by placing a base-down 10–20 diopter prism in front of one eye. Lack of alternation between the two eyes, or inability to maintain fixation with one eye, suggests amblyopia. Similarly, a child who objects strongly to occlusion of one eye but not the other can be assumed to have decreased vision in the eye that they would allow to be covered. Visual acuity can also be quantitatively assessed in nonverbal children using electrophysiologic testing, such as the visual evoked potential, or by using preferential looking (e.g., Teller acuity cards) tests.

10. **Why is it important to detect amblyopia early in childhood?**
Because the window of opportunity for initially treating amblyopia closes at 5 to 6 years. In addition, earlier detection facilitates more rapid rehabilitation, which is important for compliance. Recurrent amblyopia following initial favorable treatment can often be successfully managed until age 9 or 10 years.

11. **What is the usual presenting complaint of a child with anisometropic amblyopia and at what age?**
Anisometropic amblyopes are generally asymptomatic. The detection of these children depends heavily on effective screening programs. Because of the lack of an overt external sign, such as strabismus or ptosis, the average age at presentation is around 5–6 years, when school-initiated screening programs begin.

12. **Are the underlying neurologic/neuroanatomic changes in amblyopia reversible with treatment?**
Yes, if treatment is started within the critical period. After that, the changes are permanent. Even with early, successful treatment, there is often some minor residual functional abnormality in the amblyopic eye, and some reduction in binocularity.

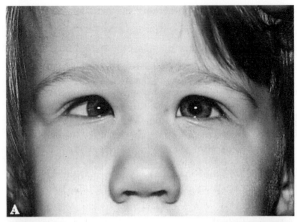

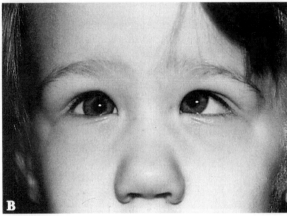

Child with esotropia showing spontaneous alternation in fixation. In *A*, the left eye is used for fixation, whereas in *B* the right eye is used. Alternating fixation is good evidence against the presence of amblyopia in children with strabismus.

13. Besides visual acuity, what other aspects of visual function may be affected in amblyopia?

Binocular vision and stereoacuity   Contrast sensitivity
Motion perception and processing   Spatial localization

14. How does anisometropia lead to amblyopia?

In anisometropia the retinal image in one eye is always defocused. If fixation is not alternated, the chronically defocused eye becomes incapable of processing high-resolution images. In addition, the binocular rivalry between the blurred image in one eye and the clear image in the other eye leads to suppression of the blurred image as a way to avoid visual confusion. This also leads to the development of amblyopia in the chronically blurred and suppressed eye. In the absence of strabismus, this process affects only a small area of the visual field in the foveal region, where high-grade visual acuity is processed and binocular rivalry is poorly tolerated. More peripheral areas of the visual field are not so severely affected. As a result, these patients often display some degree of peripheral sensory fusion and gross stereopsis (monofixation syndrome), and maintain good ocular alignment. Unilateral hyperopia or astigmatism is the most common scenario for anisometropic amblyopia.

15. Which is more likely to produce amblyopia, unilateral or bilateral ptosis, and why?

Unilateral ocular abnormalities are much more likely to lead to amblyopia than binocular ones. If one eye has a competitive advantage over the other, its afferent connections become stronger and more numerous while those of the other eye atrophy and retract. This competition also forms the basis for treating amblyopia. The amblyopic eye, by one means or another, must be given a temporary competitive advantage over the dominant eye.

16. What are the initial steps in treating amblyopia prior to patching?

The first step is to rule out any organic cause for the visual loss and identify the underlying cause for the amblyopia. The second step is to do whatever is necessary to ensure a clear visual axis. For example, this may require removal of a congenital cataract or vitreous hemorrhage. Any significant refractive errors should be corrected, particularly high degrees of astigmatism, hypermetropia, or anisometropia. It may also be helpful, in the course of treatment, to correct even relatively low degrees of hyperopia in an amblyopic eye, since the accommodative efforts of these eyes is sometimes reduced.

17. How long can a child's eye be patched full-time prior to the next follow-up visit without risking the development of amblyopia in the eye being patched (occlusion amblyopia)?

A child can receive full-time occlusion of the sound eye for up to 1 week per year of life before the next follow-up visit without significant risk of inducing occlusion amblyopia.

18. What are some of the risks associated with full-time patching?

Although full-time patching of the sound eye is the most expedient way to reverse amblyopia, there is a risk of inducing occlusion amblyopia in the sound eye if appropriate follow-up is not maintained. Also, the complete absence of any binocular interaction during the patching period may cause a phoria to decompensate into a tropia. Unfortunately, once present, the tropia does not often resolve once patching is discontinued and may require corrective surgery. Part-time patching regimens and penalization (see question 19) do not, in general, predispose to these problems.

19. What are some alternative treatments to patching?

Because the object of amblyopia treatment is to ensure that the amblyopic eye has a competitive advantage over the sound eye, it is possible to accomplish this by means other than patching. **Penalization** refers to the intentional degradation of visual acuity in the sound eye by either optical or pharmacologic means. For example, a child with high hyperopia in both eyes might have the sound eye optically penalized by wearing glasses that correct the refractive error of the amblyopic eye only. Alternatively, the sound eye of the same patient might be effectively blurred with atropine eye drops. **Translucent filters** are also available that can be placed over the spectacle lens of the sound eye in order to degrade the vision. Penalization techniques can be effective, but generally are best suited for patients with a high degree of refractive error in the sound eye who have demonstrated poor compliance with patching and whose level of visual acuity is not worse than 20/100. Penalization can often require several months or more for full efficacy.

20. How can you determine in the office if penalization is likely to work?

Penalization will be effective only if the technique chosen successfully induces the amblyopic eye to be used preferentially for fixation. It is possible to assess this fairly reliably in the office by instituting penalization and then checking whether or not a switch in fixation has indeed occurred.

21. At what point can amblyopia treatment be discontinued?

When the treated eye has a level of acuity equal to the sound eye. The decision is less clear when there is some persistent deficit in visual acuity. If poor compliance can be ruled out, many practitioners continue to patch until no further improvement is noted on three consecutive follow-up visits separated by at least 3–4 weeks. This may be modified by the particular circumstances of the case as well as by the presence of an organic lesion that might reasonably be considered responsible for the residual visual loss. It may also be beneficial to repeat the eye examination and refraction to check for any uncorrected refractive error or structural lesions that may not have been detected during the the initial or previous exams. Once treatment is stopped, the child must be checked periodically until age 8 to 9 years to detect recurrence of the amblyopia. Episodic maintenance treatment during this time is common.

22. What are some of the factors affecting the success of amblyopia treatment?

Age of onset   Compliance with treatment regimen
Depth of amblyopia   Presence of associated ocular anomalies or injuries

23. Can the vision of an amblyopic eye ever improve in adulthood?

Although the critical period has passed, significant improvements in adulthood have been reported in several cases in which the sound eye was lost to enucleation. The presence of central fixation in the amblyopic eye prior to the loss of the sound eye seemed to be the single most important predictor of the extent of visual improvement.

24. Does a compensatory chin-up head posture in a child with ptosis assure that there is no amblyopia?

No. Although somewhat reassuring, a chin-up head posture may be used to achieve peripheral fusion, in spite of amblyopia in one eye. Also, if ptosis is present bilaterally, then the chin-up head posture may serve to improve vision in one eye while still allowing for amblyopia in the fellow eye. It is important to always check for amblyopia in children with ptosis, regardless of head posture.

25. Is color vision affected in amblyopia?

Generally speaking, color vision is not affected by amblyopia, although some investigators have found mild abnormalities in color perception. Eyes with severe amblyopia, particularly those with loss of foveal fixation, tend to demonstrate such abnormalities more consistently than eyes with milder degrees of amblyopia.

26. Does amblyopia cause a relative afferent pupillary defect?

Amblyopia may cause a low-grade relative afferent pupillary defect. However, if an eye suspected of having amblyopia is found to have a relative afferent pupillary defect, it is imperative that organic causes for the visual loss that might account for this finding be carefully ruled out. Interestingly, the presence or absence of a relative afferent pupillary defect has not been found to correlate well with the visual acuity of the amblyopic eye.

27. In which of the following conditions is amblyopia most likely to occur?

(1) Congenital esotropia
(2) Accommodative esotropia
(3) Intermittent exotropia
(4) Constant exotropia

Accommodative esotropia, because patients with this condition, particularly if there is a significant degree of anisometropia, are less likely to alternate fixation than patients with congenital esotropia or exotropia. Cross-fixation is common in patients with congenital esotropia and helps to prevent amblyopia. Patients with intermittent exotropia are unlikely to develop amblyopia, since they spend a fair amount of time being bifoveal. Patients with constant exotropia may develop amblyopia but are less likely to do so than patients with accommodative esotropia because of their tendency to alternate fixation to achieve panoramic viewing.

28. What is the effect of neutral density filters on the vision of an amblyopic eye compared with a normal eye?

The visual acuity of a normal eye will be progressively reduced by neutral density filters, whereas that of an amblyopic eye may remain unchanged or even improve slightly. This has led investigators to believe that the vision in an amblyopic eye more closely resembles the type of vision normally seen under scotopic conditions, which is more dependent on rods than on cones.

29. What is the crowding phenomenon and how is it significant in amblyopia?

The crowding phenomenon refers to a loss of acuity when optotypes are presented close together rather than singly or widely separated. It is seen in both normal and amblyopic eyes but tends to be much more pronounced in amblyopia. It has been suggested that, during the course of treatment, isolated letter acuity improves faster than line acuity, and that treatment success depends on obtaining improvement in line acuity.

CONTROVERSIES

30. Should anisometropia be corrected if amblyopia is *not* present?

Although it is generally agreed that anisometropia should be treated with spectacle correction when amblyopia is present, it is not clear whether anisometropia needs to be corrected in the absence of amblyopia and, if so, what levels warrant empiric correction to prevent amblyopia. Several studies have found a positive relationship between the degree of anisometropia and incidence of amblyopia, whereas others have failed to find such a relationship. The American Academy of Ophthalmology's current preferred practice guidelines regarding amblyopia suggest that anisometropia in excess of 3 diopters myopia, 1.5 diopters hyperopia, and 1.5 diopters of astigmatism be considered for empirical correction in young children in an attempt to minimize the risk of amblyopia. Experimental data in adults suggest that even lower levels of anisometropia can significantly affect high-grade binocular interactions. The presence of anisometropia in a young child should receive sufficient follow-up to ensure that if amblyopia does develop, it is quickly detected and treated.

31. When should strabismus surgery be performed in a patient with amblyopia?

The traditional teaching has been that all amblyopia be completely treated (i.e., to the greatest extent possible) prior to performing strabismus surgery. The arguments in favor of this approach are that the presence of amblyopia will be an obstacle to fusion postoperatively, thus leading to less predictable and less favorable outcomes; that it may be more difficult to detect amblyopia postoperatively using nonverbal fixation preference techniques; and that amblyopic patients may be lost to follow-up after their eyes are aligned.

The arguments in favor of proceeding with surgery during the course of amblyopia treatment include a possible benefit to binocular vision by earlier restoration of alignment, enhanced patient satisfaction by eliminating a cosmetically troublesome condition, and the occasional spontaneous improvement in amblyopia that may occur following surgical realignment. Also, peripheral fusion may still be possible with amblyopia but bifoveal fusion is unlikely, regardless of amblyopia status. Thus, there is little to gain by delaying surgery until the amblyopia is fully treated.

It is likely that the management of any given case will need to be determined by the specifics of that case and that both practice patterns can be effectively utilized, as long as careful attention is paid to the individual patient.

BIBLIOGRAPHY

1. American Academy of Ophthalmology: Amblyopia, preferred practice pattern. San Francisco, American Academy of Ophthalmology, 1992.
2. American Academy of Ophthalmology: Comprehensive pediatric eye evaluation, preferred practice pattern. San Francisco, American Academy of Ophthalmology, 1992.
3. Brooks SE: Amblyopia. Ophthalmol Clin North Am 9:171–184, 1996.
4. Greenwald MJ, Folk ER: Afferent pupillary defects in amblyopia. J Pediatr Ophthalmol Strabismus 20:63–67, 1983.

5. Harwerth RS, Smith EL, Duncan GC, et al: Effects of enucleation of the fixing eye on strabismic ambly-opia in monkeys. Invest Ophthalmol Vis Sci 27:246–254, 1986.

6. Harwerth RS, Smith EL, Duncan GC, et al: Multiple critical periods in the development of the primate visual system. Science 232:235–238, 1986.

7. Lam GC, Repka MX, Guyton DL: Timing of amblyopia therapy relative to strabismus surgery. Ophthalmology 100:1751–1756, 1993.

8. Tongue AC, Cibis GW: Bruckner test. Ophthalmology 88:1041–1044, 1981.

9. Townsend AM, Holmes JM, Evans LS: Depth of anisometropic amblyopia and difference in refraction. Am J Ophthalmol 116:431–436, 1993.

10. Vereecken EP, Brabant P: Prognosis for vision in amblyopia after loss of the good eye. Arch Ophthalmol 102:220–224, 1984.

11. von Noorden GK: Binocular Vision and Ocular Motility, 5th ed. St. Louis, Mosby, 1996.

12. Wiesel TN, Hubel DH: Single-cell responses in striate cortex of kittens deprived of vision in one eye. J Neurophysiol 26:1003–1007, 1963.

13. Wright KW, Walonker F, Edelman P: 10-diopter fixation test for amblyopia. Arch Ophthalmol 99:1242–1246, 1981.

26. ESODEVIATIONS

Scott E. Olitsky, M.D., and Leonard B. Nelson, M.D.

1. What are esodeviations?

A convergent deviation, noted by crossing or inturning of the eyes, is designated by the prefix *eso*.

Esphoria is a latent tendency for the eyes to cross. This latent deviation is normally controlled by fusional mechanisms that provide binocular vision or avoid diplopia. The eye deviates only under certain conditions, such as fatigue, illness, stress, or tests that interfere with the maintenance of normal fusional abilities (such as covering one eye). If the amount of esophoria is large, it may give rise to bothersome symptoms, such as transient diplopia (double vision) or asthenopia (eye strain).

Esotropia is a manifest misalignment of the eyes. The condition may be alternating or unilateral, depending on the vision. In alternating strabismus, either eye may be used for definitive seeing while the fellow eye deviates. Because each eye is used in turn, each develops similar vision. In unilateral esotropia, only one eye is preferred for fixation while the fellow eye consistently crosses. The eye that is constantly crossing is prone to defective central vision during the visually immature period of life (until age 9). In cases of unilateral esotropia, the deviating eye is often part of the description of the misalignment (left esotropia).

2. How common is strabismus in infancy?

Infants are rarely born with their eyes aligned. During the first month of life, alignment may vary intermittently from esotropia to orthotropia to exotropia. Forty percent of newborn infants seem to have straight eyes, 33% may display exotropia, and approximately 3% may be esotropic. Many infants have variable alignment and cannot be neatly classified in any single category. Several large population studies have confirmed that strabismus is common in early infancy.

3. What is pseudoesotropia?

Pseudoesotropia is characterized by the false appearance of esotropia when the visual axes are actually aligned accurately. The appearance may be caused by a flat, broad nasal bridge; prominent epicanthal folds; or a narrow interpupillary distance. An observer sees less sclera nasally than expected, which creates the impression that the eye is turned in toward the nose. Pseudoesotropia can be differentiated from a true manifest deviation by use of the corneal light reflex and the cover–uncover test, when possible. Once pseudoesotropia has been confirmed, parents can be reassured that the child will "outgrow" the appearance of esotropia. As the child grows, the bridge of the nose becomes more prominent and displaces the epicanthal folds so that the sclera medially becomes proportional to the amount visible on the lateral aspect.

4. What is congenital esotropia?

Congenital esotropia describes a condition in which a child develops a convergent strabismus, with no identifiable cause, before the age of 6 months. Because few children who are eventually diagnosed with congenital esotropia are born with the condition, some authors prefer to use the term **infantile esotropia**.

5. What causes congenital esotropia?

Although the cause of congenital esotropia remains unknown, two popular theories attempt to explain its etiology:

1. Worth's "sensory" concept states that congenital esotropia results from a deficit in a purported center in the brain responsible for binocular vision. According to his theory, the goal of restoring binocularity may be hopeless, because there is no way to provide this congenitally absent function.

2. Chavasse's "motor" theory suggests that normal binocular vision may be achieved through facilitation of conditioned reflexes that depend on early ocular alignment. To Chavasse, the primary problem was mechanical. He believed that most congenital esotropes are potentially curable if the deviation can be fully eliminated in infancy. Only theoretical support was available for Chavasse's theory until several investigators began to report favorable binocular results in some infants operated on between 6 months and 2 years of age. These encouraging results became the basis for the theory of early surgery for patients with congenital esotropia.

Because it is rare for a patient with congenital esotropia to develop perfect binocular vision regardless of the age at which it is corrected, many authorities believe that both Worth's and Chavasse's theories play a role in the development of congenital esotropia.

6. What are the characteristics of congenital esotropia?

1. **Size of deviation.** The characteristic angle of congenital esotropia is considerably larger than angles of esotropia acquired later in life (see figure). Average deviations in most series reported in the literature are between 40–60 prism diopters. Some infants may measure 80 prism diopters or more. The diagnosis of congenital esotropia should be reconsidered in a child with a relatively small deviation.

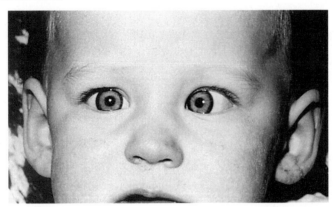

A child with congenital esotropia. Note the characteristic large angle of crossing.

2. **Refractive errors.** Children with congenital esotropia tend to have cycloplegic refractions similar to those of normal children of the same age. These observations contrast markedly with the characteristic hyperopia (farsightedness) associated with accommodative esotropia, especially of the refractive types.

3. **Ocular rotations.** Children with congenital esotropia often appear to exhibit an apparent abduction deficit (inability to turn either eye away from the nose). This pseudoparesis is usually secondary to the presence of cross-fixation. Children with equal vision have no need to abduct either eye. They use the adducted, or crossed, eye to look to the opposite field of gaze. In this case they show a bilateral pseudoparesis of abduction. If amblyopia is present, only the better seeing eye will cross-fixate, making the amblyopic eye appear to have an abduction weakness. A true unilateral or bilateral abducens nerve palsy is uncommon in infancy. To differentiate between a true abducens paralysis and a pseudoparalysis, two techniques may be used. The examiner can evaluate ocular rotations by rotating the infant's head, either with the infant sitting upright in a moveable chair or using a doll's head maneuver. The ability to abduct also can be demonstrated after the infant has worn a patch over one eye for a short time.

7. What is the differential diagnosis of an infant with esotropia?

During the first year of life, a number of conditions can simulate congenital esotropia and cause diagnostic difficulty. Because the management of these conditions may differ markedly from the treatment of congenital esotropia, clinical recognition is important. Many of the other disorders can be ruled out by a thorough ophthalmologic evaluation. For this reason, all infants presenting with esotropia require a full evaluation, including a dilated funduscopic examination. The differential diagnosis includes:

Pseudoesotropia	Congenital sixth nerve palsy
Duane's retraction syndrome	Early-onset accommodative esotropia
Möbius syndrome	Sensory esotropia
Nystagmus blockage syndrome	Esotropia in the neurologically impaired

8. How is vision evaluated in a child with congenital esotropia?

Although it is often not possible to measure absolute visual acuity in a preverbal child, it is possible to detect subtle relative differences in vision between eyes. A child with esotropia fixates with only one eye at a time. If the child constantly fixates with only one eye, it may be assumed that the fellow eye does not see as well. If the child spontaneously alternates fixation or holds fixation with either eye through a blink, the child's vision is most likely equal. The presence of cross-fixation in both eyes (as described in question 6) also may indicate equal vision.

9. How common is amblyopia in congenital esotropia?

Although the association of amblyopia (less than normal vision) and congenital esotropia is well known, it is difficult to ascertain the exact incidence of amblyopia in a disorder that occurs in preverbal children. Amblyopia may occur in as many as 40–72% of infants with congenital esotropia.

10. What are the goals in the treatment of congenital esotropia?

The primary goal of treatment in congenital esotropia is to reduce the distant and near deviation as close to orthotropia (straight eyes) as possible. Ideally, this reduction results in normal sight in each eye, in straight-looking eyes, and in development of at least a rudimentary form of binocular vision. Classically, it has been taught that patients with congenital esotropia do not develop bifoveal fixation (perfect binocular vision), regardless of their age at treatment. Clinical evidence suggests, however, that alignment within 10 prism diopters of orthotropia early in life is associated with the attainment of some degree of binocular vision and stereopsis (depth perception) and is instrumental in maintaining ocular alignment in such patients for the remainder of their lives.

11. How and when is congenital esotropia best treated?

If the child has a significant hyperopic refractive error (usually > +2 diopters), glasses should be prescribed. If the esotropia is still present with the glasses in place, surgery is necessary. Many surgeons prefer to perform a bilateral medial rectus recession. Studies have shown that early surgery is most likely to achieve the desired goals of therapy. Most surgeons attempt to operate on children with congenital esotropia between 6–12 months of age

12. What are the important features to document in the preoperative assessment of a patient with congenital esotropia?

Before contemplating surgery in a child with congenital esotropia, the angle of deviation should be stable, any possibility of accommodative esotropia should be ruled out, and amblyopia, if present, should be treated.

13. Why is it important to treat amblyopia prior to surgical correction of congenital esotropia?

Management of amblyopia in an infant is easier in the presence of large esotropia. Judgment about fixation preference is difficult in a preverbal child with straight eyes. Occlusion therapy in children at a young age generally requires only a small amount of time to equalize vision and therefore does not delay surgical correction to a significant degree. If the vision is not equal after surgery, the chance of developing binocular vision and maintaining ocular alignment is less. In addition, parental incentive to comply with the often arduous task of occlusion therapy is greatly diminished once the child's eyes are straight.

14. What other motility disorders are often associated with congenital esotropia?

Inferior oblique overaction (IOOA). IOOA causes elevation of an eye during adduction (when the eye looks toward the nose). When a patient looks to the side, the adducting eye moves upward (see figure). The incidence of overaction of one or both inferior oblique muscles in patients with congenital esotropia has been reported to be as high as 78%. The onset of IOOA is most common during the second or third year of life. If the elevation in adduction is large, surgical treatment may be indicated.

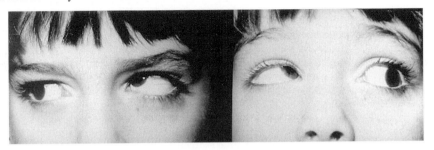

Inferior oblique overaction. As the eye adducts (moves toward the nose), it elevates.

Dissociated vertical deviation (DVD). DVD consists of a slow, upward deviation of one or alternate eyes. Latent DVD may be detected only when the involved eye is covered, whereas manifest DVD occurs intermittently or constantly. The incidence of DVD in patients with congenital esotropia is high, ranging from 46–90%, with onset greatest during the second year of life. If the DVD is large and occurs frequently, surgical treatment may be indicated.

Nystagmus. Rotary and latent nystagmus may occur in children with congenital esotropia. Latent nystagmus is more common than rotary nystagmus. It occurs in approximately 50% of patients. Latent nystagmus is a predominantly horizontal-jerk nystagmus elicited by occluding either eye. The slow phase is toward the side of the occluded eye. Latent nystagmus makes it difficult to obtain an accurate visual acuity measurement when the other eye is occluded completely. Blurring the fellow eye, however, does not manifest the nystagmus, thereby allowing accurate refraction. Both types of nystagmus tend to diminish with time.

15. What is accommodative esotropia?

Accommodative esotropia is defined as a convergent deviation of the eyes associated with activation of the accommodative reflex (see figure). When affected children attempt to focus (accommodate), they develop esotropia.

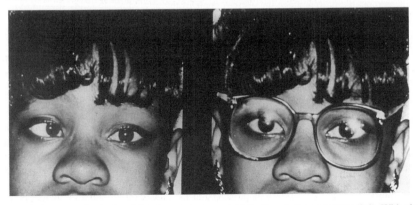

Accommodative esotropia. As the child attempts to accommodate (focus), the eyes cross (*left*). With glasses that eliminate the need to accommodate, the eyes are straight (*right*).

16. What are the three types of accommodative esotropia?
1. Refractive
2. Nonrefractive
3. Partial or decompensated

17. What three factors influence the development of refractive accommodative esotropia?
The mechanism of refractive accommodative esotropia involves uncorrected hyperopia, accommodative convergence, and insufficient fusional divergence. When a person exerts a given amount of accommodation, it is associated with a specific amount of convergence (accommodative convergence). An uncorrected hyperope must exert excessive accommodation to clear a blurred retinal image. This, in turn, stimulates excessive convergence. If the amplitude of fusional divergence is sufficient to correct the excessive convergence, no esotropia results. However, if the fusional divergence amplitudes are inadequate or motor fusion is altered by some sensory obstacle, esotropia results.

18. What is the AC:A ratio?
The AC:A—or accommodative convergence:accommodation—ratio describes how many prism diopters a person's eyes converge for each diopter that they accommodate. The normal AC:A ratio is approximately 3–5 prism diopters of convergence per diopter of accommodation.

19. How can the AC:A ratio be measured?
1. **Heterophoria method.** A strabismic deviation is recorded in prism diopters for distance of 6 meters (D) and near at $\frac{1}{3}$ meter (N). After measuring the patient's interpupillary distance in centimeters (PD), the AC:A ratio can then be calculated as follows:

$$AC:A = (PD) + \frac{N - D}{\text{Near measurement distance (in diopters)}}$$

2. **The gradient method.** A strabismic deviation is measured at distance with any refractive error fully corrected. The deviation is then remeasured at distance through a convex or concave lens. The AC:A ratio is then calculated as:

$$AC:A = \frac{\text{deviation without lens} - \text{deviation with lens}}{\text{dioptric power of lens}}$$

3. **Distance–near comparison.** Most clinicians prefer to assess the ratio using the distance–near comparison. This method is easier and quicker because it uses conventional examination techniques and requires no calculations. The AC:A relationship is derived simply by comparing the distance and near deviation. If the near measurement in an esotropic patient is > 10 prism diopters, the AC:A ratio is considered to be abnormally high.

20. How can refractive accommodative esotropia be treated?
Refractive esotropia can be treated both pharmacologically and optically. Spectacles correct the hyperopic refractive error. While wearing glasses, patients no longer need to accommodate to see well and therefore no longer cross their eyes. Miotics are anticholinesterase inhibitors that alter the AC:A ratio so that a given amount of accommodation leads to a smaller amount of accommodative convergence.

21. Why are spectacles a better option than miotics in the treatment of refractive accommodative esotropia?
Miotics control accommodation less reliably than glasses. Although 50% of patients show a similar response to miotics and spectacles, 40% respond significantly less to miotics and 10% do not respond at all. Miotics may cause pupillary cysts and, in adults, retinal detachments and cataracts. In addition, miotics may result in prolonged apnea after anesthesia if succinylcholine is used. At best, they often only delay the inevitable use of spectacles.

22. What is the relationship between accommodative esotropia and congenital esotropia?

Recurrent esotropia may occur in 28% of patients who have been successfully treated for congenital esotropia. Almost 80% respond to correction of hyperopia. The level of hyperopia leading to the recurrent deviation may be low. Patients may be prone to development of an accommodative esotropia secondary to underlying poor binocular function.

23. What is nonrefractive accommodative esotropia?

Nonrefractive accommodative esotropia is associated with a high accommodative convergence to accommodation (AC:A) ratio. The effort to accommodate elicits an abnormally high accommodative convergence response. The level of hyperopia is usually normal for the patient's age. The required amount of accommodation is not abnormal, but rather the amount of accommodative convergence associated with the accommodation. The amount of esotropia is greater at near than at distance because of the additional accommodation required to maintain a clear image at near.

24. How can nonrefractive accommodative esotropia be treated?

Nonrefractive accommodative esotropia can be treated with bifocals, miotics, or surgery. A bifocal eliminates the additional accommodative effort required at near and therefore reduces the near esotropia. Miotics may be used to reduce the AC:A ratio but have the potential side effects mentioned in question 21. Surgery may be performed to eliminate the esotropia at near and to correct the AC:A ratio permanently.

Some pediatric ophthalmologists choose simply to observe patients as long as their eyes remain straight at distance. The esotropia at near may resolve on its own as the AC:A ratio normalizes during childhood. Amblyopia rarely occurs in these patients.

25. What is partial or decompensated accommodative esotropia?

Refractive or nonrefractive accommodative esotropias do not always occur in their "pure" forms. Glasses with or without bifocals may reduce esodeviation significantly. The residual esodeviation that persists despite full hyperopic correction is called the deteriorated or nonaccommodative portion. This condition commonly occurs with a delay of months between onset of accommodative esotropia and antiaccommodative treatment. Sometimes the esotropia initially may be eliminated with glasses, but a nonaccommodative portion slowly becomes evident despite the maximal amount of hyperopic correction consistent with good vision.

Surgery for partial or decompensated accommodative esotropia may be indicated if the deviation is larger than an amount that allows development of binocular vision. Surgery is generally performed for the nonaccommodative portion of the esotropia only, not for the full deviation that is present without glasses in place.

26. What is nystagmus blockage syndrome?

The nystagmus blockage syndrome is characterized by nystagmus that begins in early infancy and is associated with esotropia. The nystagmus is reduced or absent with the fixating eye in adduction. As the fixating eye follows a target moving laterally toward the primary position and then into abduction, the nystagmus increases and the esotropia decreases. A head turn develops in the direction of the uncovered eye when the fellow eye is occluded. This abnormal head posture allows the uncovered eye to persist in an adducted position.

27. What is cyclic esotropia?

Cyclic strabismus is a relatively rare disorder of ocular motility that classically describes a large-angle esotropia alternating with orthophoria or a small-angle esodeviation on a 48-hour cycle. The duration of the cycle may be as short as 2 weeks, in which case the diagnosis may be missed, or it may persist for several years before becoming a constant deviation. It may result from an aberration in the biologic clock or a combination of defects in the clock, oculomotor nuclei, superior colliculi, or other nuclei. Cyclic esotropia is noted for its unpredictable response to various forms of therapy with the exception of surgery, which is usually curative.

28. What is acute acquired comitant esotropia (AACE)?

AACE is a rare condition that occurs in older children and adults. It is characterized by the dramatic onset of a relatively large angle of esotropia with diplopia. Patients usually have a mild hyperopic refractive error. Although there may be a brief period of intermittency, the esodeviation soon becomes constant. AACE has been reported after periods of interruption of fusion, such as occlusion therapy for amblyopia in patients in whom no deviation was initially noted or after brief occlusion for a corneal abrasion. Other patients develop AACE with no obvious exogenous cause precipitating the esotropia.

Children and adults who develop acute esotropia must undergo a careful motility analysis to rule out a paretic deviation. If the ophthalmic examination is otherwise negative and the neurologic physical examination is normal, it is still unclear whether further work-up, including computed tomographic (CT) or magnetic resonance imaging (MRI), may be warranted.

BIBLIOGRAPHY

1. Archer SM, Sondhi N, Helveston EM: Strabismus in infancy. Ophthalmology 96:133–137, 1989.
2. Hiles DA, Watson A, Biglan AW: Characteristics of infantile esotropia following early bimedial rectus recession. Arch Ophthalmol 98:697–703, 1980.
3. Ing M, Costenbader FD, Parks MM, Albert DG: Early surgery for congenital esotropia. Trans Am Ophthalmol 62:1419–1427, 1966.
4. Nelson LB: Strabismus Disorders. In Nelson LB (ed): Pediatric Ophthalmology. Philadelphia, W.B. Saunders, 1991, pp 128–143.
5. Parks MM, Wheeler MB: Concomitant esodeviations. In Tasman W, Jaegers EA (eds): Duane's Clinical Ophthalmology, vol 1 [looseleaf]. Philadelphia, Lippincott-Raven, 1990, pp 1–14.
6. Raab EL: Etiologic factors in accommodative esodeviation. Trans Am Ophthalmol Soc 80:657–694, 1982.
7. Steele MA, Furlan LE, Howard NM: Congenital esotropia. Ophthalmol Clin North Am 9:161–171, 1996.
8. Von Noorden GK: A reassessment of infantile esotropia (XLIV Edward Jackson Memorial Lecture). Am J Ophthalmol 105:1–10, 1988.

27. MISCELLANEOUS OCULAR DEVIATIONS

Janice A. Gault, M.D.

1. What is the differential diagnosis of exotropia?

- Congenital exotropia
- Sensory exotropia
- Third-nerve palsy
- Duane syndrome
- Craniofacial abnormalities with divergent orbit (e.g., Apert or Crouzon syndrome)
- Myasthenia gravis
- Thyroid disorder
- Medial wall fracture
- Slipped medial rectus muscle or excessively resected lateral rectus
- Orbital inflammatory pseudotumor
- Convergence insufficiency
- Internuclear ophthalmoplegia

2. A mother notices that her 4-month-old child seems to be "wall-eyed." What is your concern?

First, check whether deviation or pseudostrabismus is present. A wide interpupillary distance or temporal dragging of the macula from retinopathy of prematurity or toxocariasis may cause pseudoexotropia. The light reflex test or cover testing elucidates this point. Also, make sure that the eyes move normally. Have the patient follow a light or brightly colored toy to exclude paralysis or muscle restriction. If this test is normal and you notice true strabismus, quantify it at near and far. Check the cycloplegic refraction, and do a full dilated exam. Anisometropic amblyopia may cause an eye to deviate, but usually esotropia presents in the younger age group. Also, a corneal lesion, cataract, glaucoma, or retinal lesion such as a toxoplasmosis scar or retinoblastoma may cause the deviation. These conditions must be ruled out.

Once you have determined that the remainder of the exam is normal, you realize that the infant has an alternating exotropia of 40 prism diopters. Congenital exotropia is much rarer than congenital esotropia, but they have much in common. Both have a large angle of deviation and rarely develop amblyopia because of alternating fixation. The refractive error is normal. Early surgery is recommended.

3. A mother notices that her 2-year-old boy has a left eye that deviates outward when he is tired or has a fever. What is your concern?

Intermittent exotropia, which is the most common type of exotropia. The onset varies from infancy to 4 years. It may progress through three phases:

- **Phase one.** Exophoria at distance and orthophoria at near occur when the patient is fatigued or daydreaming. He has diplopia and often closes one eye. When aware of the deviation, he is easily able to straighten his eyes, often after a blink.
- **Phase two.** Exotropia at distance and exophoria at near. When the exotropia becomes more constant, suppression develops and the diplopia becomes less frequent. The exotropia remains after a blink.
- **Phase three.** The exotropia is constant at distance and near. There is no diplopia because of suppression.

Vision must be equalized by correcting any significant refractive error and patching the nondeviating eye. Surgery should be done when the patient progresses beyond phase one, but preferably before phase three.

4. An 18-year-old patient complains of blurred near vision and headaches while reading. Do you believe her, or is she jus trying to get out of doing her homework?

Check her ocular deviations at near and far. She may be experiencing convergence insufficiency, which is common in teenagers and young adults. It is often idiopathic but may be exacerbated by fatigue, drugs, uveitis, or an Adie's tonic pupil. Exodeviation is greater at near than at distance and causes asthenopia. Exophoria at near may be all that is seen. The near point of convergence is more distant than normal, and the amplitude of accommodation is reduced.

Because she is symptomatic, treat her with base-in prisms for reading to help convergence. Near point exercises or "pencil push-ups" can improve fusional amplitudes. These exercises are performed by focusing on the eraser of a pencil while slowly moving it from arm's length closer toward the face. Have the patient concentrate on maintaining one image of the eraser. Repeat 10 times several times a day. Rarely, medial rectus resection may be necessary.

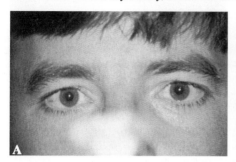

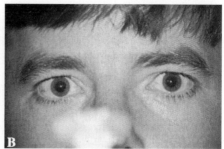

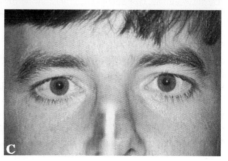

A, Convergence insufficiency. When fixating on a near target at a comfortable distance, the patient has single vision. B, However, when the target is moved closer, the left eye drifts and the patient experiences diplopia. He has a distant near point of convergence. C, By practicing near point exercises by moving a pencil target forward and backward to improve convergence ability, the symptoms may be reduced. (From Tasman W, Jaeger EA: The Wills Eye Hospital Atlas of Clinical Ophthalmology. Philadelphia, Lippincott-Raven, with permission.)

5. What if the fusional capacities are normal and there is no exodeviation?

The problem may be accommodative insufficiency, which has similar symptoms in the same age group. However, accommodation is reduced. First check the manifest and cycloplegic refraction. The patient may be underplussed and need a stronger hyperopic refraction. If refraction is normal, plus lens reading glasses will help.

6. Some patients have the opposite problem: esotropia that is worse at distance than near. What is this condition called?

Divergence insufficiency. Fusional divergence is reduced. Treatment is with base-out prisms and rarely lateral rectus resections. However, divergence insufficiency is a diagnosis of exclusion, and divergence paralysis must be ruled out because it may be associated with pontine tumors, head trauma, and other neurologic abnormalities. Neuroophthalmic evaluation is necessary.

7. What is Duane syndrome? What are the different types?

Duane syndrome is a motility disorder characterized by limited abduction, limited adduction, or both. The globe retracts, and the palpebral fissure narrows on attempted adduction. A "leash effect" may cause upward deviation at the same time. There are three types:
- Type 1—limited abduction (most common)
- Type 2—limited adduction
- Type 3—both limited abduction and limited adduction (rarest type)

There are three females to every two males afflicted with Duane syndrome. The left eye is involved in 60% of cases; in 18% of cases, both eyes are involved. Sixty percent of patients also have an associated esotropia, 15% have exotropia, and 25% are orthophoric. A and V patterns are common. Amblyopia, attributable to anisometropia, occurs in approximately one-third of cases. Surgery is done to correct a head turn, but resection should not be performed because it exacerbates the narrowing of the fissure and globe retraction.

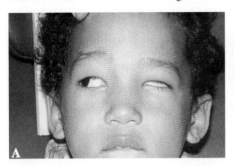 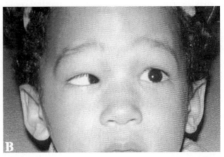

Duane syndrome, type 1, left eye. *A,* Note the narrowing of palpebral fissures on attempted adduction. *B,* The patient cannot abduct the left eye. (From Tasman W, Jaeger EA: The Wills Eye Hospital Atlas of Clinical Ophthalmology. Philadelphia, Lippincott-Raven, with permission.)

8. What is the cause of Duane syndrome?

The cause is unclear, but it appears that the lateral rectus muscle is innervated by the third nerve, causing cocontraction of the medial and lateral rectus muscle. This theory explains the globe retraction and fissure narrowing.

9. What other features may be associated with Duane syndrome?

Goldenhar's syndrome, deafness, crocodile tears, and uveal colobomas.

10. What is the differential diagnosis of hypertropia?

- Myasthenia gravis
- Thyroid eye disease
- Orbital inflammatory pseudotumor
- Orbital trauma (may cause inferior rectus entrapment)
- Fourth cranial nerve palsy
- Pseudohypertropia
- Skew deviation—any vertical deviation without restriction on forced duction testing that cannot be mapped out with the three-step test to isolate a particular muscle. The posterior fossa must be evaluated with computed tomography (CT) or magnetic resonance imaging (MRI).

11. What is Brown's syndrome?

Patients are unable to elevate the affected eye when adducted, and the eye may be hypotropic in primary gaze (see figure at top of next page). Elevation in abduction is normal. A compensatory head turn away from the affected eye with a chin-up position can be seen. The syndrome is bilateral in 10% of cases. Forced ductions reveal restriction of the superior oblique muscle.

12. What is the cause of Brown's syndrome?

Brown's syndrome may be congenital or acquired. The cause may be related to mechanical restriction of the superior oblique tendon. Examples include trauma, surgery, or inflammation in the region near the trochlea.

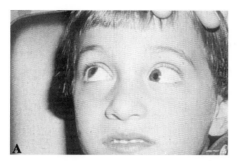

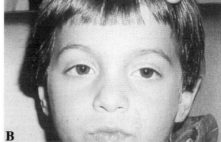

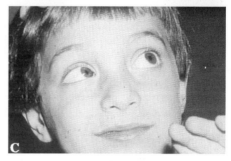

Brown's syndrome of the left eye. *A,* When looking up and to the right, the left eye is unable to elevate. *B,* In primary position, the eyes are straight; there is no compensatory head turn. *C,* When the patient looks up and to the left, both eyes elevate normally. (From Tasman W, Jaeger EA: The Wills Eye Hospital Atlas of Clinical Ophthalmology. Philadelphia, Lippincott-Raven, with permission.)

13. How is Brown's syndrome treated?

Acquired cases may be observed because they may improve spontaneously. Some improve with steroid injections near the trochlea. If no improvement is seen by 6 months, the superior oblique muscle may be weakened with a tenotomy. Some surgeons recess the ipsilateral inferior oblique at the same time to prevent an inferior oblique overaction postoperatively. Patients need to be aware that they will never be able to elevate the affected eye normally in adduction.

14. What is the differential diagnosis of Brown's syndrome?

1. **Inferior oblique palsy.** The three-step test reveals a superior oblique overaction that is not present in Brown's syndrome. In patients with diplopia, vertical deviations in primary gaze, or an abnormal head position, a superior oblique tenotomy or recession of the contralateral superior rectus is done. Forced ductions reveal no restriction.

2. **Double elevator palsy.** Patients cannot elevate the affected eye in any field of gaze. Ptosis or pseudoptosis may be seen. A chin-up position helps to maintain fusion if a hypotropia is present in primary gaze. If no chin-up position is seen with hypotropia, amblyopia is present. Treatment for a large vertical deviation or an abnormal head position is inferior rectus recession if the inferior rectus is restricted or transposition of the medial and lateral rectus toward the superior rectus (Knapp procedure) if no restriction is present.

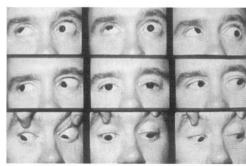

Double elevator palsy of the left eye. Because of the small hypotropia of the left eye, the patient has a small chin elevation in primary position. (From Tasman W, Jaeger EA: The Wills Eye Hospital Atlas of Clinical Ophthalmology. Philadelphia, Lippincott-Raven, with permission.)

3. **Blowout fracture with entrapment of the inferior rectus muscle.** History elucidates this injury, and forced ductions show restriction. Confirm with an orbital CT scan.

4. **Thyroid disease.** Restriction is found on forced ductions, the strabismus is acquired and incomitant, and lid retraction also may be noted. CT scan reveals enlarged extraocular muscles.

15. What is Möbius syndrome?

A congenital syndrome with varying abnormalities of the fifth through twelfth cranial nerves. Patients may have a unilateral or bilateral esotropia with inability to abduct the eyes even on doll's head maneuvers. Patients also may exhibit limb, chest, and tongue defects. They may have significant feeding difficulties.

16. A 48-year-old man undergoes medial rectus and lateral rectus resections for a sensory exotropia of 35 prism diopters in the left eye. He presents the next day with an exotropia of 60 prism diopters in primary position and an inability to abduct the eye. What is your diagnosis?

A slipped or lost medial rectus muscle. It is important to double-lock the suture through the tendon and muscle when reattaching the rectus muscle to the globe to prevent this complication. Reoperation is necessary to find the muscle and reattach it in the appropriate position. If you cannot locate the muscle, a transposition of the superior and inferior rectus muscles helps to correct the esotropia.

17. A patient complains that her right eye is hypertropic. The light reflex test and covering test show her to be orthophoric. What may be going on?

Pseudohypertropia. She may have a vertically displaced macula from retinopathy of prematurity or toxocariasis. Lid retraction of the right eye may cause the right eye to appear hypertropic. Vertical displacement of the globe superiorly by a mass, such as a mucocele, may cause a similar appearance.

18. A young boy has developed chin-up position and seems to move his head rather than his eyes to locate objects. On examination, he has poor ductions and versions in all fields of gaze as well as bilateral ptosis. Forced ductions reveal restrictions in all extraocular muscles. What is your diagnosis?

Congenital fibrosis syndrome. The normal muscle tissue is replaced by fibrous tissue to varying degrees. It may be unilateral or bilateral. The eyes may exhibit little-to-no vertical or horizontal movements, depending on the number of muscles involved as well as eso- or exotropia. Amblyopia is common. Ptosis with chin elevation is a frequent manifestation. The cause is unknown. The goal of surgery is to restore straight eyes in primary gaze.

19. A 20-year-old man with no history of strabismus complains that he cannot open his eyes well. You notice that ductions and versions are severely reduced and that he has bilateral ptosis. There is no restriction on forced ductions. What is your diagnosis?

Chronic progressive external ophthalmoplegia (CPEO). This condition begins in childhood with ptosis and progresses slowly to total paresis of the lids and extraocular muscles (see figure at top of next page). It may be sporadic or familial. Patients usually do not have diplopia. A frontalis sling procedure may be necessary to elevate the lids.

20. What other evaluations are important?

Check for retinal pigmentations, and order an electrocardiogram to check for heart block. The triad of CPEO, retinal pigmentary changes, and cardiomyopathy is known as Kearns-Sayre syndrome (see figure at bottom of next page). Patients may require pacemakers to prevent sudden death. Inheritance is by maternal mitochondrial DNA.

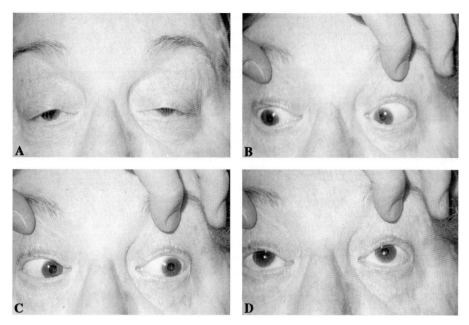

Chronic progressive external ophthalmoplegia (*A, B, C,* and *D*) with bilateral ptosis and limited extraocular movements in all directions. (From Tasman W, Jaeger EA: The Wills Eye Hospital Atlas of Clinical Ophthalmology. Philadelphia, Lippincott-Raven, with permission.)

21. What other diseases may be associated with CPEO?

1. **Abetalipoproteinemia (Bassen-Kornzweig syndrome).** Patients have retinal pigmentary changes similar to retinitis pigmentosa (RP), diarrhea, ataxia, and other neurologic signs.

2. **Refsum's disease.** Patients have an RP-like syndrome with an increased phytanic acid level. They also may have neurologic signs.

3. **Ocular pharyngeal dystrophy.** Patients have difficulty with swallowing. The condition may be autosomal dominant.

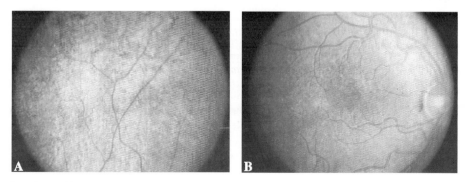

In patients with Kearns-Sayre syndrome (*A* and *B*), the pigmentary disturbance may involve the macular as well as the periphery. (From Tasman W, Jaeger EA: The Wills Eye Hospital Atlas of Clinical Ophthalmology. Philadelphia, Lippincott-Raven, with permission.)

22. A 32-year-old woman complains of intermittent double vision, which occurs more often toward the end of the day. Her lids droop significantly by evening. On awakening, she does not have these problems. What is your diagnosis?

You must be concerned about myasthenia gravis. Have the patient stare at the ceiling for several minutes and see if her ptosis worsens. Compare the orbicularis strength before and after this maneuver. The strabismus is usually variable. Myasthenia gravis is an autoimmune disease that may occur at any age. Antibodies are directed at the acetylcholine receptor. The disease may be purely ocular or systemic. Ask whether the patient has difficulty with swallowing or breathing. Diagnosis is supported with a positive Tensilon test and acetylcholine receptor antibodies. Also check thyroid functions because concurrent thyroid disease is common. A CT scan to rule out thymoma is important. Some patients with thymomas have significant improvement of symptoms once the lesion is removed. Treatment includes an oral anticholinesterase, such as pyridostigmine; corticosteroids; and immunosuppressives.

23. How is a Tensilon test performed?

Inject 0.2 ml of edrophonium chloride (Tensilon) intravenously. Observe for 1 minute. If ptosis or diplopia improves, the test is considered positive. Improvement also may be noted on electromyograph (EMG). If no untoward reaction to the medicine or improvement occurs, inject an additional 0.4 ml and wait 30 seconds. Another 0.4 ml may be injected if no response occurs. If 2 more minutes pass without reaction, the test is negative. However, a negative test does not rule out the diagnosis. Because a cholinergic crisis may occur during the test, 0.4 mg of atropine should be on hand to administer intravenously.

24. What conditions can mimic myasthenia gravis?

- Eaton-Lambert syndrome—a paraneoplastic syndrome from a carcinoma elsewhere, usually the lung
- Medications such as penicillamine and aminoglycosides
- Thyroid eye disease—incomitant strabismus
- Orbital inflammatory pseudotumor—also produces incomitant strabismus, but distinguished by pain with ocular movements and proptosis.
- Levator muscle dehiscence—a cause of ptosis but not variable with fatigue
- CPEO—no diurnal variation; Tensilon test usually negative

25. What is congenital ocular motor apraxia?

In this rare disorder patients are unable to generate normal voluntary horizontal saccades. To change horizontal fixation, a head thrust that overshoots the target is made. The head is then rotated back in the opposite direction once fixation is established. Vertical saccades are normal, but vestibular and optokinetic nystagmus are impaired. Strabismus may be associated.

26. A patient complains of diplopia. On exam, he has paresis of the third, fourth, and fifth cranial nerves on the right side. What can cause multiple ocular motor nerve palsies?

Anything that damages the cavernous sinus and/or superior orbital fissure, including the following:

- Arteriovenous fistula—carotid-cavernous or dural-cavernous
- Cavernous sinus thrombosis
- Tumors metastatic to cavernous sinus
- Skin malignancy with perineural spread to cavernous sinus
- Pituitary apoplexy—patients often have extreme headache with bilateral signs and decreased vision. They need emergent intravenous steroids and neurosurgical consultation.
- Intracavernous aneurysm
- Mucormycosis—more likely in diabetics, especially in ketoacidosis, and any debilitated or immunocompromised patient. Look for an eschar in the nose and palate. Emergent consultation with otolaryngology for debridement is imperative.

- Herpes zoster
- Tolosa-Hunt syndrome—inflammation of the superior orbital fissure or anterior cavernous sinus (diagnosis of exclusion)
- Mucocele
- Meningioma
- Nasopharyngeal carcinoma

Multiple cranial nerve palsies also may occur with brainstem lesions and carcinomatous meningitis. Other entities that can mimic multiple cranial nerve palsies include:

- Myasthenia gravis
- CPEO
- Orbital lesions such as thyroid disease, pseudotumor, or tumors
- Progressive supranuclear palsy
- Guillain-Barré syndrome

27. What is Parinaud's syndrome?

Also known as dorsal midbrain syndrome, Parinaud's syndrome is characterized by a supranuclear gaze paresis with nuclear oculomotor paresis and pupillary abnormalities. Active upward gaze is diminished, but elevation is seen with doll's head maneuver. Attempts at upward gaze cause retraction-convergence nystagmus and palpebral fissure widening (Collier's sign). Pupils are mid-dilated and do not react to light but react normally to accommodation.

28. What is the cause of Parinaud's syndrome?

In children, pinealoma and aqueductal stenosis are the most common causes. In adults, demyelination, infarct, and tumor are most common.

29. Describe the presentation of a patient with internuclear ophthalmoplegia (INO).

A young woman with a history of optic neuritis complains of double vision when looking to one side. She is unable to adduct on attempted contralateral gaze and exhibits horizontal nystagmus in the abducting eye. Adduction on convergence is normal. The condition may be unilateral or bilateral. Exotropia may be present if the condition is bilateral.

30. Where is the causative lesion?

In the medial longitudinal fasciculus. Causes include multiple sclerosis, ischemic vascular disease, brainstem tumor, and trauma.

BIBLIOGRAPHY

1. American Academy of Ophthalmology: Pediatric Ophthalmology and Strabismus. 1992.
2. Cullom RD, Chang B: The Wills Eye Manual: Office and Emergency Room Diagnosis and Treatment of Eye Disease, 2nd ed. Philadelphia, J.B. Lippincott, 1994.
3. Nelson LB, Catalano RA: Atlas of Ocular Motility. Philadelphia, W.B. Saunders, 1989.

28. STRABISMUS SURGERY

Bruce M. Schnall, M.D.

1. How are forced ductions performed?

Before beginning surgery, a lid speculum is placed in both eyes. Using one- or two-toothed forceps, the conjunctiva is grasped at the limbus. The eye is moved horizontally and vertically. The resistance encountered in moving the eye is compared with what normally would be expected as well as with the resistance encountered in performing the same forced duction on the other eye.

2. Why perform forced ductions?

Forced ductions are performed to detect "tight muscles" or restrictions in eye movement. If the forced ductions indicate that a muscle is restricted, the affected muscle should be recessed. For example, if a patient has a vertical deviation, the superior rectus on the hypertropic side or the inferior rectus on the fellow eye may be recessed. If forced ductions show resistance to elevating the fellow eye, the preferred surgery is recession of the inferior rectus.

3. When correcting a horizontal or vertical strabismus, how do you decide how many muscles to recess or resect?

The angle of the deviation determines the number of muscles to recess or resect. Whereas a small-angle strabismus (< 20 diopters) may be corrected by operating on one muscle only, a large deviation may require surgery on three or four rectus muscles. Most major texts contain tables that provide a guide as to how much surgery should be performed for the angle (measured in prism diopters) of strabismus. The tables indicate how many muscles should be operated on and the amount of recession or resection.

4. When doing a recess-resect procedure, should you first perform the recession or the resection?

The recession is performed first. In a resection the muscle is shortened and then brought forward to the insertion. This procedure creates tension on the resected muscle, making it difficult to bring the resected muscle to the insertion site. Initial recession of the yoke muscle decreases the tension pulling the globe away from the resected muscle and makes it easier to bring the resected muscle to the insertion site and to tie the sutures on the resected muscle.

5. When performing surgery on an oblique muscle and rectus muscle of the same eye, on which muscle do you operate first?

The oblique muscles are more difficult to identify and isolate on the muscle hook than the recti. Strabismus surgery creates swelling of Tenon's capsule and bleeding, which can obscure the view and make identification of the oblique muscles difficult. Therefore, it is preferable to operate on the oblique muscles first, when Tenon's capsule and the tissues surrounding the oblique muscles are the least swollen and distorted. The recti are more easily hooked and identified. There should be no difficulty in isolating the correct rectus muscle, even in the presence of significant bleeding and swelling of Tenon's capsule associated with oblique muscle surgery.

6. What type of needle is used to suture the muscle to the sclera?

A spatulated needle, which has its cutting surfaces on the side, decreases the risk of perforating the globe. The sclera is thinnest just posterior to the insertion of the rectus muscles (0.3 mm).

7. What is an adjustable suture?

Various techniques of placing and tying scleral sutures allow the muscle to be moved forward or backward during the immediate postoperative period. If a patient has an immediate overcorrection or undercorrection, the muscle can be moved to improve the alignment. This suture adjustment is performed within 24 hours of the initial surgery.

8. When should an adjustable suture be used?

The use of an adjustable suture is at the discretion of the surgeon. Some surgeons do not perform adjustable suture surgery, pointing to the fact that the correction seen immediately after strabismus surgery is variable and may not be indicative of the long-term result. Others use adjustable sutures in cases in which the results of strabismus surgery are difficult to predict, such as reoperations and restrictive or paralytic strabismus. They are used often in patients with thyroid disease.

9. What is a transposition procedure?

A transposition procedure usually involves the placement of either part or all of the tendon of the adjacent recti muscles to the insertion of the palsied or underacting muscle. For instance, in double elevator palsy the tendon of the lateral and medial recti may be sutured to the nasal and temporal borders of the superior rectus insertion.

10. When is a transposition procedure performed?

A transposition procedure is the procedure of choice when one or more recti muscles are severely limited, as with third nerve, sixth nerve, or double elevator palsy.

11. How are A and V patterns of strabismus treated?

In cases of oblique muscle overaction, the appropriate oblique muscle should be weakened. Weakening of the inferior obliques corrects a V pattern, whereas weakening of the superior obliques corrects an A pattern. In patients with no oblique muscle dysfunction, the horizontal recti are "supraplaced" or "infraplaced." The medial recti are displaced toward the point of the A or V, whereas the lateral recti are moved in the opposite direction. For example, to treat a V pattern esotropia without oblique muscle overaction, the medial recti are recessed and infraplaced (moved inferiorly) by one-half of the tendon width.

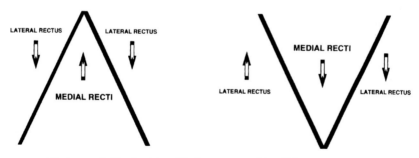

Displacement of horizontal recti in the treatment of A and V pattern strabismus.

12. What surgery can be done for Brown's syndrome?

In Brown's syndrome, a congenitally short or tight superior oblique tendon creates a mechanical restriction of elevation when the eye is in adduction, as confirmed at surgery with forced duction testing. Brown's syndrome is treated surgically by superior oblique tenotomy, recession, or a tendon expander.

13. What are the indications for surgery in Brown's syndrome?

Hypertropia in primary gaze or abnormal head position (face-turn or chin-up position).

14. List the most common complications of strabismus surgery.
- Infection
- Scleral perforation
- Granuloma at the incision site
- Adherence syndrome
- Anterior segment ischemia
- Slipped muscle
- Lost muscle
- Operating on the wrong muscle

15. What are the signs of infection after strabismus surgery?

Infection may take the form of cellulitis, subconjunctival abscess, or endophthalmitis. Cellulitis is most common with an estimated incidence between 1 case in 1000 and 1 case in 1900 surgeries. It typically occurs 2–3 days after surgery. The most common symptoms are marked swelling and pain. Suspected cellulitis requires prompt treatment with systemic antibiotics as well as careful examination to make certain that the patient does not develop endophthalmitis.

16. What should you do if you suspect that you perforated the globe when passing the scleral suture?

If a scleral perforation is suspected, indirect ophthalmoscopy should be performed in the operating room at completion of the strabismus surgery. If a retinal perforation is seen on ophthalmoscopy, retinal consultation or repeat examinations with the indirect ophthalmoscope are indicated. Treatment is controversial. Whereas some surgeons advocate treatment with cryotherapy or indirect laser, others simply observe the patient. The incidence of retinal detachment after scleral perforation is believed to be low. At the same time, cryotherapy may increase the incidence of retinal detachment by stimulating vitreous changes. In patients predisposed to retinal detachment (for example, high myopes), however, serious consideration should be given to treatment of a retinal perforation at the time of strabismus surgery. Some strabismus surgeons believe that scleral perforation increases the risk of endophthalmitis and therefore recommend sub-Tenon's injection of prophylactic antibiotics if the globe is perforated.

17. What is a slipped muscle?

The muscle is contained within a capsule. In operating on a rectus muscle, it is possible to engage only the capsule on the suture. After the muscle is reattached to the eye, it may slip back within its capsule. The result is further weakening of the muscle and consecutive deviation. For instance, if a slipped muscle occurred in recessing a medial rectus muscle for esotropia, exotropia and limited adduction will develop in the involved eye over time.

18. How is a slipped muscle prevented?

In placing the suture through the muscle, locking bites are made on either end of the muscle. Locking bites should be made by placing the suture through the muscle perpendicular to its insertion, engaging the tendon, rather than tangentially. Tangential placement may engage only the capsule.

19. What is the adherence syndrome?

The orbital fat is separated from the globe by Tenon's capsule. If an accidental opening is made in the portion of Tenon's capsule that separates the orbital fat from sclera, orbital fat may be pressed through the opening and become adherent to the globe. This adherence often results in limited eye moments. It is best treated by prevention. The orbital fat comes forward around the equator of the globe to within 10 mm of the limbus. Care should be taken not to cut Tenon's capsule more than 10 mm from the limbus.

20. How can strabismus surgery cause anterior segment ischemia?

The anterior ciliary arteries accompany the recti muscles. They penetrate the sclera at the muscle's insertion site, contributing significantly to the blood supply of the anterior segment. In standard strabismus surgery the anterior ciliary vessels are cut when the rectus muscle is disinserted.

21. How is anterior segment ischemia avoided?

By not operating on more than two recti muscles in one eye at the same time. It is also possible to dissect the anterior ciliary vessels from the rectus muscle and preserve them. Surgery to preserve the anterior ciliary vessels is performed only when the risk of anterior segment ischemia is high, such as in older patients with cardiovascular disease or patients with a history of previous rectus muscle surgery.

BIBLIOGRAPHY

1. Kivlin JD, Wilson ME, and the Periocular Infection Study Group: Periocular infection after strabismus surgery. J Pediatr Ophthalmol Strabismus 32:42–49, 1995.
2. McKeown CA, Shore JW, Lambert HM: Preservation of the anterior ciliary vessels during extraocular muscle surgery. Ophthalmology 96:498–506, 1989.
3. Parks MM: Atlas of Strabismus Surgery. New York, Harper & Row, 1983.
4. Parks MM, Bloom JN: The "slipped muscle." Ophthalmology 86:1389–1396, 1979.
5. Plager DA, Helveston EM: Transposition procedures. In Tasman W, Jaeger EA (eds): Duane's Clinical Ophthalmology, vol 6. Philadelphia, Lippincott-Raven, 1995, pp 1–10.
6. Rubin SE, Nelson LB: Complications of strabismus surgery. Ophthalmol Clin North Am 5:157–164, 1992.
7. Schnall BM: Anatomic considerations in strabismus surgery. Ophthalmol Clin North Am 5:1–8, 1992.
8. Sprunger DT, Klapper SR, Bonnis JM, Minturn JT: Management of experimental globe perforation during strabismus surgery. J Pediatr Ophthalmol Strabismus 33:140–143, 1996.

29. NYSTAGMUS

Robert D. Reinecke, M.D.

1. What is nystagmus?

A repetitive movement of the eyes, typically in a to-and-fro horizontal direction with a fast jerk in one direction. Often the nystagmus is exclusively vertical, other cases are torsional, and occasional cases are a mixture of the two. The term seems to have arisen from the sleepy-head jerk. The head of a sleepy student slowly falls to one side and then, with a start and a jerk, assumes the upright position again.

2. List the major types of nystagmus.

1. **Vestibular nystagmus**, which is caused by pathology of the vestibular system. The hallmark is the similarity of nystagmus in all fields of gaze and a slow component that is linear.

2. **Latent nystagmus** is an inherited form of nystagmus that becomes manifest only when binocularity is lost or thought by the patient to be lost. The slow phase has decreasing velocity and the fast phase beats to the fixing eye. When binocular vision is lost, the nystagmus is called **manifest latent nystagmus**.

3. **Amaurotic nystagmus** is not a true repetitive nystagmus but a roving of the eyes as if the patient is searching for something.

4. **Idiopathic infantile nystagmus** is the type that most ophthalmologists see. It is frequently associated with ocular and systemic albinism, high astigmatism, and various retinal problems. The typical natural history helps in the diagnosis.

3. What is the natural history of idiopathic infantile nystagmus?

At about 3 months of age the patient develops wide-swinging eye movements and not uncommonly is thought to be blind. At about 8 months to 1 year of age small pendular eye movements are substituted, and some control of fixation is reported. Then at about 18 months to 2 years the jerk nystagmus of adulthood is developed with its null zone.

4. What is the null zone of idiopathic infantile nystagmus?

The null zone is the direction of gaze in respect to orbital coordinates that minimizes the amplitude and frequency of nystagmus. Because a position of gaze that minimizes the nystagmus allows better vision, it is common for patients to seek out the null zone with habitual head positioning.

5. Is the null zone the same for each eye?

Yes—but there is an exception. If the patient finds that he or she can converge the eyes, cause an esotropia (the nystagmus blockage syndrome), the patient may cross-fixate and appear to have the null zone of each eye in the adducted position. Such patients are typically not stable after strabismus surgery. Over- and undercorrections are common.

6. What are the subtypes of infantile idiopathic nystagmus?

The principal and most common subtype is periodic alternating nystagmus, in which the null point drifts back and forth horizontally over a time of 30 seconds to 6 minutes (see question 21).

7. Do patients with poor vision also have the same natural history of the nystagmus wave form development?

Unfortunately, yes. Care must be taken to look for albinism, achromatopsia, Lebers congenital amaurosis, hypoplasia of the optic disc, and delayed visual development.

8. Is distinctive nystagmus associated with specific ocular pathology?

To date, only the differing nystagmus of achromatopsia seems somewhat distinctive as it evolves in an oblique direction.

9. Does nystagmus mean that the patient is blind?

No, to the contrary. You must have, or have had, some vision to develop nystagmus.

10. What is motor nystagmus?

Motor nystagmus is an archaic term used to indicate nystagmus unassociated with any visual problem. It was distinguished from sensory nystagmus, such as the nystagmus associated with albinism or cataracts. The current terminology is idiopathic infantile nystagmus, which may or may not be associated with other visual problems. Certain waveforms have been found to be diagnostic.

11. And what are the distinctive waveforms?

The slow phase of the nystagmus provides the most information. The fast phase seems to constitute a normal saccade (fixational eye movement). The slow phase may show increasing or decreasing velocity during the slow phase. If the velocity increases during a slow phase, the nystagmus is usually found to be idiopathic infantile nystagmus. If the nystagmus shows decreasing velocity of the slow phase, it is thought to be latent or manifest latent nystagmus.

12. Are some types of nystagmus present at birth?

Yes—dual jerk nystagmus. It is the most common and portends good vision.

13. You often hear of nystagmus associated with untreated congenital cataracts. Is it distinctive?

The answer is uncertain. Often the nystagmus is typical idiopathic infantile nystagmus and the course of the natural history is what is observed. If the patient develops roving eye movements, bad vision should be suspected.

14. Does a patient need vision to have nystagmus?

Yes, but the vision may be poor. The retinal or systemic conditions may worsen or cause blindness, and the typical idiopathic infantile nystagmus persists.

15. If one sees what seems to be the natural history of idiopathic infantile nystagmus, should magnetic resonance imaging (MRI) be obtained?

No. However, if the nystagmus is not symmetrical, the diagnosis of spasmus nutans should be entertained. Spasmus nutans consists of the following triad: (1) nystagmus that is unilateral or bilateral and asymmetric, (2) head nodding, and (3) torticollis. Patients develop spasmus nutans at 4–12 months of age, and symptoms usually disappear within 2 years of onset. The etiology is unknown, but patients are neurologically normal. However, because a chiasmal glioma may mimic spasmus nystagmus, an MRI is warranted.

16. If the nystagmus is vertical, will the patient develop a preferred chin-up or chin-down head position?

Yes. Patients develop a head position in relationship to the null point in the same fashion as patients with horizontal nystagmus. The null zone is in the direction of the slow phase of the nystagmus. Therefore, if the patient has obvious upbeat nystagmus, it will be worse on upgaze and the null point will be downward, with a preferred chin-up head position.

17. Do patients with torsional idiopathic infantile nystagmus exhibit a head tilt in respect to torsion?

Occasionally. One needs to look carefully for torsional nystagmus.

18. How can torsional idiopathic infantile nystagmus be observed and diagnosed?

Slit lamp observation of the iris is the most sensitive test.

19. Is the pivot of the torsion always on the visual axis?

No—and exceptions may cause some difficulty in diagnosis. If the pivot is on the visual axes, the eye rotates clockwise and counterclockwise about the fovea, and vision is only modestly degraded. In fact, it often is not noted unless an examiner studies the iris or disc. If, however, the pivot is to the left (e.g., on the left brow), the patient will have a component of horizontal and vertical nystagmus.

20. Do patients develop torsional nystagmus late in childhood or later in life?

Both. If the nystagmus is asymmetric, it is most likely due to midbrain pathology. More commonly the torsional nystagmus was present all along but not observed.

21. What is alternating in periodic alternating nystagmus?

The null point. As you watch the patient read his or her best acuity line, the patient will change the head position to maximize acuity by pointing the head in such a manner to allow the visual axis to remain in the null zone.

22. What is the time cycle of periodic alternating nystagmus?

About 90 seconds is most common, but the cycle may be as short as 30 seconds or as long as 6 minutes.

23. Is congenital periodic alternating nystagmus commonly associated with any other ocular problem?

Yes. Albinism is the most common association—and most commonly overlooked. Look for it carefully.

24. Does acquired periodic alternating nystagmus imply central nervous system pathology?

Yes, but be careful. Often the nystagmus is overlooked if the patient compensates well by changing head position. If it is truly acquired, midbrain pathology is common.

25. Does acquired periodic alternating nystagmus respond to pharmacologic treatment?

Yes. Baclofen often works.

26. Does congenital periodic alternating nystagmus respond to any drug?

None has been reported to date.

27. What is the danger of missing the diagnosis of periodic alternating nystagmus?

If a Kestenbaum or Anderson procedure is done (e.g., for a head turn accompanying an eccentric null point of idiopathic infantile nystagmus), a more severe head turn in the opposite direction will result.

28. What is the surgical treatment of periodic alternating nystagmus?

The best procedure seems to be recession of all four recti muscles by a large amount, with slightly more recession of the laterals as opposed to the medials.

29. Most patients with infantile idiopathic nystagmus have vision that is better at near than at distance. Why?

Most patients have an accommodative convergence/accommodation ratio (AC:A) that results in exophoria at near. The patient has to use fusional convergence to overcome the exophoria. Fusional convergence dampens the nystagmus and improves the vision.

30. Because convergence improves vision, should minus lenses be used to excess to stimulate accommodative convergence?

No. Only fusional convergence—i.e., overcoming exophoria—dampens nystagmus. Accommodative convergence does not dampen nystagmus and even works against the patient by increasing accommodative demands and may cause the near point to recede with reduced visual acuity at near.

31. Are bifocals helpful to a teenage patient with infantile idiopathic nystagmus?

Often yes. If the accommodation cannot provide a near point that is close to the patient (with accompanying magnification and increased exophoria), bifocals can be a big help.

32. Is photophobia common with infantile idiopathic nystagmus?

No. If photophobia is present with nystagmus, look for achromatopsia.

33. Do patients with albinism have photophobia?

For the most part, no. However, some albinos do not like excessive light, and dark tints are occasionally helpful.

34. You may have heard that contact lenses lessen nystagmus. Do they help?

For the most part, no. Remember, however, that many patients with nystagmus have considerable astigmatism. Those that do may well be helped with toric contact lenses, particularly if the null zone is eccentric at points where spectacles distort the images. Usually contact lenses seem to help for a brief period; then patients adapt to them and are back to where they were.

35. Many patients with nystagmus have vision of about 20/50 and want to pass the magic barrier of 20/40 to obtain a driver's license. What can you do to help?

For the most part, such patients are safe drivers as far as vision is concerned. If you project the full screen of letters and ask them to read the top line as you reduce the print, you will find that many read two lines or so better; hence you can endorse their improved vision.

36. Aside from using a full screen of letters, what should one do when checking visual acuity of a patient with unexpected poor vision?

Be sure to measure binocular visual acuity. If binocular vision is better, try occluding the nonfixing eye with a +4.00 lens and ask the patient to read with the opposite eye. In other words, look for latent nystagmus.

37. Clinically, how do you distinguish manifest latent nystagmus (MLN) from infantile idiopathic nystagmus (IIN)?

As you occlude each eye, with MLN the direction of the jerk changes toward the fixing eye. With IIN the direction of the nystagmus remains constant on covering either eye, but the direction of the nystagmus changes when you cross to the other side of the null zone.

BIBLIOGRAPHY

1. Gradstein L, Reinecke RD, Wizov SS, Goldstein HP: Congenital periodic alternating nystagmus. Ophthalmology 104:918–929, 1997.
2. Reinecke RD: Idiopathic infantile nystagmus: Diagnosis and treatment. AAPOS 1:67–82, 1997.

VI. Neuro-ophthalmology

30. THE PUPIL

Barry Schanzer, M.D., and Peter Savino, M.D.

1. What muscles control the size of the pupil? Describe their innervation.

The iris sphincter muscle causes pupillary constriction and is innervated by the parasympathetic nervous system. The iris dilator muscle causes pupillary dilatation and is innervated by the sympathetic nervous system. Thus, when sympathetic tone is increased, the pupil is larger, and when parasympathetic tone is increased, the pupil is smaller.

2. Trace the pathway of the parasympathetic innervation of the pupil.

Parasympathetic fibers begin in the Edinger-Westphal nucleus in the oculomotor nuclear complex. With cranial nerve (CN) III they exit the midbrain and travel in the subarachnoid space and cavernous sinus. They follow the inferior division of CN III into the orbit, where they synapse at the ciliary ganglion. Postganglionic fibers are then distributed to the iris sphincter and ciliary body via short ciliary nerves.

3. Trace the pathway of the sympathetic innervation of the pupil.

The first-order neuron begins in the posterior hypothalamus. The fibers travel caudally to terminate in the intermedial lateral cell column of the spinal cord at levels C8–T1, otherwise known as the ciliospinal center of Budge. Pupillomotor fibers exit from the spinal cord and ascend with the sympathetic chain to synapse in the superior cervical ganglion, constituting the second-order neuron. The third-order neuron begins with postganglionic fibers of the superior cervical ganglion. These fibers travel with the internal carotid artery to enter the cranial vault. In the cavernous sinus the fibers leave the carotid artery to join the ophthalmic division of CN V and enter the orbit through the superior orbital fissure. The sympathetic fibers reach the ciliary body and dilator of the iris by passing through the nasociliary nerve and long posterior ciliary nerves.

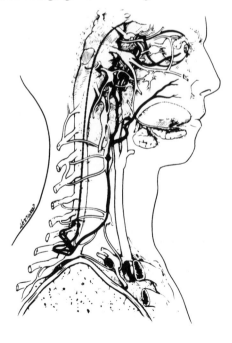

Anatomy of sympathetic pathway showing central neuron (first-order), intermediate neuron (second-order), and peripheral neuron (third-order) pathways. Note the proximity of the pulmonary apex to the sympathetic chain and lower cervical and upper thoracic nerves. (From Maloney, Younge, Moyer: Am J Ophthalmol 90:395, 1980, with permission).

4. Trace the pathway of the pupillary light reflex.

The pupillary light response begins with the rods and cones of the retina. Afferent pupillo-motor fibers travel through the optic nerves and semidecussate at the optic chiasm. They then follow the optic tracts and exit before the lateral geniculate body to enter the brainstem via the brachium of the superior colliculus. Pupillomotor fibers synapse in the pretectal nuclei, which then project equally to the ipsilateral and contralateral Edinger-Westphal nuclei. The pupillary fibers travel with CN III to innervate the iris sphincter and cause pupillary constriction, as de-scribed in question 2.

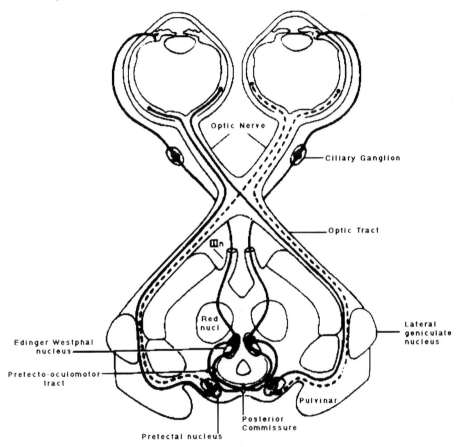

Light reflex pathway. (From Walsh F, Hoyt W (eds): Clinical Neuro-Ophthalmology, 3rd ed., vol. 1. Baltimore, Williams & Wilkins, 1969, p 473, with permission.)

5. What is an afferent pupillary defect? How should you examine for it?

The swinging flashlight test is used to elicit a relative afferent pupillary defect (rAPD). If you shine a light into one eye of a normal subject, both pupils constrict to the same degree. If you swing the light over to the other eye, the pupil stays the same size or constricts minimally. In pa-tients with rAPD, the affected eye behaves as if it perceives a dimmer light than the normal eye; therefore, both pupils constrict to a lesser degree when the light is shone in the affected eye. Thus, if you shine the light in the right eye of a patient with left rAPD, both pupils constrict. If you swing the light to the left eye, it is perceived as dimmer and the pupils dilate. Note that this is a *relative* APD and signifies a difference in the pupillary response between the two eyes. However, if both eyes are equally abnormal, there may be no rAPD.

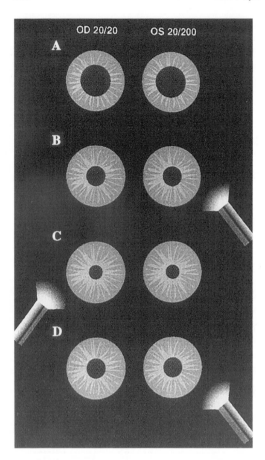

Left rAPD. *A,* The pupils in dim light are equal. *B,* Light directed into the left eye results in partial and sluggish constriction in each eye. *C,* Light directed into the right eye results in a brisk and normal reaction in each eye. *D,* The light quickly directed into the left eye results in a dilatation of both pupils. (From Tasman W, Jaeger EA (eds): The Wills Eye Hospital Atlas of Clinical Ophthalmology. Philadelphia, Lippincott-Raven, 1996, p 297, with permission.)

6. A lesion in which anatomic areas may cause an afferent pupillary defect?

A lesion anywhere in the afferent pupillary pathway may cause an rAPD—that is, retina, optic nerve, optic chiasm, optic tract, or along the course of pupillary fibers from the optic tract to pretectal nuclei. Pupillary fibers leave the optic tract prior to the lateral geniculate body. Therefore, any lesion from the lateral geniculate body posteriorly does not cause an rAPD. A retinal lesion causes an rAPD only if it is rather large. An optic nerve lesion causes an rAPD in the ipsilateral eye. A lesion in the optic chiasm may cause an rAPD if one optic nerve is affected more than the other. An optic tract lesion causes an rAPD in the eye with the most visual field loss. Typically, in patients with a mass lesion of the optic tract, an rAPD is produced in the ipsilateral eye, but an ischemic lesion causes an rAPD in the contralateral eye. A lesion in the brainstem in the area of the pretectal nuclei may cause an rAPD without visual defects.

7. What is anisocoria? How should one examine a patient with anisocoria?

Anisocoria is a difference in the size between the two pupils. In anyone who has anisocoria the pupil size should be measured in both bright and dim light. If the anisocoria is greater in bright light, the larger pupil is abnormal and constricts poorly, usually because of a defect in parasympathetic innervation. If the anisocoria is greater in dim light, the smaller pupil is abnormal because it dilates poorly, usually because of a defect in pupillary sympathetic innervation. If the difference in the size of the two pupils remains the same in bright and dim light, the anisocoria is physiologic and not pathologic.

8. What is the differential diagnosis of a unilateral dilated, poorly reactive pupil?
1. Third-nerve palsy
2. Pharmacologic paralysis (an anticholinergic medication such as atropine)
3. Adie's tonic pupil
4. Iris damage (such as sphincter tears secondary to trauma or posterior synechiae secondary to inflammation)

9. What are the clinical findings in a third-nerve palsy?
CN III innervates the superior, medial, and inferior recti and inferior oblique and levator palpebrae muscles. Therefore, in a complete CN III palsy, ptosis is complete, and the eye is in the down-and-out position; it does not move up, down, or medially. The parasympathetic nerves that innervate the pupillary sphincter travel with CN III; therefore, if those fibers are affected, the pupil will be dilated and unreactive.

10. What are possible causes of the third-nerve palsy?
In adults the most common causes are (1) microvascular ischemia in the nerve, (2) aneurysm (usually of the posterior communicating artery), (3) trauma, and (4) neoplasm. In children, aneurysm is rare, and consideration must be given to ophthalmoplegic migraine.

11. What is the significance of pupil involvement or pupil sparing in third-nerve palsy?
Pupil involvement in third-nerve palsy suggests a compressive lesion such as aneurysm or tumor. Pupil sparing is suggestive of microvascular ischemia. The parasympathetic fibers are on the outer portion of CN III and are more susceptible to external compression and less susceptible to ischemia, which is usually axial in the nerve.

12. What is the appropriate work-up for an isolated third-nerve palsy with pupillary sparing?
In patients in the vasculopathic age group, the most likely cause is microvascular ischemia. Patients may simply be followed with the expectation that the ocular misalignment will improve. Certainly a medical work-up for hypertension or diabetes is appropriate. If there is no improvement in 3–6 months, neuroimaging should be performed. Patients under the vasculopathic age should have an MRI scan. If the scan is negative, they should be observed.

13. What is the appropriate work-up for an isolated third-nerve palsy with pupillary involvement?
The first step is to perform an emergent MRI scan. If the MRI scan is negative, a cerebral arteriogram must be performed to rule out an aneurysm. If the MRI scan is negative in children under the age of 10, an arteriogram is not necessary because the likelihood of an aneurysm is very low. Ten years is an arbitrary age based on the principle that aneurysms are rare in young children.

14. What is an Adie's tonic pupil? What is its natural history?
Adie's tonic pupil is a postganglionic defect in the parasympathetic innervation to the pupil. The clinical findings are a dilated pupil that is usually slightly irregular and shows segmental iris constriction at the slit lamp. There also may be light-near dissociation, with characteristically slow and tonic constriction and redilation phases. This condition is benign and most commonly affects women in their second to fourth decade (see figure, next page).

15. How do you test for an Adie's pupil?
An Adie's tonic pupil constricts to dilute pilocarpine ⅛%, whereas a normal pupil does not. This is a result of denervation hypersensitivity.

16. What is Horner's syndrome?
Horner's syndrome is a clinical syndrome characterized by ptosis, miosis, and occasionally anhidrosis (see figure, next page). It is caused by any lesion in the sympathetic innervation to the eye.

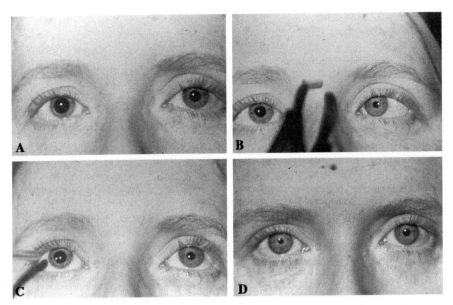

Adie's tonic pupil right eye. *A,* Anisocoria with right pupil larger than left pupil. *B,* Right pupil constricts with near response. *C,* Right pupil reacts poorly to light. *D,* Right pupil constricts markedly in response to 1/8% pilocarpine, whereas the left pupil does not. (From Tasman W, Jaeger EA (eds): The Wills Eye Hospital Atlas of Clinical Ophthalmology. Philadelphia, Lippincott-Raven, 1996, p 298, with permission.)

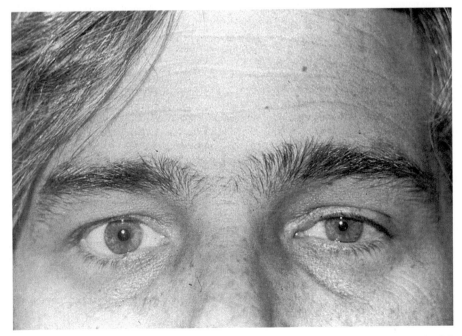

Horner's syndrome with ptosis and miosis on the left. Note that the left lower lid is higher than the right lower lid. This inverse ptosis is due to interruption of sympathetic innervation to the analog of Mueller's muscle in the lower lid.

17. What is the cause of the ptosis in Horner's syndrome?

Ptosis in Horner's syndrome is caused by decreased sympathetic tone in Mueller's muscle. Mueller's muscle is responsible for about 2 mm of elevation of the upper lid. Thus, the ptosis in Horner's syndrome is mild (only about 2 mm).

18. What are the possible causes of Horner's syndrome?

The course of the sympathetic innervation to the eye was discussed in question 3. A lesion anywhere along this course may cause Horner's syndrome. Isolated third-order neuron lesions are generally benign. Second-order neuron lesions are more ominous and may be caused by apical lung tumors or carotid artery dissection. First-order neuron lesions are uncommon in isolation. They are found in demyelinating disease, cerebrovascular accidents, and neoplasms.

19. How do you test for Horner's syndrome?

Cocaine test. Cocaine blocks the reuptake of norepinephrine. A normal pupil dilates in response to a drop of cocaine, whereas in Horner's syndrome the pupil fails to dilate.

20. What pharmacologic testing helps to localize the lesion in Horner's syndrome?

Localization is important because the etiology and focus of the work-up are quite different, depending on whether the lesion is first- or second-order or third-order neuron. Hydroxy-amphetamine 1% causes release of epinephrine from the third-order neuron junction with the iris. Thus, in third-order neuron lesions there is no pupillary response to hydroxyamphetamine drops. In a first- or second-order neuron lesion, the pupil dilates in response to hydroxyamphetamine drops.

21. What is light/near dissociation? What are its possible causes?

In light/near dissociation a pupil does not constrict to light but will constrict as part of the near response. Causes include (1) Adie's syndrome, (2) dorsal midbrain syndrome (Parinaud's syndrome), (3) Argyll-Robertson pupils, and (4) blindness from any anterior afferent cause.

22. What is an Argyll-Robertson pupil?

Argyll-Robertson pupils are small, often irregular pupils that do not react to light but have a brisk near response. The cause of Argyll-Robertson pupils is tertiary syphilis.

23. What is Parinaud's syndrome?

Found in dorsal midbrain disease, the syndrome is composed of (1) light/near dissociation of the pupils, (2) paralysis of upward gaze, and (3) lid retraction.

BIBLIOGRAPHY

1. Burde RM, Savino PJ, Trobe JD: Clinical Decisions in Neuro-Ophthalmology, 2nd ed. St. Louis, Mosby, 1992, pp 321–338.
2. Miller NR: Walsh and Hoyt's Clinical Neuro-Ophthalmology, 4th ed, vol 2. Baltimore, Williams & Wilkins, 1995, pp 400–556.
3. Newell FW: Ophthalmology: Principles and Concepts, 8th ed. St. Louis, Mosby, 1996, pp 165–174.

31. DIPLOPIA

Julian D. Perry, M.D.

1. What is diplopia?

Diplopia is a symptom in which the patient perceives two images of a single object. Diplopia may be monocular or binocular. You should check if the double vision resolves with each eye closed. If it does not, the patient has monocular diplopia. If it does, the patient has binocular diplopia.

2. List the causes of monocular diplopia.

Start with glasses and work your way posteriorly through the ocular tissues to obtain this differential:

- Refractive error: astigmatism is the most common cause of monocular diplopia
- Chalazion or other eyelid tumor producing irregular astigmatism
- Keratopathy: keratoconus, irregular astigmatism (use a retinoscope to see scissoring reflex)
- Iris atrophy, polycoria, large nonreactive pupil
- Cataract, subluxated lens, intraocular lens decentration, capsular opacity
- Retinal disease may produce metamorphopsia or aniseikonia

Also consider a psychogenic etiology.

3. What are the causes of binocular diplopia?

Causes of binocular diplopia may be grouped into three general categories:

1. Neuropathic. The pathology may be supranuclear, nuclear, or infranuclear. Signs and symptoms can often localize the lesion, and specific etiologies often affect certain anatomic areas of the nervous system. Specific neuropathic causes include vasoocclusive infarction, compression, inflammation, demyelination, and degeneration.

2. Myopathic. The pathology may exist within the extraocular muscles. Myopathic causes of diplopia include inflammatory pseudotumor or myositis and thyroid-related eye disease (TED).

3. Neuromuscular junction disorders. The major etiology in this category is myasthenia gravis (MG).

4. What are some causes of intermittent diplopia?

The most common causes of intermittent double vision are MG, TED, decompensated phoria, and multiple sclerosis (MS). Other causes include spasm of the near reflex, convergence retraction nystagmus, and ocular neuromyotonia.

5. What is the most important sign to check for in a third nerve (oculomotor) palsy?

The presence or absence of a dilated, nonreactive pupil. A pupil-involving oculomotor palsy is an emergency. An aneurysm must be ruled out.

6. What is the work-up of a pupil-involving III nerve palsy?

In adults, perform MRI/A or spiral CT angiography. If the results are consistent with an aneurysm or even if the results are negative, perform an angiogram. In children, perform MRI/A regardless of the state of the pupil. If the results are negative, children usually do not need an angiogram.

7. Why do aneurysms involve the pupil in oculomotor nerve palsies while infarctions generally do not?

Pupillary parasympathetic fibers travel superficially and dorsomedially in the third nerve as it traverses the subarachnoid space. These fibers are often affected first in a compressive lesion. Ischemic infarction often occurs in the center of the nerve, so the superficial fibers remain unaffected.

8. What is the work-up of an isolated pupil-sparing but otherwise complete oculomotor nerve palsy in the vasculopathic age group?

A lesion that compresses the central third nerve fibers sufficiently to produce a complete paresis should affect the peripheral pupillary fibers sufficiently to produce at least some degree of pupil involvement. If not, the likelihood of an aneurysm or other compressive etiology is extremely low. The patient may be treated for an assumed vasoocclusive etiology. Diagnostic work-up includes at least the measurement of systemic blood pressure and a 2-hour postprandial glucose. If the patient has symptoms of giant cell arteritis (GCA), check erythrocyte sedimentation rate, administer corticosteroids, and perform a temporal artery biopsy; otherwise, the patient may be seen again in 6 weeks. Some physicians reexamine the patient within 5 days to ensure the pupil remains uninvolved.

9. What are the causes of isolated cranial neuropathies?

Many cranial neuropathies are idiopathic, but the causes of isolated cranial neuropathies are as follows:

Cranial Neuropathy	Etiology _giant cell arteritis_
III (pupil-sparing)	Adults: infarction, trauma, GCA, tumor; rarely, an aneurysm Children: congenital, trauma, tumor, aneurysm, migraine
III (pupil-involving)	Usually posterior communicating artery (rarely, basilar artery) aneurysm
IV	Adults: trauma, infarction, congenital, GCA Children: congenital, trauma
VI	Adults: infarction, tumor, trauma, MS, Wernicke's, sarcoid, GCA, herpes zoster, Lyme disease, increased intracranial pressure as in pseudotumor cerebri Children: trauma, tumor, postviral

10. How do you test for a trochlear nerve palsy in the presence of an oculomotor nerve palsy?

It is important to specifically test trochlear, abducens, and trigeminal nerve function in a patient with an oculomotor nerve palsy in order to localize the lesion. Because the third nerve palsy may prevent adduction, it may be difficult to test fourth nerve function. When the patient attempts to look down and in with the paretic eye, you will observe intorsion if the trochlear nerve is intact.

11. What else should you know about oculomotor nerve palsy?

1. Aberrant regeneration of the third nerve does not occur after a vasoocclusive (e.g., diabetic) third nerve palsy.

2. Primary oculomotor aberrant regeneration is highly suggestive of a lesion that is slowly compressing the third nerve, often an intracavernous meningioma or aneurysm.

3. Divisional paresis of the third nerve can occur from a lesion anywhere from the midbrain to the orbit. A superior division palsy involves ptosis and an inability to elevate the eye. An inferior division palsy consists of an inability to look nasally or inferiorly and the pupil is involved. An inferior division involving the pupil should warrant emergent work-up as in question 6.

4. Always consider MG and TED in the evaluation of diplopia, even if the palsy "maps out" to a specific cranial nerve.

12. Describe the 3-step test.

This is a test to determine if a hypertropia is due to superior oblique palsy or other causes.

Step 1: Which eye is hyperdeviated? A right hyperdeviation could be caused by palsy of any of the muscles circled in Step 1. Determine which muscles might cause this.

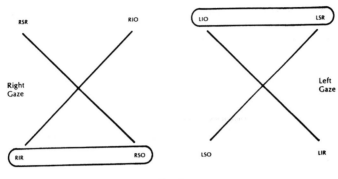

Step 1

Step 2: Is the hyperdeviation worse in right gaze or left gaze? Isolate these muscles. A right superior oblique palsy reveals worsening of the right hyperdeviation in the left gaze.

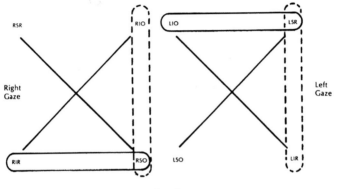

Step 2

Step 3: Is the hyperdeviation worse on right head tilt or left head tilt? The muscle isolated in all 3 steps is the palsied muscle. A right superior oblique palsy reveals increased hyperdeviation upon head tilt to the right. A double Maddox rod can then be used to determine if the trochlear nerve palsy is bilateral. If excyclotorsion is more than 10°, bilateral superior oblique palsies exist.

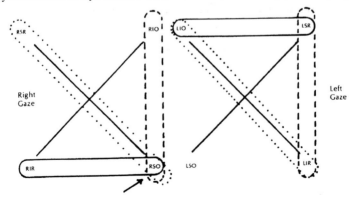

Step 3

(Figures from American Academy of Ophthalmology: Pediatric Ophthalmology and Strabismus, Section 6. San Francisco, American Academy of Ophthalmology, 1992–1993, with permission.)

13. What is the best procedure to treat unresolved superior oblique palsy, and do I have to memorize Knapp's Rules?

Knapp published his treatment scheme several years ago, and many surgeons use similar schemes. You do not need to memorize his particular scheme, but you should understand the principles. Generally, there are three possible surgical approaches:

1. Strengthen (tuck) the palsied superior oblique muscle.
2. Weaken the antagonist ipsilateral inferior oblique muscle.
3. Weaken the yoke contralateral inferior rectus muscle.

Typically, the surgeon operates on the muscle or muscles that act in the field of gaze where the diplopia is worst. For example, if the left hyperdeviation in a left superior oblique (LSO) palsy is worst in downgaze, one would consider an LSO tuck or a right inferior rectus recession. The latter procedure may be favored because an adjustable suture technique can be used and there is no chance of producing an iatrogenic Brown's syndrome.

14. Explain the Harada-Ito procedure.

The Harada-Ito procedure involves anterior and lateral displacement of the anterior portion of the palsied superior oblique muscle. This procedure is used primarily for correction of excyclotorsion but will correct a small degree of hyperdeviation. The amount of incyclotorsion created is variable, but the procedure is generally successful.

15. What else should you know about trochlear nerve palsy?

1. The trochlear nerve is the longest and most commonly injured cranial nerve in trauma.
2. Patients of all ages with trochlear nerve palsy and increased vertical fusional amplitudes do not need further evaluation; they have decompensated "congenital" trochlear nerve palsies.
3. Always consider MG and TED in the evaluation of diplopia, even if the palsy "maps out" to a specific cranial nerve.

16. List the major causes of abduction deficit other than cranial neuropathy.

Restricted medial rectus muscle
   Trauma (entrapment, damage)
   Inflammatory pseudotumor or myositis
   Thyroid related eye disease
Spasm of the near reflex
Myasthenia gravis

17. How do you treat an unresolved abducens nerve palsy?

1. Weaken the ipsilateral medial rectus with strengthening of the ipsilateral lateral rectus muscle.
2. Vertical transposition procedure.
3. Botulinum toxin (Botox) injections may be used with the above procedures.

18. What else should you know about abducens nerve palsy?

1. Abducens palsy may occur as a nonspecific sign of increased intracranial pressure. Abducens palsy may also occur after lumbar puncture.
2. In the case of bilateral abducens paresis, you must consider tumor, MS, subarachnoid hemorrhage, or infection. Do not "write it off" as being due to infarction without a work-up.
3. In children with bilateral abducens paresis, reconsider strabismus and check for "doll's eyes." "Doll's eyes" should be incomplete in a paretic disorder.
4. Third-order sympathetic fibers briefly join the abducens nerve in the cavernous sinus. Horner's syndrome with an abducens nerve palsy localizes to this region.
5. Always consider MG and TED in the evaluation of diplopia, even if the palsy "maps out" to a specific cranial nerve (sound familiar?).

19. What are the localizing symptom complexes of nerve palsy?

Symptoms/Signs	Syndrome	Anatomic Location
Ipsilateral III nerve palsy with a contralateral fascicle hemiplegia	Weber's	Midbrain third nerve fascicle and cerebral peduncle
Ipsilateral III nerve palsy with contralateral choreiform movements	Benedickt's	Midbrain third nerve fascicle and red nucleus
Ipsilateral VI nerve palsy with hearing loss and facial pain	Gradenigo's	Petrous apex
Ipsilateral gaze palsy with facial palsy, Horner's syndrome and deafness	Foville's, Anterior inferior cerebellar artery syndrome	Dorsolateral pons
Ipsilateral VI and VII nerve palsies with contralateral hemiparesis	Millard-Gubler	Anterior paramedial pons
III, IV, VI (V_1, V_2) nerve palsies with Horner's syndrome, and primary aberrant regeneration	Cavernous sinus syndrome	Cavernous sinus
III, IV, VI (V_1) nerve palsies, often with proptosis	Superior orbital fissure syndrome	Superior orbital fissure
V, VI, VII, VIII nerve palsies	Cerebellopontine angle tumor	

20. What is internuclear ophthalmoplegia (INO)?

The medial longitudinal fasciculus carries nerve fibers from the abducens nucleus on each side to the contralateral medial rectus subnucleus to coordinate horizontal gaze. This area of the brainstem may be damaged by demyelination, ischemia, or tumor. Ipsilateral decreased adduction and contralateral abduction nystagmus are observed on attempted contralateral gaze. Saccadic velocity may be decreased in the adducting eye and may be the only sign of a subtle INO. Bilateral INO is common, often presenting with exotropia and upward beating nystagmus on attempted convergence in addition to the above findings.

21. Tell me all I need to know about ocular myasthenia gravis.

Intermittent diplopia and ptosis are common symptoms of this condition, and diurnal variability increases suspicion. On exam, ptosis will frequently worsen with prolonged upgaze, and orbicular strength is frequently affected. Myasthenia may mimic any isolated ocular motor nerve palsy or an INO. A Tensilon test (edrophonium chloride) is a short-acting anticholinesterase that can cause improvement of symptoms and signs of MG. A positive acetylcholine receptor antibody test supports the diagnosis. Placing an ice compress for 2–3 minutes over the ptotic lid frequently improves the ptosis and supports the diagnosis. Once the diagnosis is made, work-up includes MRI of the chest and thyroid studies to rule out associated thymoma and hyperthyroidism. Myasthenia that is purely ocular after two years is likely to remain so. Treatment includes the long-acting cholinesterase inhibitors, corticosteroids, and plasmapheresis.

22. How is the Tensilon test performed?

Ten mg of Tensilon is drawn into a syringe. A 2-mg IV is given initially to observe for adverse reactions or a positive response. If neither occur after 2 minutes, then the remainder is given either incrementally or as a single bolus. A positive test shows improved facial expression, lid position, or double vision within 3 minutes of injection. A positive test is quite specific for MG; however, false-negative tests occur. An EMG may also show improvement after Tensilon administration. Atropine must be readily available in case adverse reactions occur (abdominal cramps and bradycardia are common).

23. What is convergence insufficiency?

Typical convergence insufficiency presents with asthenopia and double vision at near. It is diagnosed by observing an exotropia at 33 cm, an abnormally remote near point of convergence (> 3–6 cm for patients under 20 years; > 12 cm for patients over 40 years) and inadequate amplitudes of fusion. Patients can fully adduct during conjugate gaze movements, and the deviation is comitant for a given distance. The isolated condition is rarely associated with tumor or other serious pathology.

Patients are treated with near point exercises such as focusing on the end of a pencil while moving from arm's length toward the face.

24. What is skew deviation?

Skew deviation is a vertical deviation that cannot be isolated to a single extraocular muscle or muscles. It is almost always associated with other manifestations of posterior fossa disease.

25. What other supranuclear conditions commonly produce diplopia?

Progressive supranuclear palsy produces a variety of systemic and ocular motility disturbances, including bradykinesia, axial rigidity, and difficulty with vertical eye movements. If diplopia is present, it is typically caused by convergence difficulty. Similarly, patients with parkinsonism, Huntington's disease, and Parinaud's dorsal midbrain syndrome may also have diplopia at near due to convergence difficulty.

26. Explain divergence paresis.

Patients with divergence paresis present with an esodeviation at distance causing diplopia. Patients are able to fuse at near. The esodeviation is comitant, and horizontal versions are normal. This condition tends to be benign and self-limited; however, it may be associated with infection, demyelinating disease, and tumor. MRI should be performed.

BIBLIOGRAPHY

1. Brazis PW, Masdeu JC, Biller J: Localization in Clinical Neurology, 3rd ed. Boston, Little, Brown, 1994.
2. Burde RM, Savino PJ, Trobe JD: Clinical Decisions in Neuro-ophthalmology, 2nd ed. St. Louis, Mosby–Year Book, 1992.
3. Cone RA: Diplopia. Amsterdam, Excerpta Medica, 1973.
4. Harada M, Ito Y: Surgical correction of cyclophoria. Jpn J Ophthalmol 8:88–92, 1964.
5. Mein J, Trimble R: Diagnosis and Management of Ocular Motility Disorders, 2nd ed. London, Blackwell Scientific Publications, 1991.
6. Miller NR, Newman NJ: Walsh and Hoyts' Clinical Neuro-Ophthalmology, 5th ed. Baltimore, Williams & Wilkins, 1998.
7. Walsh TJ: Neuroophthalmology: Clinical Signs and Symptoms, 2nd ed. Philadelphia, Lea & Febiger, 1985.
8. von Noorden GK: Binocular Vision and Ocular Motility: Theory and Management of Strabismus, 5th ed. St. Louis, Mosby, 1996.

32. OPTIC NEURITIS

Barry Schanzer, M.D., and Peter Savino, M.D.

1. What is optic neuritis?

Optic neuritis is any inflammation of the optic nerve. It may be idiopathic or associated with systemic disease.

2. Which systemic diseases are associated with optic neuritis?

The most common disease associated with optic neuritis is multiple sclerosis. However, syphilis, sarcoidosis, Lyme disease, and other collagen vascular diseases, such as Wegener's granulomatosis and systemic lupus erythematosus, are less commonly associated.

3. Who most commonly gets optic neuritis?

Women between the ages of 15 and 45 years are most commonly affected.

4. What are the typical clinical findings in optic neuritis?

Optic neuritis causes acute or subacute visual loss that may progress over 10–14 days. Visual acuity may range from 20/20 to no light perception. However, even if visual acuity is 20/20, the patient usually has a defect in color vision, contrast sensitivity, and visual field. If the neuritis is unilateral, an afferent pupillary defect is present. The optic disc may be normal or swollen.

5. Which clinical test is most sensitive for patients with optic neuritis?

The most sensitive test—that is, the test that is most likely to be abnormal in a patient with optic neuritis—is contrast sensitivity.

6. How common is pain on eye movement in patients with optic neuritis?

Pain around the eye or pain exacerbated with eye movement was present in 92% of patients in the Optic Neuritis Treatment Trial (ONTT).

7. What visual field defects are found in patients with optic neuritis?

The classic visual field defect in optic neuritis is central scotoma. However, the ONTT found that any optic nerve visual field defect is compatible with optic neuritis, including altitudinal defects and arcuate defects as well as diffuse visual field defects.

8. What is the natural history of optic neuritis?

The visual loss of optic neuritis may progress over 10–14 days. At that point it should stabilize and shortly thereafter begin to improve.

9. What is the expected visual outcome for patients with optic neuritis?

The ONTT found that at 12 months 93% of patients were 20/40 or better; 69% were 20/20 or better; and 3% were 20/200 or worse.

10. Are there any predictors of poor visual outcome?

The ONTT found that the only predictor for poor visual outcome was poor visual acuity at presentation. Nevertheless, all patients with an initial visual acuity of 20/200 or less showed some improvement. However, 5% of the patients were still 20/200 or less at 6 months.

11. What were the objectives of the ONTT?

The ONTT was a multicentered, randomized, prospective clinical trial to determine whether corticosteroid treatment of optic neuritis was beneficial. A secondary objective was to determine the risk of developing multiple sclerosis in patients with optic neuritis. The patients in the ONTT were randomized to three treatment arms. One group of patients received oral placebo; one group received oral prednisone, 1 mg/kg for 14 days; and one group received IV solumedrol, 250 mg every 6 hr for 3 days, followed by oral prednisone, 1 mg/kg for 11 days.

12. What were the conclusions of the ONTT regarding treatment of optic neuritis?

No treatment group had statistically significant better visual acuity at 6 months. However, patients treated with IV solumedrol began to recover vision more quickly. The surprising result was that patients treated with oral prednisone, 1 mg/kg for 14 days, had an increased incidence of recurrence of optic neuritis in the affected or contralateral eye. The researchers concluded that oral prednisone in a dose of 1 mg/kg is contraindicated in the treatment of optic neuritis.

13. What was the strongest predictor for the development of multiple sclerosis?

An abnormal MRI scan was found to be the strongest predictor for development of clinically definite multiple sclerosis (MS) at 2 years. Placebo-treated patients whose MRI scan at study entry showed two or more periventricular white matter lesions ≥ 3 mm had a 36% chance of developing multiple sclerosis within 2 years. Patients with 1 lesion had a 17% chance, and patients with no signal abnormalities had only a 3% chance.

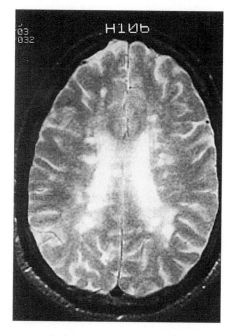

Abnormal MRI in a patient with multiple sclerosis. Classic periventricular white matter lesions appear bright on T2-weighted image.

14. What were the other predictors for development of MS?

Previous optic neuritis in the fellow eye, previous nonspecific neurologic symptoms, white race, and family history of MS were associated with an increased risk of developing MS. Although young age and female gender have been reported to be risk factors for MS, they were not shown to increase the risk within 2 years in the ONTT.

15. What were the conclusions of the ONTT about the effect of treatment on the risk of developing MS?

The results of the ONTT showed that IV solumedrol significantly decreased the risk of developing MS at 2 years. Most of the beneficial effect was seen in patients with abnormal MRI scans because patients with normal MRI scans had a low incidence of MS, regardless of treatment. Among patients with two or more signal abnormalities on MRI, MS developed in 36% treated with placebo, 32% treated with prednisone, and 16% treated with IV solumedrol. Thus the risk of developing MS at 2 years was cut in half by treatment with IV solumedrol. After 2 years the beneficial effect seemed to wear off, and at 3 years the three groups had a similar incidence of MS.

16. Describe the appropriate work-up and treatment for patients with optic neuritis.

Patients presenting with optic neuritis should have an MRI scan. If the scan is normal, no further work-up is warranted and sequential follow-up is indicated. If the scan shows two or more typical white matter lesions, the patient should be offered treatment with IV solumedrol to decrease the risk of developing MS over the next 2 years. The ONTT found no significant benefit in blood tests for antinuclear antibody or fluorescent titer antibody in patients with typical optic neuritis and no other signs of collagen vascular disease.

BIBLIOGRAPHY

1. Beck RW, Cleary PA, Anderson MM Jr, et al: A randomized, controlled trial of corticosteroids in the treatment of acute optic neuritis. N Engl J Med 326:581–588, 1992.
2. Beck RW, Clearly PA, Trobe JD, et al: The effect of corticosteroids for acute optic neuritis on the subsequent development of multiple sclerosis. N Engl J Med 329:1764–1769, 1993.
3. Beck RW, Trobe JD: What we have learned from the Optic Neuritis Treatment Trial. Ophthalmology 102:1504–1508, 1995.
4. Burde RM, Savno PJ, Trobe JD: Clinical Decisions in Neuro-Ophthalmology, 2nd ed. St. Louis, Mosby, 1992, pp 41–49.

33. MISCELLANEOUS OPTIC NEUROPATHIES AND NEUROLOGIC DISTURBANCES

Janice A. Gault, M.D.

1. A young woman complains of headaches. Her vision is 20/20 in each eye with no evidence of afferent pupillary defect. She has a bitemporal visual field cut. What do you suspect?
A chiasmal lesion. Get a scan to evaluate.

2. What may simulate a bitemporal field defect?
Sector retinitis pigmentosa, coloboma, or a tilted disc.

3. A patient has 20/20 vision in her right eye and 20/400 in her left. The left eye has an afferent pupillary defect and decreased color plates. What should you evaluate in her right eye?
Check visual fields in both eyes. A central scotoma in one eye may be accompanied by a superior temporal field loss in the other. This condition, called a junctional scotoma, is also found in chiasmal lesions.

4. Describe the underlying anatomy.
At the chiasm, the ganglion cells representing the contralateral nasal retina loop forward in the other optic nerve (Willebrand's knee). Injury at this site causes a central scotoma on the same side as the damage with a contralateral superotemporal visual field defect.

5. What is the differential diagnosis of a lesion causing chiasmal visual field defect?
- Pituitary tumor
- Pituitary apoplexy
- Craniopharyngioma (often in children)
- Meningioma
- Glioma
- Aneurysm
- Trauma
- Infection
- Optic nerve glioma
- Other rare tumors

6. Is there a difference in the treatment of secreting and nonsecreting pituitary tumors?
Yes. A prolactinoma secretes prolactin and may be treated successfully with bromocriptine. A nonsecreting tumor probably requires surgery. Of course, the patient should be fully evaluated by an endocrinologist for other hormonal imbalances.

7. What visual field is often seen in a toxic or metabolic optic neuropathy?
Bilateral central or centrocecal scotomas. Optic nerves show temporal pallor. Alcohol, tobacco, and vitamin B12 deficiency as well as drugs such as chloramphenicol, ethambutol, digitalis, chloroquine, and isoniazid have been implicated. Check for heavy metals also.

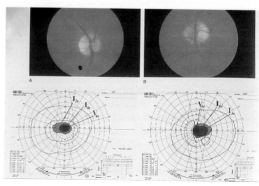

Patients with nutritional toxic optic neuropathies often have temporal pallor of the optic nerves (top) with bilateral centrocecal scotomas (bottom) on Goldmann visual field exam. (From Tasman W, Jaeger EA: The Wills Eye Hospital Atlas of Clinical Ophthalmology. Philadelphia, Lippincott-Raven, 1996, with permission.)

8. What may cause a constricted visual field?

- Retinitis pigmentosa
- End-stage glaucoma
- Thyroid ophthalmolopathy
- Optic nerve drusen
- Vitamin A deficiency
- Occipital strokes
- Panretinal photocoagulation
- Hysteria

9. How do you differentiate hysteria from real disease?

Have the patient do a tangent screen at two different distances. The closer the patient stands, the smaller the field should be. Hysteric patients rarely know this fact. Patients also may demonstrate spiraling with kinetic visual field testing (see visual field chapter).

10. A 65-year-old man notices that the vision in his left eye has worsened suddenly. He has 20/50 vision in his right eye and 20/100 in his left eye. The left eye also shows an afferent pupillary defect and decreased color plates. Visual field exam reveals an inferior altitudinal defect on the left with a normal full field on the right. On fundus exam, the left optic nerve appears pale and swollen superiorly. What is your concern?

Ischemic optic neuropathy (ION). An altitudinal defect is classic with ION. The two types are arteritic and nonarteritic. Because they are treated differently, you must differentiate the two. First, it is important to ask about symptoms of giant cell arteritis, such as weight loss, anorexia, fevers, jaw claudication, headache, scalp tenderness, and proximal joint and muscle pain. Check for a palpable, tender, nonpulsatile temporal artery. Immediately order an erythrocyte sedimentation rate (ESR) if you believe that giant cell arteritis is a consideration.

The patient denied any of the symptoms, and his ESR was 20. He was diagnosed with nonarteritic ION. Because 50% of these patients have cardiovascular disease, diabetes, and/or hypertension, he was sent to his internist. He was told that his prognosis for improved vision was low and that he should remain stable. Unfortunately, there is no proven treatment. A study recently showed no improvement with optic nerve sheath decompressions. With time, his optic nerve should atrophy in the area of damage. He has a 35% risk of involvement of the other eye.

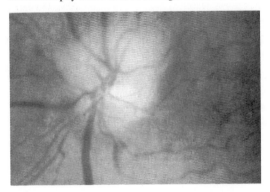

Superior segmental pale swelling of the optic disc in a patient with nonarteritic ischemic optic neuropathy. (From Tasman W, Jaeger EA: The Wills Eye Hospital Atlas of Clinical Ophthalmology. Philadelphia, Lippincott-Raven, 1996, with permission.)

11. An 80-year-old man presents with the same history of sudden vision loss and the same visual field. However, his vision is counting fingers at 10 feet, and his optic nerve is pale and swollen with flame-shaped hemorrhages. He admits to pain in his jaw when he chews, weight loss of 10 pounds, and difficulty in getting up from a chair. He has a tender temporal artery without pulses. The ESR is 120. What do you do?

First, you make a diagnosis of giant cell arteritis and place him on 250 mg of methylprednisolone every 6 hours IV for 3 days. Evidence suggests that such high doses can prevent the same process in the other eye. There is a 30% risk of involvement of the second eye. The patient is then scheduled for temporal artery biopsy.

12. Should the biopsy be done before the steroids are started to ensure that the diagnosis can be made?

Absolutely not. The steroids will not affect the biopsy results for at least 7 days. The therapeutic effect of the steroids is necessary immediately.

13. What biopsy finding makes the diagnosis?

Disruption of the internal elastic lamina. Giant cells are often present but are not necessary for the diagnosis.

14. What if the temporal artery biopsy is normal?

Giant cell arteritis is a diagnosis based mainly on symptoms. The ESR may be normal, and your suspicion should be extremely high because of the patient's history. Because skip areas also occur, make sure to get a significant length of artery for biopsy. Sometimes it is necessary to biopsy the other side in addition.

15. What else may herald giant cell arteritis?

Amaurosis fugax, cranial nerve palsies, or central retinal artery occlusion.

16. What is the differential diagnosis of optociliary shunt vessels?
- Meningioma
- Glaucoma
- Old central retinal vein occlusion
- Optic nerve glioma
- Chronic papilledema
- Idiopathic disease

17. An obese 30-year-old woman presents with severe headaches and occasional double vision. Her vision is 20/20 in both eyes. How do you evaluate her?

Check pupillary responses, color plates, visual fields, and extraocular motility; do a full slit-lamp and dilated exam. You notice that she has bilateral swollen optic nerves.

18. What do you do now?

You must emergently evaluate the patient for increased intracranial pressure. First, she needs a CT or MRI of the head to rule out a mass. Provided the scan is normal, a lumber puncture should follow. If the only abnormality is an increased opening pressure, the diagnosis is pseudotumor cerebri, also known as idiopathic intracranial hypertension.

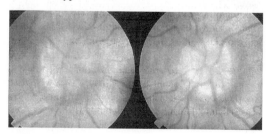

Papilledema in a 24-year-old obese woman with pseudotumor cerebri. The patient complained of severe headaches and transient visual obscurations. (From Tasman W, Jaeger EA: The Wills Eye Hospital Atlas of Clinical Ophthalmology. Philadelphia, Lippincott-Raven, 1996, with permission.)

19. What may cause pseudotumor cerebri?
- Obesity
- Pregnancy
- Steroids
- Oral contraceptives
- Tetracycline
- Nalidixic acid
- Vitamin A
- Idiopathic disease

20. How should the patient be treated?

If she has no optic nerve damage on visual fields, encourage her to lose weight. If the headaches continue or she has evidence of decreased visual acuity or visual field loss, treatment is indicated. Medications include a diuretic, such as acetazolamide, or systemic steroids. Optic nerve sheath decompression is used for worsening visual fields, and lumboperitoneal shunts have been used for headaches. The intraocular pressure should be treated if elevated.

21. Why did the patient have double vision?

Increased intracranial pressure may cause sixth-nerve palsies.

22. A mother brings in her first born for his first exam. He is 6 months old and appears not to see well. Dilated exam reveals optic nerve hypoplasia. What is the differential diagnosis?

Optic nerve hypoplasia seems to occur in the first born of young mothers who may have diabetes or who may have used lysergic acid diethylamide (LSD), phenytoin, or alcohol during pregnancy. Patients also may have optic nerve hypoplasia in association with Goldenhar's syndrome or septooptic dysplasia of de Morsier. The latter patients have see-saw nystagmus and chiasmal anomalies. Because of the risk of growth retardation, diabetes insipidus, and other pituitary abnormalities, patients with optic nerve hypoplasia should have a scan of the optic chiasm and an endocrine evaluation.

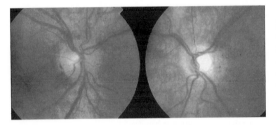

Hypoplasia of the left optic nerve. A small amount of optic nerve tissue is present nasally. Note the double ring sign. The right optic nerve is normal. (From Tasman W, Jaeger EA: The Wills Eye Hospital Atlas of Clinical Ophthalmology. Philadelphia, Lippincott-Raven, 1996, with permission.)

23. How do you differentiate between papilledema and pseudopapilledema?

Pseudopapilledema is not true disc swelling. The vessels surrounding the disc are not obscured, the disc is not hyperemic, and the peripapillary nerve fiber layer is normal. Spontaneous venous pulsations, if present, strongly suggest pseudopapilledema. Nerve fiber layer hemorrhages are not present in pseudopapilledema. Causes of pseudopapilledema include optic nerve drusen and congenitally anomalous discs.

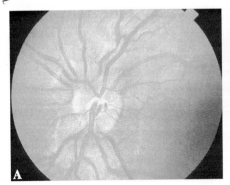
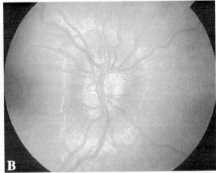

Pseudopapilledema (*A* and *B*) with no cupping. The vessels emerge from the center of the nerve and course into the retina without obscuration by edema, hemorrhage, or exudate. (From Tasman W, Jaeger EA: The Wills Eye Hospital Atlas of Clinical Ophthalmology. Philadelphia, Lippincott-Raven, 1996, with permission.)

24. A patient has a bilateral right-sided superior field defect. Where do you suspect the lesion is located?

A "pie-in-the-sky" defect is located in the temporal lobe. The inferior fibers loop around the temporal lobe (Meyer's loop).

25. What other symptoms may the patient have?

Formed hallucinations, déjà vu experiences, or uncinate fits.

26. What if the patient has a bilateral inferior right-sided visual field loss?

This "pie-on-the-floor" defect is typical for the parietal lobe. Patients have spasticity of conjugate gaze and optokinetic nystagmus abnormalities.

27. A patient presents with the visual field illustrated below. Where is the lesion located?

The right occipital lobe. The more congruous the defects, the more posterior their location. In addition, the nasal retina is larger and allows a temporal crescent in the visual field in the contralateral eye. Macular sparing or splitting also may occur.

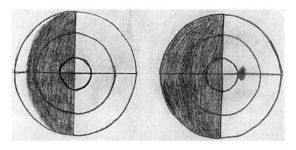

28. What else may the patient experience?

Patients with occipital lobe lesions often do not experience other neurologic abnormalities. If they do, they may have unformed hallucinations, dyschromatopsia, prosopagnosia, and alexia without agraphia.

29. What causes pseudo-Foster-Kennedy syndrome?

Pseudo-Foster-Kennedy syndrome is optic atrophy with contralateral optic disc edema. True Foster-Kennedy syndrome is due to a frontal lobe tumor. The pseudosyndrome is usually due to an acute ischemic optic neuropathy in one eye with contralateral atrophy due to a past episode of the same process. An olfactory groove meningioma also may cause the pseudosyndrome.

30. An 18-year-old man presents with sudden vision loss in one eye and then in the other within days. He denies pain. He has 20/20 vision in both eyes with decreased color plates and bilateral mild disc swelling with peripapillary telangiectatic microangiopathy. Affected vessels do not leak on fluorescein angiography. What does he have?

Leber's hereditary optic neuropathy. The patient's history is typical. The disorder is transmitted by mitochondrial DNA; all female carriers transmit it to their offspring. Ten percent of daughters and 50–70% of sons manifest the disease. All daughters are carriers. None of the sons are carriers. No effective treatment is known, but some mutations are more likely to have spontaneous improvement in the future; thus, genetic evaluation of the mitochondria is worthwhile.

BIBLIOGRAPHY

1. Burde RM, Savino PJ, Trobe JD: Clinical Decisions in Neuro-ophthalmology, 2nd ed. St. Louis, Mosby, 1992.
2. Cullom RD Jr, Chang B: The Wills Eye Manual, 2nd ed. Philadelphia, J.B. Lippincott, 1994.
3. Kline LB, Bajandas FJ: Neuro-ophthalmology Review Manual, 4th ed. Thorofare, NJ, Slack, 1996.

VII. Oculoplastics

34. TEARING AND THE LACRIMAL SYSTEM

Nancy G. Swartz, M.D., and Marc S. Cohen, M.D.

1. Describe the anatomy of the tear drainage system.

Tears travel across the cornea and conjunctiva to the medial canthus, where they enter the puncta of the upper and lower eyelids. The lacrimal puncta are small openings in the eyelid located approximately 6–7 mm from the medial canthus. They sit in small elevations of the soft tissue called the lacrimal papillae and are directed posteriorly toward the globe.

The tears then enter the canaliculi, which are mucosa-lined ducts approximately 10 mm in length that carry the tears to the lacrimal sac. The first portion of the canaliculus is a 2-mm dilated, vertical segment called the ampulla. The canaliculus then bends acutely and runs just below the eyelid margin toward the medial canthus, where, in most patients, the upper and lower canaliculi join to form the common canaliculus. In some patients, the canaliculi enter the lacrimal sac separately. The common canaliculus measures 3–5 mm in length and dilates to form the sinus of Maier just before entering the lacrimal sac on its posterolateral wall. A fold of mucosa of the lacrimal sac (the valve of Rosenmüller) covers this ostium, preventing the reflux of tears. The pretarsal orbicularis muscle surrounds the canaliculi and attaches to the wall of the lacrimal sac. Contraction and relaxation of this muscle help draw the tears into the canaliculus and the sac, and eventually force the tears down the nasolacrimal duct.

The lacrimal sac lies in a bony fossa of the medial orbital wall formed by the maxillary and lacrimal bones. It is generally in a collapsed state. The superficial head of the medial canthal tendon passes anterior to the sac, whereas the deep head passes posteriorly. The sac extends vertically for approximately 10 mm beginning a few millimeters superior to this medial canthal tendon and extending inferiorly to the nasolacrimal duct.

The nasolacrimal duct travels through a 12-mm bony canal and then continues inferiorly for 3–5 mm before opening into the inferior meatus of the nose. This ostium also gets protection from reflux by a fold of mucosa, the valve of Hasner. The ostium is located 30 mm from the external nares in an adult. In young children, this distance is approximately 20 mm.

2. What causes tearing?

Tearing, also called epiphora, can be caused by an increase in the amount of tears produced or by a problem with the tear drainage system. Excess tears are produced as a reflex when there is corneal irritation. Corneal irritation can be mechanical or can be be from a tear film deficiency. Inadequate tear drainage can result from a blockage in the tear drainage system, as in punctal stenosis, canalicular stenosis, and nasolacrimal duct obstructions. Eyelid malpositions (e.g., ectropion or punctal ectropion) and laxity of the lower eyelid with resultant poor tear pump function will also cause inadequate drainage of tears. For many patients, tearing is multifactorial.

3. What is the tear pump, and how does lower eyelid laxity reduce its function?

The excretion of tears is facilitated by a muscular "pump" in the eyelids that forces the tears by peristalsis through the lacrimal drainage system and into the nose. Normal drainage of tears requires normal structure and function of the eyelids, as well as a patent lacrimal drainage system.

The peristalsis of tears happens as follows. It is believed that tears first enter the punctum/ampulla by capillary action. In the resting state, the lacrimal sac is collapsed and tears do not enter at this time. During a blink, the orbicularis oculi muscle contracts, causing the puncta to close, the canaliculi to shorten and move medially, and the lacrimal sac to expand. This forces the tears medially through the canaliculi and creates a negative pressure in the sac, drawing the tears into it. When the muscle relaxes, the lacrimal sac again collapses. A valve between the canaliculi and sac, the valve of Rosenmüller, prevents the tears from reentering the canaliculi, so they are forced down the nasolacrimal duct into the nose. When lower eyelid laxity is present, the lacrimal pump mechanism cannot function adequately.

4. How can I tell if a patient has lower eyelid laxity?

Stretching of the medial and/or lateral canthal tendon causes lower eyelid laxity. This can be evaluated by the distraction test. If the lower eyelid can be pulled more than 6 mm from the globe, it is lax. Lateral canthal tendon laxity causes a rounding or blunting of the lateral canthal angle. When there is a stretching of the medial canthal tendon, the punctum can be pulled at least as lateral as the nasal corneal limbus. Poor orbicularis oculi tone, most obvious in patients with CN VII palsy, also causes laxity of the lower eyelid. This is best demonstrated with the snap back test. In this test, the lower eyelid is pulled down inferiorly and allowed to "snap back" into place. If the eyelid returns to its correct position immediately, the muscle tone is good. If the patient must blink in order to place the eyelid back in its normal position, eyelid tone is poor.

5. How do you correct lower eyelid laxity?

If there is laxity of the lateral canthal tendon, a horizontal lid shortening procedure is performed laterally. In this procedure, the inferior limb of the lateral canthal tendon is disinserted from the periosteum of the lateral orbital rim, and a new lateral canthal tendon is created from the lateral portion of the tarsus. The newly formed lateral canthal tendon is sutured back to the periosteum of the lateral orbital rim. This effectively shortens the lower eyelid.

Horizontal shortening is usually performed laterally when there is mild medial canthal tendon laxity as well, because medial canthal tendon plication can result in bunching of the canaliculus, with poor tear drainage postoperatively. However, if the medial canthal tendon laxity is severe, plication of the tendon or a medial wedge resection with canalicular reanastomosis over silicone stents can be performed.

6. Why do patients with dry eyes complain of tearing?

Patients tear when they have dry eyes for the same reason that they tear when cutting an onion. Onion fumes cause corneal irritation. Corneal irritation, in turn, causes reflex tearing. Likewise, abnormalities in the tear film coating the cornea cause an irritation of the cornea. Tear abnormalities can be due to a decrease in the overall production of tears or to an imbalance in the composition of the tears. Tears are composed of three layers. Mucin, made by the conjunctival goblet cells, covers the epithelium, assuring a smooth, uniform tear film. The middle layer of aqueous, made by the main and accessory lacrimal glands, provides the oxygen and nutrients to the cornea. The surface lipid layer made in the meibomian glands of the eyelids prevents rapid evaporation of the tears and provides a smooth surface for the eyelids to move across the cornea. Inadequacies in any of these causes a tear film deficiency. Staining with fluorescein or rose bengal occurs when corneal or conjunctival epithelium is affected by inadequate tears.

7. How can I determine if a patient produces enough tears?

The volume of tears can be assessed with direct visualization of the tear meniscus or by the Schirmer test. The tear meniscus, the tear layer between the lower eyelid and globe, should be approximately 1 mm in height. The Schirmer test is performed by gently drying the palpebral conjunctiva with a cotton swab and then placing the small folded end of a 5 mm wide strip of Whatman #41 filter paper into the inferior conjunctival fornix at the junction of the middle and lateral third of the lower eyelid for 5 minutes. The amount of wetting of the filter paper is then measured. If performed on an anesthetized cornea, basal tear secretion is measured. A normal result is at least 10 mm. If performed on a nonanesthetized cornea, both basal and reflex tearing are measured. In this setting, less than 15 mm of wetting is abnormal.

8. How do I know if the tear composition is inadequate?

A decrease in the tear break-up time or the presence of protein, mucus, or debris in the tears indicates a tear inadequacy. The tear break-up time is the time between a blink and the development of a dry spot on the cornea. It is measured by touching the palpebral conjunctiva with a moistened fluorescein strip and observing the tear film through the slit lamp with a cobalt-blue filter. It is important not to use other eye drops mixed with fluorescein, as this will change the composition of the tear film you observe. Once the patient blinks, time is measured until the tear film begins to break up on the cornea, causing a dry spot. Less than 10 seconds is considered abnormal.

9. What are ectropion and entropion, and how are they repaired?

Ectropion is an outward rotation of the eyelid margin. Involutional ectropion is due to stretching of the canthal tendons and is managed similarly to horizontal eyelid laxity without ectropion. If a punctal ectropion is present that does not resolve with a horizontal lid shortening procedure, this can be corrected by shortening the posterior lamella. This procedure, called a medial spindle procedure, involves excising a spindle-shaped portion of the conjunctiva and lower eyelid retractors inferior to the punctum. A horizontal mattress suture is then placed to reappose the edges of the tissue. The ends of the suture are brought out through the skin inferiorly and tied so that the everted punctum is brought back to its correct anatomic position.

Entropion is an inward rotation of the eyelid margin. Involutional entropion is caused by a constellation of eyelid abnormalities: eyelid laxity, attenuation or disinsertion of the lower eyelid retractors, orbicularis override (the preseptal orbicularis muscle overrides the pretarsal orbicularis muscle), and involutional enophthalmos. Correction of this necessitates not only a horizontal shortening procedure to address the eyelid laxity, but also a repair of the lower eyelid retractors and orbicularis. These can be addressed either by directly reattaching or plicating the retractors, or by a Wies procedure in which a full-thickness horizontal eyelid incision is made and then reapproximated. Here, the retractors and orbicularis are held in the correct position by the scar that forms postoperatively.

Repair of **cicatricial** ectropions and entropions usually requires grafting to replace the contracted tissue.

10. What causes obstructions in the lacrimal system?

Punctal obstructions can be due to a congenital agenesis, inflammation, infection, or trauma, or they can result from iatrogenic closure in the treatment of dry eyes.

Canalicular stenoses can occur in one or both canaliculi or in the common canaliculus. These can be congenital or acquired from trauma, infections, inflammation, or the long-term use of topical medications.

Lacrimal sac obstructions occur most frequently from scarring due to a prior infection. Dacryoliths may develop from infections or chronic use of topical medications. Lacrimal sac tumors are rare.

Nasolacrimal duct obstructions can be congenital, traumatic, inflammatory, or infectious. However, primary acquired nasolacrimal duct obstruction is the most common cause of obstructions in this location. The cause of these is poorly understood, although likely relates to obstruction of the ostium of the duct due to inflammation of the nasal mucosa.

11. How do I evaluate the lacrimal system for obstructions?

Obstructions can occur anywhere in the lacrimal system. Punctal obstructions can be visualized on examination. To determine the presence and location of the obstructions in the canaliculus, lacrimal sac, and nasolacrimal duct, a dye disappearance test is first performed. In the dye disappearance test, a drop of fluorescein is placed in the inferior conjunctival fornix and after 5 minutes the amount present in the tear lake is assessed using a cobalt-blue light. The presence of little or no fluorescein indicates a normally functioning system. If most of the fluorescein remains, the system is not functioning properly.

A primary Jones dye test can then be performed in which fluorescein is placed in the inferior conjunctival fornix and a cotton-tipped applicator is placed under the inferior turbinate at 2 minutes and 5 minutes. If dye is recovered on the cotton-tipped applicator, the system is patent and functioning well. If no dye is recovered, this indicates a poorly functioning system. This can be further evaluated with a secondary Jones dye test. In this test, the inferior fornix is then irrigated to remove all residual fluorescein. Clear saline is then irrigated through the canaliculus with a cannula. If fluorescein-stained fluid is recovered from the nose, the fluorescein must have passed freely through the punctum, canaliculus, and to the lacrimal sac during the primary Jones test, indicating a partial block of the nasolacrimal duct. If clear fluid is recovered, a partial obstruction or functional disorder of the punctum or canaliculus is indicated. If no fluid is recovered from the nose, but instead regurgitates from the adjacent punctum, an obstruction at or distal to the common canaliculus is present.

Obstruction in the canaliculus can be determined by probing the canaliculus and feeling for stenoses and complete obstructions. Imaging techniques of the lacrimal system, including ultrasound, CT scans, contrast dacryocystography, and radionuclide dacryoscintigraphy, are rarely necessary.

12. How do I treat obstructions of the lacrimal system?

When the punctum is not patent, this can frequently be opened with a sharp probe or cutdown procedure to find the proximal canaliculus. The punctum can be dilated, if needed. In some patients, placement of a temporary silicone stent is helpful to prevent the punctum from reclosing. This office-based procedure is performed with local infiltrative anesthesia.

The majority of lacrimal system obstructions occur in the nasolacrimal duct, which connects the lacrimal sac to the nose. When the obstruction is in the nose or nasolacrimal duct, a dacryocystorhinostomy (DCR) is performed. In this procedure, the lacrimal sac is marsupialized to the nasal passages, so the tears can bypass the blocked nasolacrimal duct and drain directly from the lacrimal sac into the nose.

Canalicular stenoses and obstructions are more difficult to manage. Dilation of a stenosis may be helpful, but the stenoses frequently recur. If obstruction is distal in the canaliculus, a canaliculo-dacryocystorhinostomy (CLDCR) is performed. In this surgery, a fistula is created between the canaliculi and the nasal mucosa. When the canaliculi are obstructed proximally, a conjunctivo-dacryocystorhinostomy (CJDCR) is needed. A fistula from the caruncle to the nasal mucosa is created, and a permanent glass tube (Jones tube) is placed in this tract to maintain its patency.

These procedures are generally performed on an outpatient basis. General anesthesia or local anesthesia with sedation can be used.

13. Describe acute dacryocystitis.

An acute infection of the lacrimal sac is called dacryocystitis. Patients typically present with a painful, erythematous swelling in the medial canthus just inferior to the medial canthal tendon. A purulent discharge from the punctum may be seen with gentle pressure on the lacrimal sac. If not adequately treated, an orbital cellulitis may develop. Systemic antibiotics should be given, and warm compresses should be applied to the medial canthus. Patients should be watched carefully to assure improvement. Once a dacryocystitis develops, a nasolacrimal duct obstruction is typically present and a DCR is usually needed to prevent recurrent infection and treat epiphora.

14. What are the signs of congenital nasolacrimal duct obstructions?

Approximately 6% of newborns have a congenital obstruction of the nasolacrimal system. Infants may present with epiphora, conjunctivitis, amniocele formation, or a dacryocystitis. The lacrimal drainage system begins embryologically as a cord in the medial canthus that expands laterally to the punctum and inferiorly to the nasal mucosa of the inferior meatus. The lumen also forms first in the medial canthus, and canalization develops laterally and inferiorly. The distal end of the duct is the last portion to canalize. This may not yet be patent at birth and is the most common site of congenital obstructions. However, developmental anomalies can occur anywhere in the lacrimal drainage system.

15. How are congenital obstructions first managed?

Most clinicians recommend massaging the infant's lacrimal sac (in the medial canthus) in an inferior direction to increase the hydrostatic pressure in the nasolacrimal duct and hopefully force open any obstruction. If there is an associated conjunctivitis or discharge, topical antibiotics are also used. Systemic antibiotics are used when a dacryocystitis is present.

16. What if this doesn't work?

When the problem persists, a probing of the system can be performed. Some clinicians probe infants as early as 3 months of age to avoid chronic inflammation, which can worsen the obstruction. Others feel that this should be postponed until 12 months of age, as most obstructions will resolve spontaneously by this time, thus avoiding unnecessary procedures. Katowitz and Welsh have shown that the success rates of probing drop significantly if performed after 13 months of age.

Approximately 90–95% of infants who undergo a probing enjoy a resolution of their symptoms. For those that do not, a second probing may be successful. When the problem persists after two probings, intubation with silicone tubes is indicated. Tubes are generally left in place for approximately 6 months and serve to keep the passageway open. Durso et al. reported an 84% success rate for patients intubated for nasolacrimal duct obstruction.

When probing and intubation are unsuccessful, DCR is performed. Unless complicated by recurrent dacryocystitis, surgery is usually delayed until the child is 18 months of age. Success rates for DCR surgery in children are similar to those for adults, usually between 90 and 95%.

BIBLIOGRAPHY

1. Durso F, Hand SI Jr, Ellis FD, Helveston EM: Silicone intubation in children with nasolacrimal obstruction. J Pediatr Ophthalmol Strabismus 17:389, 1980.
2. Kanski JJ: Clinical Ophthalmology. Oxford, Butterworth Heineman, 1989, pp 45–60.
3. Katowitz JA, Welsh MG: Timing of initial probing and irrigation in congenital nasolacrimal duct obstruction. Ophthalmology 94:698–705, 1987.
4. Wellham RAN, Hughes SM: Lacrimal surgery in children. Am J Ophthalmol 99:27, 1985.

35. ORBITAL IMAGING

Patrick De Potter, M.D.

1. What is required when you order orbital MR studies?
1. Surface coil (orbital or head coil) for better visualization of structures of the orbit
2. Precontrast axial, coronal, and sagittal T1-weighted images
3. Axial, coronal T2-weighted images (fast spin-echo sequences)
4. Postcontrast axial coronal T1-weighted images with fat suppression techniques
5. Sedation in children

2. What is the strategy in ordering imaging studies in a child with the diagnosis of retinoblastoma?
The first goal of imaging studies is to confirm the diagnosis suspected clinically. The presence of calcification is highly suggestive of retinoblastoma, and documentation by imaging studies confirms the diagnosis. The second goal of imaging studies is to evaluate the possible extraocular extension of the tumor. Ultrasonography should be the first imaging tool. A- and B-scan ultrasonography is cheap and allows the eye to be evaluated in the office without general anesthesia. If calcification is documented on ultrasonography, orbital MRI is recommended to evaluate the optic nerve and orbital tissue and rule out extraocular extension of retinoblastoma. Initial MRI of the brain is recommended in patients with bilateral and/or familial retinoblastoma to detect an associated early asymptomatic midline cerebral malignancy (pinealoblastoma). As the second imaging step, orbital CT is recommended only if calcification is not visualized on ultrasonography.

3. What is the strategy in ordering imaging studies in an adult with the diagnosis of intraocular neoplasm?
A- and B-scan ultrasonography is the first imaging tool to evaluate an adult with an intraocular neoplasm. The role of CT is limited because of its poor tissue definition. Therefore, there is no indication for CT in the evaluation of an elevated choroidal or subretinal mass. If ultrasonography, fluorescein angiography, and indocyanine green angiography do not help in the differential diagnosis, pre- and postcontrast-enhanced MR studies with fat suppression techniques are most helpful in detecting and diagnosing intraocular lesions.

4. What are paramagnetic agents?
Paramagnetic agents produce proton relaxation enhancement by shortening the intrinsic T1 and T2 relaxation times of the tissue in which they are present. Therefore, paramagnetic agents increase the signal intensity of the tissues. Melanin, methemoglobin, protein, and gadolinium are the most common paramagnetic agents. For example, a dermoid cyst with a high proteinaceous content shows a higher signal intensity on T1- and T2-weighted images than a clear inclusion cyst.

5. In which clinical situations are contrast-enhanced MR studies most helpful in the evaluation of a child with leukocoria?
To differentiate retinoblastoma from Coats' disease.

6. In which clinical situations are contrast-enhanced MR studies most helpful in the evaluation of an adult with vitreous hemorrhage?
To differentiate a malignant melanoma of the choroid from a hemorrhagic retinal detachment in age-related macular/extramacular degeneration. These two conditions are the most

common causes of vitreous hemorrhage when an elevated subretinal mass is detected by ultra-sonography. Although in precontrast studies both lesions may show the same MR features, the choroidal melanoma shows enhancement after contrast administration, whereas the hemorrhagic detachment does not.

7. What are the indications for ordering CT orbital studies as a first choice?
1. Evaluation of orbital trauma
2. Detection of foreign body
3. Detection of calcification
4. Evaluation of osseous, cartilaginous, and fibroosseous lesions
5. Evaluation of orbital soft tissue lesion with suspicion of bony erosion or detection
6. Contraindication to MRI

8. What are the indications for ordering MR orbital studies as a first choice?
1. Acute proptosis
2. Suspicion of optic nerve sheath complex lesion
3. Intraocular tumor with extraocular extension
4. Detection of wood foreign body
5. Contraindications to CT

9. Name the most common orbital lesions showing a well-circumscribed and sharply de-lineated appearance on CT and MRI.

Children	Adults
1. Dermoid cyst	1. Cavernous hemangioma
2. Lymphangioma	2. Neurofibroma
3. Rhabdomyosarcoma	3. Neurilemoma
4. Optic nerve glioma	4. Fibrous histiocytoma
	5. Lymphoproliferative disorders

10. Name the most common orbital lesions showing an ill-defined appearance on CT and MRI.

Children	Adults
1. Capillary hemangioma	1. Idiopathic orbital inflammation
2. Idiopathic orbital inflammation	2. Metastasis
3. Plexiform neurofibroma	3. Leukemic infiltrate
4. Leukemic infiltrate	4. Primary malignant tumor
5. Eosinophilic granuloma	5. Lymphoproliferative disorders

11. Which are the ocular and orbital tissues that do not normally enhance on postcontrast MR studies?
1. Lens
2. Vitreous
3. Sclera
4. Orbital fat
5. Optic nerve sheath complex

12. In which clinical situation are contrast-enhanced MR studies most helpful in the evaluation of a patient with proptosis?
In general, the soft tissue definition of MRI does not allow a definite histopathologic diagnosis. Ill-defined inflammatory tissues may share the same MR features as solid infiltrative neoplastic lesions on pre- and postcontrast studies. Well-circumscribed solid tumors may share the same MR characteristics as well-defined cystic lesion on precontrast studies. MRI becomes the most helpful tool for the clinician when a well-circumscribed lesion is found. After contrast

administration, a solid neoplastic tumor always shows enhancement, whereas a cystic lesion does not enhance (except intralesional septae and capsule).

13. What are the indications for MR angiography and carotid angiography when imaging orbital lesions?

None.

14. How can you differentiate optic nerve from optic nerve sheath lesions with CT and MR studies?

Differentiation is almost impossible with CT. MRI is the relevant study. First of all, a normal optic nerve does not demonstrate any enhancement on MRI studies after contrast injection. The localization of the enhancement (best seen on T1-weighted images with fat suppression techniques) helps to differentiate a neoplastic or inflammatory optic nerve from an optic nerve sheath process. An optic nerve tumor or inflammation demonstrates central enhancement, whereas an optic nerve sheath neoplasm or inflammation demonstrates peripheral enhancement. A cystic or hemorrhagic lesion does not enhance.

MR Features of Normal Ocular and Orbital Tissues

	SIGNAL INTENSITY T1-WEIGHTED IMAGES	SIGNAL INTENSITY T2-WEIGHTED IMAGES	ENHANCEMENT AFTER GADOLINIUM-DTPA INJECTION
Lens	High	Low	−
Vitreous	Low	High	−
Choroid	High	High	+++
Retina	Not detected	Not detected	−
Sclera	Low	Low	−
Optic nerve	Low	Low	−
Orbital fat	High	Low	−
Extraocular muscle	Low	Low	+++
Lacrimal gland	Low	Low	+++
Cortical bone	Low	Low	−

BIBLIOGRAPHY

1. De Potter P, Shields JA, Shields CL: MRI of the Eye and Orbit. Philadelphia, J.B. Lippincott, 1995.
2. Newton TH, Bilaniuk LT: Radiology of the Eye and Orbit. New York, Raven Press, 1990.
3. De Potter P, Shields CL, Shields JA, Flanders AE: The role of magnetic resonance imaging in children with intraocular tumors and simulating lesions. Ophthalmology 103:1774–1783, 1996.
4. De Potter P, Flanders AE, Shields JA, et al: The role of fat-suppression technique and gadopentetate dimeglumine in magnetic resonance imaging evaluation of intraocular tumors and simulating lesions. Arch Ophthalmol 112:340–348, 1994.
5. De Potter P, Shields JA, Shields CL: Computed tomography and magnetic resonance imaging of intraocular lesions. Ophthalmol Clin North Am 7:333–346, 1994.

36. PROPTOSIS

David G. Buerger, M.D.

1. What is proptosis?

Proptosis is a forward protrusion of one or both eyeballs. Unilateral proptosis is frequently defined as asymmetric protrusion of one eye by at least 2 mm. Normal upper limits for proptosis are approximately 22 mm in Caucasians and 24 mm in African-Americans (see table, p. 244).

2. How is proptosis diagnosed?

Clinically, proptosis can be recognized by observing the globes from above, over the patient's forehead. It is measured with an exophthalmometer, which is usually based at the lateral orbital rim. The amount of proptosis can also be quantified by measuring globe protrusion on a CT scan.

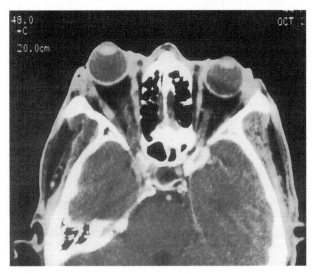

CT scan demonstrating proptosis of the right globe secondary to thyroid-related enlargement of the rectus muscles.

3. List common problems associated with proptosis.

1. **Exposure keratopathy** frequently develops secondary to a poor blink mechanism over the protruding globe. Patients can have mild symptoms of irritation and foreign body sensation, or more severe symptoms associated with corneal abrasions and ulcers (see figure, next page).

2. **Diplopia** (double vision) can result from unilateral or bilateral proptosis from displacement of the globes or poor extraocular muscle function.

3. **Optic nerve compression** can occur with space-occupying lesions of the orbit, which cause proptosis. Indications of nerve compression include decreased visual acuity, relative afferent pupillary defect, color vision deficit, and visual field defect of the affected eye. This is a medical emergency and requires prompt therapeutic intervention, surgically or medically.

4. What is the most common cause of unilateral proptosis?

Thyroid eye disease (Graves' ophthalmopathy).

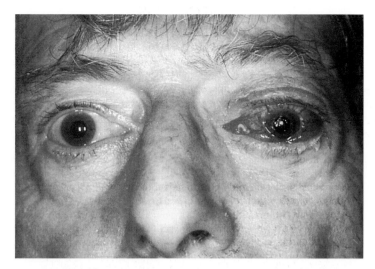

Severe conjunctival chemosis and injection with corneal erosion secondary to proptosis caused by an orbital lymphoma.

5. What is the most common cause of bilateral proptosis?
Thyroid eye disease.

6. What are other causes of proptosis?
Orbital inflammatory pseudotumor

Orbital infectious cellulitis

Orbital tumors (benign or malignant)

Lacrimal gland tumors

Trauma (retrobulbar hemorrhage)

Orbital vasculitis (i.e., polyarteritis nodosa, Wegener's granulomatosis)

Mucormycosis

Carotid–cavernous fistula

Orbital varix

7. List the causes of pseudoproptosis.
1. Unilateral high axial myopia can mimic proptosis owing to the increased length of the myopic eye.

2. Actual enophthalmos of one eye may cause apparent proptosis of the contralateral eye (see figure).

3. Upper lid retraction produces a more prominent appearing eye. This often coexists in cases of thyroid ophthalmopathy.

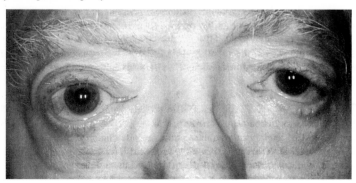

Patient with enophthalmos of the left eye secondary to old trauma, which is causing apparent proptosis of the right eye.

.euroimaging test is best to evaluate the etiology of proptosis?

‿ı scans are superior in most cases of proptosis because the relationship of the orbital process to the orbital bones is better visualized. MRI may be desirable in certain cases when optic nerve dysfunction is present. Plain films are not used for diagnostic accuracy in cases of proptosis.

9. Which clinical entity is frequently associated with unilateral or bilateral painless proptosis, eyelid retraction, eyelid lag on downward gaze, and motility disturbances?

Thyroid ophthalmopathy associated with Graves' disease is a complex, multisystem, autoimmune disorder. Patients can be hyperthyroid, hypothyroid, or euthyroid to manifest the ophthalmic symptoms. Eye problems develop as a result of inflammation and enlargement of various extraocular muscles (most frequently the inferior rectus and medial rectus) and peribulbar tissues. CT scan or MRI often shows fusiform enlargement of the involved extraocular muscles with sparing of the tendon that attaches the muscle to the globe. Proptosis and eyelid retraction cause corneal problems, and muscle enlargement in the orbit causes diplopia and possibly optic nerve compression. Treatment is in stages depending on the severity of the eye disease. Systemic and laboratory evaluation is mandatory.

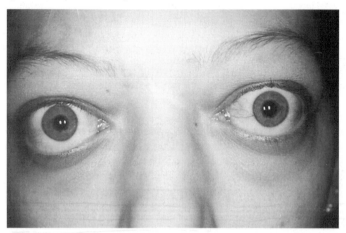

Proptosis and eyelid retraction caused by thyroid ophthalmopathy.

10. Which clinical entity is frequently associated with unilateral proptosis, pain, conjunctival injection, and motility disturbances in an adult?

Orbital inflammatory pseudotumor is a nonspecific idiopathic inflammatory disease of the orbit. Inflammation may be localized to a muscle, the lacrimal gland, sclera, or may be diffuse. Other possible signs include eyelid erythema or edema, palpable mass, decreased vision, uveitis, hyperopic shift, and optic nerve edema. Bilateral disease is more common in children. CT scan may show thickening of one or more extraocular muscles (including the tendons), lacrimal gland enlargement, or thickening of the posterior sclera. Treatment is primarily with corticosteroids and possibly radiation therapy.

11. Which clinical entity is characterized by unilateral proptosis, pain, fever, decreased ocular motility, erythema, and edema of the eyelids?

Infectious orbital cellulitis involves an infection (usually bacterial) that has extended posterior to the orbital septum. Once past the orbital septum barrier, infection can spread rapidly and cause serious complications such as meningitis or cavernous sinus thrombosis. The most common organisms include staphylococci, streptococci, anaerobes, and *Haemophilus influenzae* (in children under 5 years of age). The most common source of infectious spread to the orbit is an ethmoid sinusitis. Treatment is with intravenous antibiotics.

12. What should be done for persistent proptosis or progression of infect **quate antibiotic treatment in a case of orbital cellulitis?**

The situation is highly suggestive of an orbital subperiosteal abscess. CT sc\: performed to confirm this diagnosis and locate the abscess. Definitive treatment \(cal drainage and continued intravenous antibiotics.

13. Which clinical entity is characterized by a child less than 6 years of age with gradual, painless, progressive, unilateral axial proptosis with visual loss?

Optic nerve glioma (juvenile pilocytic astrocytoma) is a slow-growing tumor of the optic nerve that causes axial proptosis. Decreased visual acuity is usually associated with a relative afferent pupillary defect. CT scan or MRI shows fusiform enlargement of the optic nerve. Many cases are associated with neurofibromatosis and may be bilateral. Systemic evaluation and genetic counselling for neurofibromatosis is essential.

14. Which clinical entity is characterized by a child with rapidly progressive unilateral proptosis, displacement of the globe inferiorly, and edema of the upper eyelid?

Rhabdomyosarcoma is the most common primary orbital malignancy of childhood. This malignant growth of striated muscle tissue typically produces a rapidly progressive mass in the superior orbit with proptosis, globe displacement, and eyelid swelling. The average age of presentation is 7 years. Prompt diagnosis with orbitotomy and biopsy is crucial, because **overall mortality is 60%** once the disease has extended to orbital bones. Current treatment strategies with radiation and chemotherapy have lowered mortality rates to 5 to 10% for orbital rhabdomyosarcoma.

15. What is the most common benign orbital tumor in adults that causes unilateral proptosis?

The cavernous hemangioma is a slow-growing vascular tumor that is usually diagnosed in young adulthood to middle age. CT scan usually shows a well-defined orbital mass within the ocular muscle cone. Visual acuity is often not affected. Treatment is observation or surgical excision.

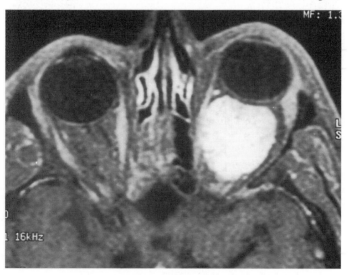

Cavernous hemangioma of the left orbit causing proptosis.

16. What is the most common malignant orbital tumor in adults that causes unilateral proptosis?

Orbital lymphomas typically develop in the superior orbit with a slow onset and progression. These lesions may be associated with a subconjunctival "salmon-colored" mass in the fornix. CT

.n shows a poorly defined mass conforming to the shape of the orbital bones and globe without bony erosion. Diagnosis is made following orbital biopsy, and definitive treatment is radiation therapy. Orbital lymphoma can be associated with systemic lymphoma; therefore, a medical consult and systemic evaluation are necessary for all patients.

17. Of the various orbital tumors causing proptosis, list those tumors that are encapsulated or appear well circumscribed on neuroimaging.

Cavernous hemangioma	Schwannoma
Fibrohistiocytoma	Neurofibroma
Hemangiopericytoma	

BIBLIOGRAPHY

1. Dolman PJ, Glazer LC, et al: Mechanisms of visual loss in severe proptosis. Ophthal Plast Reconstr Surg 7:256, 1991.
2. Frueh BR: Positional effects on exophthalmometric readings in Graves' eye disease. Arch Ophthalmol 103:1355, 1985.
3. Frueh BR: Exophthalmometer readings in patients with Graves' eye disease. Ophthalmic Surg 17(1):37, 1986.
4. Henderson JW: Orbital Tumors. New York, Raven Press, 1994.
5. Hornblass A: Oculoplastic, Orbital and Reconstructive Surgery. Baltimore, Williams & Wilkins, 1988.
6. Rootman J: Diseases of the Orbit. Philadelphia, J.B. Lippincott, 1988.
7. Zimmerman RA, Bilaniuk LT, et al: Orbital magnetic resonance imaging. Am J Ophthalmol 100:312, 1985.

37. THYROID-RELATED OPHTHALMOPATHY

Robert B. Penne, M.D.

1. What is thyroid-related ophthalmopathy?

Thyroid-related ophthalmopathy (TRO) is a chronic inflammatory disease of the orbits that often occurs in patients with systemic thyroid imbalance. Chronic inflammation results in scarring and dysfunction of the orbit. The course and severity are variable.

2. Who develops TRO?

TRO may occur in a wide range of ages. It has been reported from 8 to 88 years of age, with the average age in the 40s. Females are affected 3–6 times more often than males. Children are rarely affected.

3. Is everyone with TRO hyperthyroid?

Eighty percent of patients who develop TRO do so while they are hyperthyroid or after they are diagnosed with hyperthyroidism. Ten percent of patients have some form of hypothyroidism, and up to 10% may not develop a clinically detectable thyroid abnormality. A recent study found that as many as one-third of patients do not develop clinical hyperthyroidism for more than 6 months after onset of symptoms of TRO. This finding suggests that a significant number of patients who present with TRO have not yet developed hyperthyroidism.

4. What causes TRO?

We do not know. TRO appears to be an immunologically mediated process with the extraocular muscles as the end organs. Many theories link the orbit and thyroid gland by shared antigens, with some defect in immune surveillance initiating the process. Research continues.

5. Do environmental factors affect TRO?

The one environmental factor that has been shown definitely to affect TRO is smoking. Multiple studies have shown a higher incidence of smoking in patients with TRO than in patients with Graves' disease who do not have TRO. Evidence also suggests that smokers with TRO have more severe disease than nonsmokers. The effects of second-hand smoke can only be speculated.

6. Does eye disease improve when systemic thyroid imbalance is treated?

Treatment of the systemic thyroid dysfunction has little predictable effect on the course of TRO. An equal number of patients improve, worsen, or stay the same. The effects of systemic treatment on TRO are still debated. Also debated is whether radioactive iodine, surgery, and medical treatment have different effects on the course of TRO. To date, the type of treatment does not seem to affect the course of TRO.

7. What are the early signs of TRO?

Many patients initially present with intermittent lid swelling along with nonspecific ocular irritation, redness, and swelling. All of these symptoms are so nonspecific that early onset is usually missed. The disease is not recognized until the appearance of more obvious clinical signs such as lid retraction, lid lag, or early proptosis (see figure, next page). Suspecting TRO in patients with the above nonspecific symptoms is important, especially if they have symptoms or history of a thyroid imbalance.

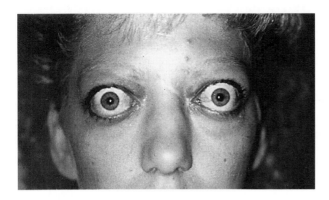

Thyroid-related ophthalmopathy
with proptosis and lid retraction.

8. What studies need to be done in the work-up for TRO?

The most effective screening tool for systemic thyroid imbalance in patients with TRO is the level of thyroid-stimulating hormone (TSH). Further evaluation and work-up can be done by an internist or endocrinologist. A complete ophthalmic exam is needed. Special attention is paid to visual function, including acuity, pupils, color vision, and visual fields, if indicated. Ocular motility with note of any diplopia needs evaluation, along with corneal exposure, proptosis, and eyelid position.

9. Which patients require orbital imaging?

Not all patients with TRO require orbital imaging. Indications for imaging include suspicion of optic nerve compression, evaluation for orbital decompression surgery, unclear diagnosis, and need to rule out other orbital processes. I prefer a CT scan in patients with TRO who require imaging.

10. What findings are present on orbital imaging?

Enlargement of the rectus muscle belly with sparing of the tendon is the classic finding. The inferior rectus is the most commonly involved muscle, followed by the medial rectus and the superior rectus. The lateral rectus is least likely to be involved.

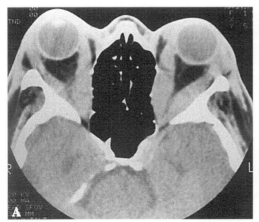
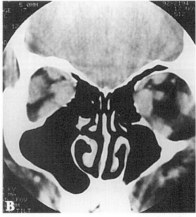

Axial *(A)* and coronal *(B)* CT scans showing enlargement of all four rectus muscles.

11. Does everyone with proptosis have TRO?

No. TRO is the most common cause of both unilateral and bilateral proptosis in adults, but it is not the only cause. Patients with systemic thyroid disease may develop orbital tumors and non-thyroid orbital inflammation. TRO is a bilateral disease, whereas most orbital tumors are unilateral. TRO may present asymmetrically and appear unilateral, especially early in the disease. In rare cases the disease may remain unilateral. If the entire clinical picture is not consistent with TRO, orbital imaging is indicated.

12. How do the tissues of the orbit change in TRO?

The extraocular muscles are the main target for TRO. Infiltration by inflammatory cells results in fibroblasts that produce mucopolysaccharides in early disease and collagen in later stages. Orbital and eyelid swelling is common early in the disease. Late in the disease, the inflammation resolves and the enlarged muscles become fibrotic and scarred.

13. How long does the disease last?

Most patients go through a period of active inflammation and changes in their eyes. This period lasts from 6 months to more than 2 years. In some patients the process may involve slow, mild changes over many months, whereas in others the process is more acute with rapid changes over weeks. Once the disease activity has quieted and the eyes are stable, reactivation is rare. Careful examinations that note changes in motility, eyelid position, proptosis, and general inflammation help to determine disease activity.

14. Is everyone who develops TRO affected in the same way?

No. There is a wide variation from mild irritation and lid retraction that resolve totally to severe orbital infiltration with visual loss. Visual loss may result from optic nerve compression or corneal scarring due to corneal exposure. More severe disease involves older patients (average age of 52 vs. 36 for milder disease) and has less of a gender difference (female-to-male ratio of 1.5:1 in severe disease vs. 8.6:1 in mild disease).

15. What can be done to treat TRO?

Many patients do not require any treatment, but monitoring during the active phase of the disease is important. Systemic steroids decrease inflammation. They are best used as a temporizing measure until more definitive treatment is given because of their side effects. Cessation of steroids generally results in return of orbital inflammation. Orbital irradiation decreases inflammation in the orbit. Surgical treatment is also used.

16. When are systemic steroids used?

Systemic steroids are used to decrease orbital inflammation acutely, usually on a temporary basis until other treatment can be started. The most common indication is visual loss from optic nerve compression. Severe proptosis with resultant corneal exposure is a second indication. Both short-term and long-term side effects of steroids limit their usefulness as long-term treatment.

17. How does orbital irradiation affect TRO?

The exact mechanism of action of irradiation in the orbit is unclear. Multiple theories of localized immunosuppression in the orbit have been postulated, but all remain unproved. Most patients have a definite decrease in orbital inflammation and edema after orbital irradiation.

18. Does orbital irradiation work immediately?

No. It takes from 2–4 weeks to see the effects of irradiation, and improvement may continue well beyond that time. If steroids are stopped immediately after completion of irradiation, inflammation may recur rapidly.

19. Which patients require surgery?

Surgery may be indicated on an emergent basis because of optic nerve compression or corneal exposure. More often patients require nonemergent surgery because of severe disfiguring proptosis, double vision from restrictive myopathy, or eyelid retraction.

20. What kinds of surgery are done in patients with TRO?

Surgery falls into three basic categories: orbital decompression, eye muscle surgery, and eyelid surgery. Surgery needs to be done in this order because earlier surgeries affect the results of later surgeries. Decompression should be done before eye muscle surgery. Decompression affects ocular motility and may alter muscle surgery. Likewise, muscle surgery should be completed before eyelid surgery is done.

21. What is orbital decompression?

Orbital decompressive surgery involves removal of bone and/or fat to allow the eye to settle back in the orbit. Bone is removed from the inferior and medial walls of the orbit to let the expanded orbital tissue move partially into the sinus space. Removal of orbital fat has a decompressive effect to a much lesser degree. The amount of decompression is related to the amount of fat removed.

22. Which patients require orbital decompression?

Patients with optic nerve compression require decompressive surgery to relieve pressure on the optic nerve. Patients with severe proptosis resulting in corneal exposure or disfigurement are also candidates for orbital decompressive surgery.

23. What is optic nerve compression?

Optic nerve compression is squeezing of the optic nerve at the apex of the orbit. When the extraocular muscles swell in TRO, there is relatively little space at the apex of the orbit; therefore, enlargement of muscles exerts pressure on the nerve lying in the center of the muscles. Pressure decreases vision because the function of the optic nerve is affected.

24. What are the complications of orbital decompression?

The most common complication is worsening of existing diplopia or new double vision. Patients with preexisting motility problems have a much higher risk of postoperative diplopia. Many patients have infraorbital hypesthesia postoperatively, but it usually improves with time. Risk of visual loss is small. Bleeding and infection, as with any surgery, must be considered.

25. When do patients require muscle surgery?

Patients with double vision in their functional field of vision require muscle surgery. Every effort must be made to ensure that the inflammation is quiet and the patient's motility pattern stable. Repeated stable measurements over months help to ensure that motility is stable.

26. What are the alternatives to muscle surgery?

The use of prisms in glasses works for patients with double vision and relatively small deviations. Larger deviations or patterns of diplopia in which the deviation changes with small changes in the direction of gaze are poor candidates for prisms. It is also important that the motility is stable before prisms are prescribed. Temporary Fresnel prisms may be helpful during periods of instability.

27. What type of muscle surgery is required?

Recession of muscles, usually on an adjustable suture. Because the muscles are tight and scarred, resection is not done. The inferior and medical rectus muscles are the most common targets of surgery. Surgery can be done under local or general anesthesia with adjustment of the sutures on the following day.

28. Does eye muscle surgery affect the eyelids?

Recession of the tight inferior rectus often improves upper eyelid retraction. The superior rectus muscle has to work against the tight inferior rectus; thus the associated levator muscle is overactive, causing eyelid retraction. When the inferior muscle is recessed, the overactivity ends and often the upper lid retraction is less. Large recessions of the inferior rectus muscle may worsen inferior lid retraction.

29. What kind of eyelid surgery is done?

Eyelid retraction is the main problem in patients with TRO. In patients undergoing orbital decompression, the eye is lowered, often improving the lower lid retraction. For mild lid retraction, recession of the eyelid retractors (upper or lower) is adequate. For more severe retraction, spacers are needed, such as hard palate in the lower lids and fascia in the upper lids. Patients also may require a blepharoplasty and/or brow lift to deal with the excessive skin that results from stretching due to chronic swelling. This goal may be met at the time of eyelid repositioning or at at later date.

30. How many surgeries do patients with TRO require?

Most patients with TRO do not require surgery. Patients needing surgery may need from 1 to as many as 8–10 operations. Patients with severe disease may require many operations over 2–3 years of reconstruction.

BIBLIOGRAPHY

1. Bartley GB, Fatourechi V, Kadrmas EF: The chronology of Graves' ophthalmopathy in an incidence cohort. Am J Ophthalmol 121:426–434, 1996.
2. Char DH: The ophthalmology of Graves' disease. Med Clin North Am 75:97–119, 1991.
3. Char DH: Thyroid Eye Disease, 2nd ed. New York, Churchill Livingstone, 1990.
4. Hornblass A: Oculoplastic, Orbital, and Reconstructive Surgery. Baltimore, Williams & Wilkins, 1990.
5. McCord CD, Tanenbaum M, Nunery WR: Oculoplastic Surgery, 3rd ed. New York, Raven Press, 1995.
6. Nunery WR, Martin RT, Heintz GW: The association of cigarette smoking with subtypes of ophthalmic Graves' disease. Plast Reconstr Surg 9(2):77–82, 1993.
7. Rootman J: Diseases of the Orbit. Philadelphia, J.B. Lippincott, 1988.
8. Rootman J, Stewart B, Goldberg RA: Orbital Surgery: A Conceptual Approach. Philadelphia, Lippincott-Raven, 1995.
9. Shorr N, Seiff SR: The four stages of surgical rehabilitation of the patient with dysthyroid ophthalmopathy. Ophthalmology 93:476, 1986.
10. Tasman W: Duane's Clinical Ophthalmology, vol. 2. Philadelphia, Lippincott-Raven, 1995.

38. ORBITAL INFLAMMATIONS

Marlon Maus, M.D., F.A.C.S.

1. What diseases affect the orbit? Which are inflammatory in nature?

Only about 60% of orbital disease is inflammatory in nature. Of the remainder, 20% is neoplastic, 15% structural, 3% vascular, and about 2% degenerative. Over 85% of inflammatory disease is thyroid-related, whereas less than 15% is due to other types of inflammation.

2. What is inflammation?

The classic signs of inflammation are dolor, calor, rubor, tumor, and functio laesa—in simpler terms, pain, heat, redness, swelling, and loss of function. All of these signs are normally seen in acute inflammation, which is defined as a localized protective response elicited by injury or destruction of tissues and serving to sequester both the injurious agent and the injured tissue. Inflammation is **acute** when it is sudden in onset. **Chronic** inflammation, on the other hand, represents a slow progression that may be a continuation of the acute form or a prolonged low-grade form. Chronic inflammation has a greater tendency to cause permanent tissue damage. Orbital inflammation can affect any or all of the structures within the orbit.

3. What is a complete orbital exam?

Orbital symptoms include proptosis, diplopia, visual impairment, and pain. A complete orbital exam addresses each and includes basic evaluative procedures.

Proptosis. Usually proptosis is measured with a Hertel exophthalmometer from the lateral orbital rim to the corneal apex (see table). A normal measurement is < 20 mm. A difference of 2 mm between the eyes is considered significant. Proptosis is defined according to race and gender. The different types of proptosis are (1) axial, which represents an intraconal process (i.e., within the conc formed by the extraocular muscles), the most common example of which is Graves' disease, and (2) nonaxial, which represents an extraconal process and is seen in 95% of orbital tumors. Proptosis may have different properties; for example, it may increase with the Valsalva maneuver or have pulsations.

Hertel Exophthalmometry Values—Normal Adults

	MEAN PROTRUSION	UPPER LIMITS OF NORMAL
White men	16.5 mm	21.7 mm
White women	15.4 mm	20.1 mm
Black men	18.5 mm	24.7 mm
Black women	17.8 mm	23.0 mm

Adapted from Migliori ME, Gladstone GJ: Determination of the normal range of exophthalmometric values for black and white adults. Am J Ophthalmol 98:438–442, 1984.

Diplopia. Extraocular movement problems usually present with symptoms of diplopia. Ocular movements should always be checked. A forced duction test may be used to diagnose restriction of the extraocular muscles.

Visual impairment. Vision may be impaired by optic nerve compression due to raised intraorbital pressure. One of the earliest signs is decreased color vision. Color vision is measured with Ishihara color plates. Other causes of impairment include raised intraocular pressure, exposure keratopathy, choroidal folds, and pseudohypermetropia.

Pain. Do not forget to palpate for masses or local swellings (e.g., lacrimal gland). Check for tenderness and test retropulsion. Decreased retropulsion may be seen in space-occupying lesions or swelling.

Auscultation. Listen for bruits (for example, in the case of a carotid-cavernous fistula).

Slit lamp exam. Check tear film, cornea (for example, superior limbic keratoconjunctivitis is seen in Graves' disease), and conjunctival vessels, which may be arterialized in a dural shunt or tortuous at the muscle insertion in Graves' disease. Record intraocular pressure, particularly in upgaze, which may be raised in Graves' disease.

Ophthalmoscopy. Check for (1) disc pallor, (2) disc swelling, (3) optociliary shunt vessels, and (4) choroidal folds.

A complete general exam may give hints of systemic disease.

4. What tests help in the diagnosis of orbital disease, in particular Graves' disease?

A computed tomography (CT) scan is obtained to evaluate causes of proptosis and patients for whom decompression surgery is contemplated. The CT scan shows enlarged extraocular muscles that spare the tendon when Graves' disease is a concern; if the tendon is involved, pseudotumor may be a possibility. Be sure to get both axial and coronal cuts.

Magnetic resonance imaging (MRI) is increasingly used to evaluate the orbit; however, it is not preferable to CT in patients scheduled for surgery because the orbital bones are not visible. MRI may be used to detect acute muscle inflammation early in Graves' disease. Other tests include color Doppler exam of the orbit to show reversed flow in the superior ophthalmic vein when there is crowding in the apex of the orbit. Doppler can be used to support the effects of surgical decompression. New tests under development to help diagnose thyroid-associated ophthalmopathy, particularly in cases of euthyroid Graves' disease, include single-photon emission computed tomography (SPECT) and various blood antibody tests.

5. What about orbital inflammations not caused by Graves' disease?

Of inflammations not due to Graves' disease, 40% are infections, 40% are nonspecific inflammations, and 20% are specific inflammations.

6. How do we recognize infections of the orbit?

Infections of the orbit present a continuum of disease that ranges from mild preseptal cellulitis to orbital cellulitis, abscess of the orbit, and cavernous sinus thrombosis.

Preseptal cellulitis, the mildest infection, presents anterior to the orbital septum. By definition, it does not affect any of the structures within the orbit. It may be seen in cases of trauma, infected styes, or insect bites.

Orbital cellulitis is most often seen in children less than 5 years old. The signs and symptoms show the involvement of the structures of the orbit. Examples include chemosis, proptosis, and decreased motility of the eye. The most common cause is spread from the adjacent sinuses, most often the ethmoid sinuses. In children, systemic symptoms also may be found, such as malaise or fever. Usually, the infection is caused by *Staphylococcus aureus* or streptococci; in children less than 3 years old, however, *Hemophilus influenzae* should be considered.

Orbital abscess represents a collection of pus either subperiosteally or within the orbit. Again, it usually results from sinus disease. Complications include central retinal artery or vein occlusion from increased pressured and optic nerve compression resulting in visual loss.

Cavernous sinus thrombosis is the most serious complication from infections of the orbit. It always has systemic symptoms, including fever, nausea, headache, extraocular nerve palsies, and loss of vision. It may be bilateral and accompanied by a brain abscess. It has an extremely high mortality rate.

7. How do we diagnose orbital infections?

After a complete orbital exam shows some of the signs and symptoms mentioned above, diagnostic measures should include a CT scan to check the sinuses (air-fluid levels) and to rule out an orbital abscess. In the cases of chronic or long-standing disease, an MRI also may be useful. A complete blood count with differential should be done, and if a wound is present, cultures and sensitivities should be obtained. Blood cultures also may be done. In young children a lumbar tap should be performed if meningitis is suspected.

8. How do we treat orbital infections?

In adults with preseptal cellulitis, oral antibiotics may be used initially. Lid abscesses should be drained, and in patients with a history of trauma, foreign bodies, particularly organic in nature, should be suspected and evaluated with a CT scan. Admission to the hospital should be seriously considered for young children, particularly if they have systemic involvement, and intravenous antibiotics should be started. Patients with orbital cellulitis or an abscess should be admitted to the hospital and started on intravenous antibiotics. Possible combinations include the use of intravenous vancomycin or nafcillin, in addition to cefuroxime or ceftriaxone (check with an infectious disease specialist for the appropriate antibiotics for your area). In adults, gram-negative bacteria or anaerobic bacteria should be considered; thus, metronidazole may be added to their regimen. If an orbital abscess does not respond to intravenous antibiotics, surgical drainage needs to be performed. If chronic sinus disease is the cause of the cellulitis, an ear-nose-throat specialist may need to perform a sinusotomy to prevent future recurrences.

9. Are there other kinds of orbital infections?

Yes. Fungal infections are most often seen in immunocompromised patients. *Aspergillus* sp. infections have been increasing and are seen in patients with AIDS and patients treated with immunosupressants. Mucor is a particularly devastating infection if it is not caught early; it usually is seen in debilitated patients or diabetics in ketoacidosis. A complete exam of the palate and nose should be done to find areas of eschars. The treatment is amphotericin B. Other chronic orbital infections are more rare, such as tuberculosis, syphilis, and infestations with cysticercosis, trichinosis, or hydatid disease. Infestations are seen much more commonly in third-world countries.

10. What is nonspecific inflammation of the orbit?

Nonspecific inflammations of the orbit have no known cause; they are a diagnosis of exclusion. They may present as acute or subacute inflammations, showing all of the signs previously discussed. On further investigation, however, they have no infectious or neoplastic etiology. The general term is **idiopathic inflammatory orbital pseudotumor**. Orbital pseudotumor can affect any or all soft-tissue components of the orbit. Examples include dacryoadenitis (lacrimal gland inflammation), myositis, or optic neuritis. Pain is a common complaint. In children orbital pseudotumor may be bilateral and present with systemic symptoms. Depending on the location of the inflammation, it may affect the orbital apex and present as an orbital apex syndrome. Inflammation may affect vision by compression of the optic nerve or cause extraocular muscle paralysis. A rare sclerosing type may become a chronic problem and ultimately lead to blindness. The orbital exam can show all of the signs of orbital disease, including redness, proptosis, decreased extraocular muscle function, visual problems, and decreased retropulsion.

11. How do we diagnose and treat inflammatory orbital pseudotumor?

Orbital pseudotumor is a diagnosis of exclusion. A CT scan should be performed to exclude a mass, abscess, or other signs of infection such as sinusitis. If an abnormal area suggestive of a mass is found, it may be necessary to do a biopsy to rule out a neoplasm such as orbital lymphoma. Orbital pseudotumor is treated with oral steroids, usually 40–60 mg of prednisone with a slow taper. Recurrences are common, particularly when the steroids are decreased to a low dose. If the disease recurs, again it may be necessary to perform an orbital biopsy to exclude lymphoma. The usual histopathologic findings of inflammatory orbital pseudotumor include a polymorphous infiltration of inflammatory cells. Specimens from the sclerosing type also may show areas of fibrosis. If the recurrences continue, low-dose radiotherapy to the orbit may be considered. Late sequelae include fibrosis, which may lead to diplopia, exophthalmos, and, in rare patients, blindness.

The response to oral steroids should be extremely fast, and the patient should show significant improvement in signs and symptoms within 24–48 hours of institution of treatment. Some authorities suggest that this in itself is a test for the disease. Although neoplastic disease may have some response to steroids, it is rarely as impressive as the response of orbital pseudotumor.

12. What other inflammations affect the orbit?

Orbital inflammation may be associated with systemic or local disease and usually must be diagnosed with biopsy. Examples include sarcoidosis, which is a multisystem granulomatous disease (intraocular and lacrimal disease is more common than purely orbital disease); Sjögren's syndrome, an autoimmune disease that presents with keratoconjunctivitis sicca (dry eye), xerostomia (dry mouth); and various vasculitides, which destroy the blood vessels and have an immunologic cause. Examples include polyarteritis nodosa, Wegener's syndrome, giant cell arteritis, Kawasaki's disease, and Buerger's disease.

BIBLIOGRAPHY

1. Gold SC, Arrigg PG, Hedges TR: Computerized tomography in the management of acute orbital cellulitis. Ophthal Surg 18:753, 1987.
2. Harris GJ: Subperiosteal abscess of the orbit. Age as a factor in the bacteriology and response to treatment. Ophthalmology 101:585, 1994.
3. Kennerdell JS: The management of sclerosing nonspecific orbital inflammation. Ophthal Surg 22:512, 1991.
4. McCord CD: Current trends in orbital decompression. Ophthalmology 92:21, 1985.
5. Paris GL, Waltuch GF, Egbert PR: Treatment of refractory orbital pseudotumors with pulsed chemotherapy. Ophthal Plast Reconstr Surg 6:96, 1990.
6. Rootman J, Nugent R: The classification and management of acute orbital pseudotumors. Ophthalmology 89:1040, 1982.
7. Siatkowski RM, Capo H, Byrne SF, et al: Clinical and echographic findings in idiopathic orbital myositis. Am J Ophthalmol 343:118, 1994.

39. PTOSIS

Carolyn S. Repke, M.D.

1. How is ptosis classified?

Ptosis is classified by either time of onset or etiology. By onset, ptosis is either congenital or acquired. By etiology, ptosis may be neurogenic, aponeurotic, mechanical, myogenic, or traumatic.

2. What is the most common cause of acquired ptosis?

Acquired ptosis is most often the result of disinsertion or attenuation of the levator aponeurosis, which is most commonly related to aging but can be related to chronic ocular inflammation or eyelid edema.

3. What are the features of aponeurotic ptosis (levator dehiscence)?

Features of levator dehiscence include an abnormally high lid crease, a moderate degree of ptosis (3–4 mm), good levator function (generally > 10 mm), no lid lag on downgaze, and thin eyelid tissue, through which the dark color of the cornea and iris can sometimes be visualized.

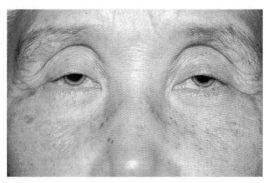

Involutional (aponeurotic) ptosis characteristically is mild to moderate with high lid creases. Levator function is usually normal. (From Tasman W, Jaeger EA: The Wills Eye Hospital Atlas of Clinical Ophthalmology. Philadelphia, Lippincott-Raven, 1996, with permission.)

4. What clinical findings help to differentiate congenital ptosis from acquired aponeurotic ptosis?

Patients with aponeurotic ptosis have a ptotic eyelid in all positions of gaze. In downgaze, the ptotic eyelid remains ptotic. Patients with congenital ptosis, however, demonstrate lid lag in downgaze. The ptotic eyelid frequently appears higher than the normal eyelid as the patient moves toward downgaze. This finding is due to the maldevelopment of the levator muscle, with poor ability to contract in elevation as well as inability to relax as the lid moves to downgaze.

5. What are the features of congenital ptosis?

Congenital ptosis is dystrophy or maldevelopment in the levator muscle/superior rectus complex (see figure, next page). Most patients demonstrate poor levator function on examination and, at surgery, have fatty infiltration of the levator muscle. This myogenic abnormality causes an inability of the levator to relax on downgaze, resulting in lid lag. Patients may or may not demonstrate motility defects due to superior rectus dysfunction. Approximately 75% of cases are unilateral.

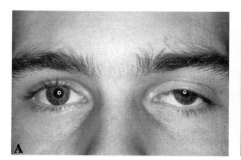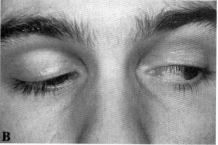

A, Congenital ptosis in the left eye of an adult. *B,* Note the lagophthalmos in downgaze typical of congenital ptosis. (From Tasman W, Jaeger EA: The Wills Eye Hospital Atlas of Clinical Ophthalmology. Philadelphia, Lippincott-Raven, 1996, with permission.)

6. What causes pseudoptosis?

Causes of pseudoptosis include lid retraction on the opposite side, hypotropia on the ptotic side, enophthalmos, anophthalmos, microphthalmos, and phthisis bulbi. Severe dermatochalasis with excessive skin overhanging the eyelid margin also gives a false appearance of ptosis.

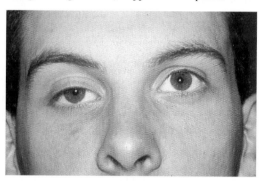

Pseudoptosis in a patient with a blow-out fracture of the right eye. (From Tasman W, Jaeger EA: The Wills Eye Hospital Atlas of Clinical Ophthalmology. Philadelphia, Lippincott-Raven, 1996, with permission.)

7. What is the primary cause of ptosis after intraocular surgery?

Ptosis related to previous intraocular surgery is thought to be due to levator dehiscence. The exact etiology is uncertain; however, it has been linked to superior rectus bridal sutures, lid speculums, and other draping maneuvers associated with manipulation of the eyelids. Affected patients probably had a tendency toward levator dehiscence preoperatively.

8. What is the anatomic cause for the lid crease?

The lid crease is formed by the levator aponeurotic attachments that travel through the orbicularis muscle to the skin. With aponeurotic ptosis, these attachments are disinserted, causing the eyelid crease to elevate.

9. What neurologic conditions are associated with ptosis?

Neurologic conditions that must be considered in a ptosis evaluation include third-nerve palsy, Horner's syndrome, myasthenia gravis, Marcus Gunn jaw winking syndrome, ophthalmoplegic migraine, and multiple sclerosis.

10. What are the myogenic causes of ptosis?

Muscular abnormalities associated with ptosis include myasthenia gravis, muscular dystrophies, chronic progressive external ophthalmoplegia, oculopharyngeal dystrophy, and congenital maldevelopment of the levator.

11. What are the features of blepharophimosis syndrome?

Blepharophimosis syndrome is a congenital autosomal dominant disorder characterized by ptosis, epicanthus, blepharophimosis (narrowing of the palpebral fissure in all dimensions), and telecanthus (widening of the distance between the medial canthi). Some patients also may demonstrate a flat nasal bridge, lower lid ectropions, and hypoplastic orbital rims.

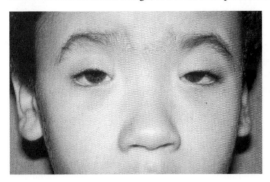

Blepharophimosis with congenital ptosis, lid phimosis, telecanthus, and epicanthus inversus. (From Tasman W, Jaeger EA: The Wills Eye Hospital Atlas of Clinical Ophthalmology. Philadelphia, Lippincott-Raven, 1996, with permission.)

12. What are the signs and symptoms of myasthenia gravis?

The history of any patient with acquired ptosis should include questions searching for symptoms of myasthenia gravis. Patients may comment on variability in the degree of ptosis from day to day. They also may notice increased ptosis during periods of fatigue or toward the end of the day. They may give a history of diplopia or difficulty with swallowing as well as other muscular weakness. On examination, they may demonstrate eyelid fatigue on sustained upgaze, with curtaining of the eyelid on returning to the primary position. They also may demonstrate a Cogan's lid twitch after attempted upgaze. On return to primary position, the lid may show an upward twitch before it settles to its final resting place. Orbicularis strength may be weak, allowing the examiner to open the patient's lids even during attempted forceful closure.

13. What measurements should be taken during the preoperative examination of patients with ptosis?

A complete evaluation of ptosis usually consists of a description of the palpebral fissure height in millimeters, the marginal reflex distance, measurement of levator function, and an evaluation of the lid crease height. The **palpebral fissure** measurement alone cannot be used as an accurate measurement of ptosis, because lower eyelid position can affect this value. In particular, patients with Horner's syndrome demonstrate a reverse ptosis of the lower eyelid, which has a higher than normal position. The **marginal reflex distance** is the distance from the corneal light reflex to the upper eyelid margin. It is a more reliable measure of ptosis than the palpebral fissure because it evaluates the distance of the upper eyelid from the visual axis. The amount of **levator function** is critical in planning the surgical procedure. If levator function is poor or absent, consideration may be given to a frontalis suspension rather than a levator resection or Müller's muscle resection.

Other critical parts of the preoperative evaluation include a careful pupillary examination for anisocoria, a cover test for strabismus, and evaluation of corneal sensation and tear film. Frequently, a Schirmer test is performed to measure basal tear production. The lid position is carefully evaluated in primary position with the action of the frontalis muscle negated. The eyelid position is also evaluated in downgaze, looking for lid lag that suggests congenital ptosis or previous thyroid ophthalmopathy. The lid is evaluated in upgaze for signs of muscle fatigue and curtaining, which suggest myasthenia gravis. Finally, it is important to document the presence of a good Bell's phenomenon (upshoot of the cornea with eyelid closure).

14. How is levator function determined?

Levator function is measured in millimeters from extreme downgaze to upgaze. The action of the frontalis muscle must be negated by placing manual pressure above the eyebrows. This maneuver eliminates the small amount of eyelid elevation associated with eyebrow elevation. The patient is then asked to look into extreme downgaze. A millimeter rule is held in front of the lid as the patient looks to upgaze. Levator function is the measurement of the entire excursion of the lid. Normal levator function is considered to be 15 mm or greater. Levator function is considered good if > 8 mm, fair if 5–7 mm, and poor if < 4 mm.

15. How does Herring's law affect ptosis?

Herring's law of equivalent innervation of yoke muscles applies to the two levator muscles. It needs to be considered during the preoperative evaluation to determine accurately the degree of ptosis on each side. The normal eyelid in a patient with unilateral ptosis may become ptotic when bilateral stimulation is broken. The degree to which Herring's law contributes to ptosis is affected by the eye with which the patient prefers to fixate. If the ptotic eye is preferred for fixation, the opposite eyelid may develop a retracted position due to increased stimulation during attempts to open the ptotic lid. Upon occluding the ptotic fixating eye, the previously retracted lid may resume a more normal position.

16. What is the Neosynephrine test?

The Neosynephrine test is an evaluation of the effect of Müller's muscle contraction on the degree of ptosis. One drop of 2.5% phenylephrine is placed in the eye. After 5 minutes the degree of ptosis is reevaluated. The phenylephrine causes contraction of the sympathetic Horner's muscle, sometimes causing dramatic improvement in the degree of ptosis. If phenylephrine corrects the ptosis completely, many surgeons elect to perform a Müller's muscle resection as opposed to a levator resection.

17. What are the surgical and nonsurgical approaches to the correction of ptosis?

The most common surgical approaches to ptosis correction include levator resection, either from an internal or external approach; Müller's muscle resection; and frontalis suspension. A nonsurgical option is ptosis eyelid crutches, which may be secured to spectacle lenses. Although rarely used, spectacle adaptations are a reasonable option for patients with neurologic ptosis who have a poor Bell's phenomenon and are considered to be at high risk for exposure keratopathy.

18. What are the complications of ptosis surgery?

The most common complication is over- or undercorrection of the ptosis and/or abnormalities in eyelid contour. Other complications include lid lag on downgaze and lagophthalmos on eyelid closure. These complications may result in corneal exposure and superficial keratopathy or even corneal ulceration and scarring. Abnormalities in the lid crease and eyelid fold, loss of eyelashes, conjunctival prolapse, and upper eyelid ectropion also may complicate surgery. In addition, retrobulbar hemorrhage is a risk with all eyelid surgery, and, although rare, infection is a potential complication.

19. What is the Marcus Gunn jaw winking syndrome?

The Marcus Gunn syndrome is a unilateral congenital ptosis with synkinetic innervation of the levator and ipsilateral pterygoid muscle. Patients demonstrate retraction of the ptotic eyelid on stimulation of the ipsilateral pterygoid muscles by either opening the mouth or moving the jaw to the opposite side.

BIBLIOGRAPHY

1. Gonnering RS (chairman) Orbit, Eyelids, and Lacrimal System: Basic and Clinical Science Course. San Francisco, American Academy of Ophthalmology, 1992, pp 160–168.
2. McCord CD Jr, Tannebaum M, Nunery WR: Oculoplastic Surgery, 3rd ed. Philadelphia, Lippincott-Raven, 1995, pp 175–220.
3. Schaefer AJ, Schaefer DP: Classification and correction of ptosis. In Stewart WB (ed): Surgery of the Eyelid, Orbit, and Lacrimal System, vol 2. San Francisco, American Academy of Ophthalmology, 1994, pp 84–133.

40. EYELID TUMORS

Janice A. Gault, M.D.

1. What clues are helpful in determining whether a lid lesion is benign or malignant?

The size, location, age of onset, rate of growth, presence of bleeding or ulceration, any color change, history of malignancy, or prior radiation therapy are important. A thorough examination is necessary. Malignant or inflammatory lesions may cause loss of eyelashes and distortion of meibomian gland orifices, but only malignant lesions destroy the orifices. If a lesion is near the lacrimal punctum, evaluate for invasion to the lacrimal system. Probing and irrigation may be necessary. Palpate lesions for fixation to deep tissues or bone. Regional lymph nodes also should be examined for enlargement. Restriction of extraocular motility and proptosis are clues to localized invasion. If a sebaceous adenocarcinoma or melanoma is diagnosed, system evaluation should target lung, liver, bones, and neurologic systems. Any lesion to be treated or observed needs photographic documentation.

2. What is the difference between seborrheic keratosis and actinic keratosis?

Both are papillomas, an irregular frond-like projection of skin with a central vascular pedicle. These lesions are more common in the elderly. Seborrheic keratosis is pigmented, oily, and hyperkeratotic. It appears stuck onto the skin. A shaved biopsy is all that is needed to diagnose and treat. It has no increased risk for malignant change. Actinic keratosis is found in sun-exposed areas and appears as flat, scaly, or papillary lesions. This premalignant lesion may evolve into either a basal cell or squamous cell carcinoma.

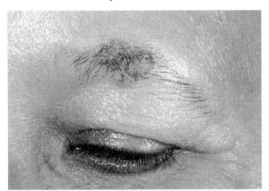

Seborrheic keratosis is a light-brown, greasy lesion that appears to be "stuck" onto the skin. (From American Academy of Ophthalmology: Basic and Clinical Science Course, Section 8. San Francisco, CA, American Academy of Ophthalmology, 1992, with permission.)

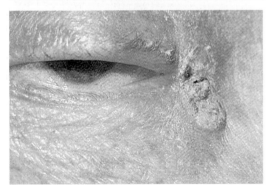

Actinic keratosis is a dry, scaly lesion due to sun exposure occurring in fair-skinned elderly people. (From Spalton DJ, Hitchings RA, Hunter PA: Atlas of Clinical Ophthalmology, 2nd ed. St. Louis, Mosby, 1994, with permission.)

3. **What lid lesion is associated with a chronic follicular conjunctivitis?**
Molluscum contagiosum. The multiple waxy nodules with an umbilicated center are caused by a virus. They may resolve spontaneously but frequently require surgical excision or cautery to prevent reinfection.

4. **What blood tests should you order in young patients with the lesions shown below?**

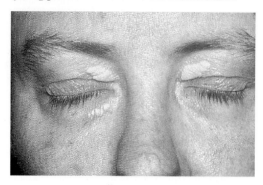

Patient with xanthelasma in all four lids. (From Tasman W, Jaeger EA: The Wills Eye Hospital Atlas of Clinical Ophthalmology. Philadelphia, Lippincott-Raven, 1996, with permission.) (See Fig. 12, Color Plates.)

The appropriate tests are cholesterol level, triglyceride level, and fasting blood sugar. Xanthelasma are yellowish plaques found at the medial canthal area of the upper and lower lids. They are collections of lipid. In older patients, they are common and no cause for concern. In younger patients, they may be a sign of hypercholesterolemia, a congenital disorder of cholesterol metabolism, or diabetes mellitus. Cosmetically, they may be removed easily but may recur.

5. **What is a keratoacanthoma? What malignancy does it simulate?**
A keratoacanthoma is a rapidly growing lesion that appears over several weeks. It is hyperkeratotic with a central crater that often resolves spontaneously. Clinically, the lesion simulates a "rodent ulcer" basal cell carcinoma. Pathologically, the lesion appears similar to squamous cell carcinoma. It may occur near the edge of areas of chronic inflammation, such as a burn, or on the periphery of a true malignant neoplasm. If you are sure of the diagnosis, it is reasonable to observe. However, because it may cause destruction of the lid margin, lesions in this area are often removed surgically. They also may be injected with steroids.

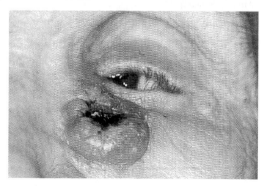

Keratoacanthoma that developed over 4 months. Note the central keratin-filled crater. (From Tasman W, Jaeger EA: The Wills Eye Hospital Atlas of Clinical Ophthalmology. Philadelphia, Lippincott-Raven, 1996, with permission.)

6. **What is the most common malignant eyelid tumor?**
Basal cell carcinoma, which is most common in middle-aged or elderly patients.

7. **What are its two clinical presentations?**
Nodular and morpheaform tumors. A nodular tumor is a firm, raised, pearly, discrete mass, often with telangiectasias over the tumor margins. If the center of the lesion is ulcerated, it is

called a "rodent" ulcer. Morpheaform tumors are firm, flat lesions with indistinct borders. They tend to be more aggressive and have a worse prognosis than the nodular variety.

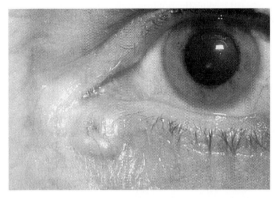

Nodular basal cell carcinoma, well-circumscribed with raised edges and central ulceration, has arisen over a much longer period in comparison with acanthoma. The location near the medial canthus is worrisome for invasion. (From Tasman W, Jaeger EA: The Wills Eye Hospital Atlas of Clinical Ophthalmology. Philadelphia, Lippincott-Raven, 1996, with permission.)

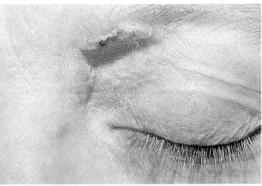

Morpheaform basal cell carcinomas have less clearly defined surgical margins. (From Spalton DJ, Hitchings RA, Hunter PA: Atlas of Clinical Ophthalmology, 2nd ed. St. Louis, Mosby, 1994, with permission.)

8. In order of frequency, where do basal cell carcinomas present?

The most common location is the lower lid, followed by the medial canthus, lateral canthus, and upper lid.

9. Do basal cell carcinomas metastasize? If not, are they dangerous?

Lesions grow only by local extension. They can be dangerous, especially if near the medial canthus. Tumors at this site may invade the orbit via the lacrimal drainage system. Ocular adnexal basal cell carcinomas have a 3% mortality rate; the vast majority of patients had canthal area disease, prior radiation therapy, or clinically neglected tumors.

10. How do you treat tumors with a suspicious lesion?

First, do an incisional biopsy of the lesion to confirm the diagnosis. Permanent sections must be done, not merely frozen sections. If basal cell is found, there are several possibilities:

1. A large surgical resection with frozen sections to confirm the entire tumor has been removed. If the lacrimal system must be removed, do not do a dacryocystorhinostomy at the same time as the primary surgery. Wait at least 1 year to prevent iatrogenic seeding of the nose.

2. Mohs' lamellar resection. The complete tumor is removed, sparing as much healthy tissue as possible. The excised bits of tissue are sent to pathology during the procedure to confirm the presence or absence of tumor and therefore direct the subsequent course of the surgery. This procedure preserves a larger amount of normal tissue, allowing improved function and cosmesis. Sometimes it even saves the globe, whereas conventional surgery may require exenteration. This time-consuming procedure is not available everywhere.

3. Radiation. Basal cell carcinoma is radiosensitive, but treatment is not curative, only palliative (see question 9). Radiation should be reserved for elderly patients who are unable to undergo surgery.

4. Cryotherapy. This treatment is not curative and should be used only palliatively.

11. How do you treat a recurrent tumor that has limited the extraocular motility from invasion of the orbit?

Exenteration.

12. Describe basal cell nevus syndrome.

This autosomal dominant disease is characterized by development of multiple basal cell carcinomas at an early age. Patients also have skeletal, endocrine, and neurologic abnormalities.

13. What are the complications of radiation to the area around the eye?

Keratitis sicca, cataracts, radiation retinopathy (if over 3000 rads are used), optic neuropathy, entropion, lacrimal stenosis, and dermatitis. In young children, the bones of the orbit may not grow normally, causing a significant cosmetic deformity.

14. Where do squamous cell carcinomas usually present around the eye?

The upper eyelid. However, basal cell carcinomas are 40 times more common.

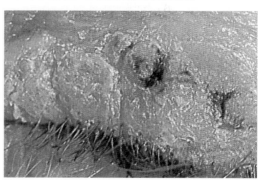

Squamous cell carcinoma of the upper eyelid. (From American Academy of Ophthalmology: Basic and Clinical Science Course, Section 8. San Francisco, CA, American Academy of Ophthalmology, 1992, with permission.) (See Fig. 13, Color Plates.)

15. How are patients with squamous cell carcinomas treated?

Similarly to patients with basal cell carcinomas. However, squamous cell carcinomas are more aggressive locally and metastasize via the blood or lymph system. Exenteration is suggested for recurrences.

16. A 60-year-old man has had a chalazion removed from his left upper lid three times. It has recurred again. How do you treat?

A sebaceous gland carcinoma must be suspected. Lesions arise from the meibomian glands in the tarsal plate, Zeis glands near the lashes, and sebaceous glands in the caruncle and brow. Any recurrent chalazia must be biopsied for pathologic evaluation. The lesion can mimic benign ocular diseases such as chronic blepharoconjunctivitis, corneal pannus, and superior limbic keratitis. Patients who do not respond to treatment should be biopsied, especially those with loss of lashes and destruction of meibomian gland orifices.

17. How is the biopsy performed? How is the specimen sent to the lab? What stains should be requested?

Sebaceous cell carcinoma is multicentric and undergoes Pagetoid spread. Multiple sites must be biopsied, including bulbar and palpebral conjunctiva, even if they appear uninvolved. A full-thickness lid biopsy may be necessary to make the diagnosis because the lesion originates deep in the tissues. The tissue should not be placed in alcohol, which will dissolve the fat from the specimen and make the diagnosis more difficult. Oil-red-O stain will stain the fat red.

18. How are patients with sebaceous cell carcinoma treated?

Because sebaceous cell carcinoma is an aggressive and potentially fatal disease, wide surgical excision is mandatory. Some physicians prefer exenteration as a primary treatment. Mohs' microsurgery should be used with caution because the disease is multicentric with skip areas and some lesions may be missed. The tumor may spread hematogenously, lymphatically, or by direct extension.

19. What is the most common type of malignant melanoma of the lid?

Superficial spreading melanoma accounts for 80% of cases; lentigo maligna and nodular melanoma each occur in 10% of cases. However, all are rare and represent less than 1% of eyelid tumors. Superficial spreading melanoma occurs in both sun-exposed and nonexposed areas. Lentigo maligna, also known as Hutchinson's melanotic freckle, is sun-induced. Both have a long horizontal growth phase before invading the deeper tissues. Nodular melanoma is more aggressive with earlier vertical invasion. Treatment is wide surgical excision and lymph node dissection if microscopic evidence of lymphatic or vascular involvement is noted.

20. How do you follow a patient who has had an eyelid malignancy?

Once the patient has healed from the initial treatment, reevaluate every 6–12 months. Patients are at risk for additional malignancies. A thorough examination by a dermatologist may reveal cutaneous malignancies elsewhere.

BIBLIOGRAPHY

1. Albert DM, Jakobiec FA: Principles and Practice of Ophthalmology, vol 3. Philadelphia, W.B. Saunders, 1994, pp 1713–1812.
2. American Academy of Ophthalmology Basic and Clinical Science Course on Orbit, Eyelids, and Lacrimal System.
3. Cullum RD, Chang B: The Wills Eye Manual, 2nd ed. Philadelphia, J.B. Lippincott, 1994.

VIII. Uveitis

41. GRANULOMATOUS UVEITIS

Caroline R. Baumal, M.D., F.R.C.S.C.

1. Define granulomatous uveitis.

Uveitis may be classified based on the anatomic, etiologic, clinical, or pathologic features. Pathologically, uveitis is classified as granulomatous or nongranulomatous. Granulomatous uveitis is intraocular inflammation characterized by nodular collections of epithelioid cells and giant cells surrounded by lymphocytes. In contrast, nongranulomatous uveitis consists of a cellular infiltrate of lymphocytes and plasma cells.

2. What are the symptoms of granulomatous uveitis?

Symptoms may include blurred vision, floaters, and scotomata. The presence and severity of pain are variable, and the external eye has mild inflammation.

3. What are the clinical features of granulomatous uveitis?

Granulomatous uveitis is typically chronic and can involve any portion of the uveal tract. Anterior segment examination may reveal any of the following: large, greasy **mutton-fat** keratic precipitates, iris infiltration with nodules at the pupillary border (**Koeppe nodules**) or over the iris surface (**Busacca nodules**), dense posterior synechiae (adhesions between the iris and anterior lens capsule). Examination of the posterior segment may reveal focal areas of inflammation.

4. Differentiate the features of granulomatous and nongranulomatous uveitis.

This distinction is not always useful clinically because some forms of granulomatous uveitis (e.g., sarcoidosis) may occur at times with nongranulomatous features. Nongranulomatous conditions do not present in a granulomatous fashion.

Features of Granulomatous and Nongranulomatous Uveitis

FEATURES	GRANULOMATOUS	NONGRANULOMATOUS
Onset	Often insidious	Acute (usually)
Course	Chronic	Acute or chronic
Anterior Segment:		
Injection	+	+++ (usually)
Pain	+/–	+++ (usually)
Iris nodules	+++	–
Keratic precipitates	Large, mutton-fat	Small, fine
Other	Dense posterior synechiae	+/– posterior synechiae, hypopyon

+ = present, – = absent

5. What are mutton-fat keratic precipitates?

Mutton-fat keratic precipitates are collections of epithelioid cells plus lymphocytes, macrophages, inflammatory multinucleated giant cells, or pigment on the posterior surface of the cornea. These are larger than keratic precipitates in nongranulomatous uveitis and have a greasy, stuck-on appearance.

6. Can iris nodules occur in nongranulomatous uveitis?

Koeppe nodules are white-gray, round nodules at the pupil border and may be present in granulomatous and nongranulomatous disease. Busacca nodules in the iris stroma only occur in granulomatous uveitis.

7. List the *infectious* causes of granulomatous uveitis.

Infectious agent	Disease
Mycobacterium tuberculosis	Tuberculosis
Mycobacterium leprae	Leprosy
Treponema pallidum	Syphilis
Borrelia burgdorferi	Lyme disease
Brucella melitensis/abortus	Brucellosis
Herpesviruses	Acute retinal necrosis
Toxoplasma gondii	Toxoplasmosis
Propionibacterium acnes	Chronic postoperative endophthalmitis
Fungal infections	Multiple (e.g., cryptococcus, aspergillus)

8. What are the *immune-mediated* causes of granulomatous uveitis?

Ocular	*Systemic*
Sympathetic ophthalmia	Sarcoidosis
Phacoanaphylactic endophthalmitis	Vogt-Koyanagi-Harada (VKH) syndrome

9. What other entities should be considered in the differential diagnosis of uveitis?

Masquerade syndromes are conditions that mimic uveitis. These include the following:

Malignancies—retinoblastoma, leukemia, malignant melanoma, large cell sarcoma, lymphoma
Intraocular foreign body

Juvenile xanthogranuloma
Peripheral retinal detachment
Multiple sclerosis

10. Name the most common causes of granulomatous uveitis.

Toxoplasmosis and sarcoidosis.

11. What tests may be useful for the work-up of granulomatous uveitis?

All cases of granulomatous uveitis should be evaluated for a specific cause. Target diagnostic tests based on clinical history and ocular and physical examination.

Skin tests—purified protein derivative (PPD) for tuberculosis, anergy screen to make sure patient can mount immune response
Blood tests—antibody titers, culture, polymerase chain reaction, HLA typing, HIV testing
Radiologic evaluation—chest x-ray, gallium scan
Ocular tests—fluorescein angiography, ultrasound
Surgical procedures—skin biopsy, lumbar puncture
Ocular specimens from aqueous humor, vitreous fluid, conjunctiva, iris, retina, choroid

12. What is toxoplasmosis?

Toxoplasmosis is caused by the obligate intracellular parasite *Toxoplasma gondii*. The cat is the definitive host, and humans are incidental hosts. Infection may be congenital, or acquired by ingestion of oocysts or bradyzoites from contact with cat feces or from contaminated undercooked meat. Infection has rarely been acquired after organ transplant or leukocyte transfusion.

13. Describe the ocular features of toxoplasmosis.

Ocular toxoplasmosis manifests as a focus of necrotizing retinochoroiditis surrounded by edematous retina with overlying vitreous inflammation. The lesion may be isolated or adjacent to a pigmented retinal scar. A diffuse vitritis that obscures fundus detail (referred to as "headlight in the fog") may occur. Additional features may include uveitis that is granulomatous or nongranulomatous, papillitis, retinal vasculitis, and elevated intraocular pressure.

14. How is the diagnosis of ocular toxoplasmosis made?

Diagnosis is based on clinical history and fundus examination, and is supported by serologic evidence of acute or previous *Toxoplasma gondii* exposure. Interpretation of serologic results may be confounded by the high prevalence of positive titers in the population. Positive toxoplasma serology, even in undiluted serum, should be present to corroborate the diagnosis. There is no correlation between toxoplasma antibody titers and activity of recurrent ocular toxoplasma.

15. What is the treatment for ocular toxoplasmosis?

Therapy is based on the location of the lesion in the retina. Observation is recommended for small peripheral lesions, which usually heal spontaneously. Treatment is recommended when visual acuity is reduced, inflammatory lesions threaten the macula, papillomacular bundle, or optic nerve, or when there is moderate to severe vitreous inflammation. Antibiotic therapy is directed against the tachyzoite replication that occurs during active retinitis, but is ineffective against the cysts that persist in the retina. Combination antibiotic therapy with sulfadiazine (2 gm oral loading dose, followed by 1 gm four times daily), pyrimethamine (75 mg oral loading dose, followed by 25 mg daily), and folinic acid (3 to 5 mg two times per week) is given for 4 to 6 weeks. Alternative regimens include clindamycin (300 mg four times daily) alone or with sulfadiazine and/or pyrimethamine in the above doses or trimethoprim-sulfamethoxazole (160 mg/800 mg) alone or with clindamycin. Systemic corticosteroids to limit inflammatory retinal destruction may be considered for lesions that threaten vision in immunocompetent patients only with concomitant antibiotic therapy. Topical steroids, cycloplegics, and antiglaucoma medications are used to treat anterior uveitis and elevated intraocular pressure. Surgical vitrectomy is rarely required to remove persistent vitreous opacities.

16. What potentially serious side effects may occur with oral antibiotic therapy for toxoplasmosis?

Clindamycin-associated pseudomembranous colitis
Pyrimethamine-induced hematologic toxicity, which is counteracted by folinic acid administration

17. Define sarcoidosis.

Sarcoidosis is a multisystem granulomatous disorder of unknown etiology, and may affect the lungs, skin, and eye. The eye is involved in up to 30% of patients. Uveitis is the most common ocular manifestation.

18. What are the ocular features of sarcoidosis?

Uveitis—often but not exclusively bilateral and granulomatous
Posterior segment inflammation—granulomas, vitritis, vasculitis, neovascularization
Conjunctival and eyelid nodules
Lacrimal gland enlargement

19. Which systemic findings corroborate the diagnosis of sarcoidosis?

Anergy on skin testing, abnormal chest x-ray, positive gallium scan, elevated angiotensin converting enzyme, and serum calcium.

20. Describe the features of ocular tuberculosis.

Mycobacterium tuberculosis, an aerobic acid-fast bacilli, is the major causative agent of human tuberculosis. Ocular involvement may occur without signs of active pulmonary involvement. In addition to uveitis, which is often chronic and granulomatous, other features may include choroiditis, choroidal granulomas, retinal vasculitis, optic neuritis or atrophy, eyelid nodules, dacryoadenitis, conjunctivitis, scleritis, phlyctenulosis, interstitial keratitis, and orbital disease.

21. Describe the treatment of ocular tuberculosis.

Antituberculosis therapy requires a combination of systemic antibiotics for a prolonged duration. Current regimens include isoniazid, rifampin, and pyrazinamide for 6 to 9 months. Ethambutol or streptomycin may be added if drug resistance is suspected. A toxic optic neuropathy is a potentially serious side effect that may occur secondary to isoniazid, ethambutol, or streptomycin therapy of pulmonary or extrapulmonary tuberculosis.

22. In what stage does uveitis occur in syphilis?

Syphilitic uveitis occurs in the secondary, latent, and tertiary stages and may be the sole finding of syphilis.

23. What are the ocular features of syphilis?

In congenital syphilis, ocular signs include chorioretinitis with a salt and pepper fundus, vitritis, uveitis, and interstitial keratitis.

Acquired primary syphilis may manifest with a periocular or conjunctival chancre. In later stages, a variety of findings have been described, including uveitis (granulomatous or nongranulomatous), vitritis, choroiditis, retinitis, vasculitis, panophthalmitis, macular edema, choroidal neovascularization, optic nerve disease, pupillary abnormalities, conjunctivitis, scleritis, interstitial keratitis, and gummatous involvement of the conjunctiva and optic nerve.

24. Which diagnostic tests are used to assess for syphilitic uveitis?

Treponema pallidum may be identified from a cutaneous lesion, if present, by dark-field microscopy or immunofluorescent techniques. The two commonly used nontreponemal tests are the Venereal Disease Research Laboratory (VDRL) and the Rapid Plasma Reagin (RPR). Serial VDRL titers are useful to monitor response to therapy but may be negative in late-stage syphilis. Specific treponemal tests include the fluorescent treponemal antibody absorption test (FTA-ABS) and the microhemagglutination test (MHA-TP), and are more sensitive in late-stage syphilis. Because syphilitic uveitis may occur in late stages and the screening VDRL can be negative, it is mandatory to perform a FTA-ABS or MHA-TP test in the evaluation for ocular syphilis. Examination of cerebrospinal fluid for elevated protein, lymphocytic pleocytosis, or VDRL serology may reveal concomitant neurosyphilis.

25. How is syphilitic uveitis treated?

Ocular syphilis is treated similarly to neurosyphilis, with high-dose intravenous penicillin (12 to 24 million units/day of penicillin G for 14 days) followed by intramuscular benzathine penicillin G (2.4 million units/week for 3 weeks). Doxycycline, tetracycline, or erythromycin have been used in penicillin-allergic patients. Patient contacts at risk for syphilis should be assessed and treated accordingly. Patients and contacts should also be tested for other sexually transmitted diseases.

26. What is Vogt-Koyanagi-Harada (VKH) syndrome?

This is an idiopathic multisystem disorder that primarily affects heavily pigmented individuals, and is associated with a severe, often bilateral granulomatous uveitis. Clinical manifestations may include:

Cutaneous—alopecia, vitiligo, poliosis

Neurologic—meningeal symptoms, encephalopathy, dysacousis, cerebrospinal fluid lymphocytosis

Ocular—granulomatous uveitis, exudative retinal detachment

27. What is sympathetic ophthalmia and what immune response is responsible?

This is a bilateral, diffuse granulomatous T cell-mediated uveitis that develops from 5 days to many years after perforating ocular injury or ocular surgery. Ninety percent of cases occur within 2 weeks to 1 year after the inciting event. Sympathetic ophthalmia is mediated by a delayed type 4 hypersensitivity reaction of the uvea to antigens localized on the RPE or on uveal melanocytes.

28. Name the ocular features of Lyme disease.

Lyme disease is caused by the spirochete *Borrelia burgdorferi*, which is transmitted to humans by the bite of an infected *Ixodes* tick from infested deer, birds, or field mice. Ocular involvement is usually bilateral. In stage one, a nonspecific self-limiting conjunctivitis may occur. In stages two and three, there may be a pars planitis-like syndrome, which is atypical owing to the presence of granulomatous keratic precipitates and posterior synechiae. Other potential findings include uveitis, which may be granulomatous, vitritis, choroiditis, neuroretinitis, retinal vasculitis, panophthalmitis, branch retinal artery occlusion, pseudotumor cerebri, optic nerve disorders, cranial nerve palsies, episcleritis, conjunctivitis, and keratitis.

29. How is Lyme disease diagnosed?

1. A clinical history of outdoor activity in an endemic area in the late spring or summer. A migratory rash (erythema migrans) or arthritis may be described.

2. Positive antibody serology to *Borrelia burgdorferi*. Serology is most often performed with indirect immunofluorescent antibody (IFA) or the enzyme-linked immunosorbent assay (ELISA). False-negative results may occur in the early stages of infection before sufficient antibody responses occur or owing to incomplete antibiotic treatment. Serology is more likely to be positive as duration of disease increases. Because only one of the serologic tests may be positive, it is recommended to perform both IFA and ELISA and to interpret these tests based upon specific laboratory criteria. The spirochete may be identified by evaluation of biopsied skin rash or cerebrospinal fluid.

30. Describe the acute retinal necrosis (ARN) syndrome.

Acute retinal necrosis (ARN) is a clinical syndrome caused by herpes virus infections (varicella-zoster, herpes simplex types 1 and 2). Although initially described in healthy patients, ARN has subsequently been reported in immunocompromised patients. Features include a rapidly progressive peripheral retinitis, vasculitis, vitritis, elevated intraocular pressure, granulomatous uveitis, scleritis, optic neuropathy, retinal artery or vein occlusion, and macular edema. Long-term complications include retinal detachment and neovascularization, glaucoma, cataract, and optic atrophy.

31. Why is long-term ocular evaluation recommended in ARN patients?

Acute retinal necrosis may occur in the contralateral eye in approximately one-third of patients at an average interval of 4 weeks. It has been reported in the fellow eye after an interval as long as 34 years.

32. What options are available for treatment of ARN?

Antiviral therapy with acyclovir is effective to limit retinal necrosis, as well as the occurrence of ARN in the contralateral eye. Intravenous acyclovir for 10 to 14 days, followed by 3 months of oral therapy, is recommended. Ganciclovir is also effective against varicella-zoster (VZV) and herpes simplex viruses (HSV) and may be considered as alternative therapy in cases unresponsive to acyclovir. Systemic corticosteroids may be used to limit inflammation, but only with concomitant antiviral therapy. Topical steroids and cycloplegics are used for anterior segment inflammation. Prophylactic laser photocoagulation applied to the junction of necrotic and healthy retina to form a chorioretinal adhesion is recommended if not precluded by vitritis.

33. What difficulties may arise in interpreting serology for infectious causes of granulomatous uveitis?

Due to its localized nature, an active intraocular infection is not always accompanied by a rise in systemic antibody titers. Serology may be unreliable in immunocompromised patients secondary to altered antibody responses.

34. What is the indication for surgical sampling of intraocular fluids or tissue for diagnostic purposes?

Progressive sight-threatening uveitis that is unresponsive to present therapy is an indication for surgical sampling. The results should be expected to alter clinical therapy. Another indication is severe unresponsive disease in one eye and early disease in second eye.

35. How is granulomatous uveitis treated?

Timely diagnosis and therapy are imperative to prevent irreversible ocular damage.

Treatment principles

1. Treat the underlying cause if one is identified.

2. Prevent vision-threatening complications that may be secondary to the disease process or the medications used for therapy.

3. Relieve ocular discomfort and improve vision.

Medical treatments available

1. Topical eye drops—corticosteroid eye drops to counteract intraocular inflammation; pupil-dilating drops to prevent formation of synechiae and relieve ciliary spasm

2. Periocular corticosteroid injection

3. Systemic agents—antibiotics, antivirals, corticosteroids, immunosuppressive agents

BIBLIOGRAPHY

1. Aaberg TM: The expanding ophthalmologic spectrum of Lyme disease. Am J Ophthalmol 107:77–80, 1989.
2. Blumenkranz MS, Duker JS, D'Amico DJ: Acute retinal necrosis. In Albert DM, Jakobiec FA (eds): Principles and Practice of Ophthalmology: Clinical Practice. Philadelphia, W.B. Saunders, 1994, pp 945–962.
3. Duker JS, Blumenkranz MS: Diagnosis and management of the acute retinal necrosis (ARN) syndrome. Surv Ophthalmol 35:327–343, 1991.
4. Engstrom RE Jr, Holland GN, Nussenblatt RB, Jabs DA: Current practices in the management of ocular toxoplasmosis. Am J Ophthalmol 111:601–610, 1991.
5. Helm CJ, Holland GN: Ocular tuberculosis. Surv Ophthalmol 38:229–256, 1993.
6. Holland GN, and the Executive Committee of the American Uveitis Society: Standard diagnosis for the acute retinal necrosis syndrome. Am J Ophthalmol 117:663–667, 1994.
7. Margo CE, Hamed LH: Ocular syphilis. Surv Ophthalmol 37:203–220, 1992.
8. Martin DF, Chan C, de Smet MD, et al: The role of chorioretinal biopsy in the management of posterior uveitis. Ophthalmology 100:705–714, 1993.
9. Opremcak EM, Scales DK, Sharpe MR: Trimethoprim-sulfamethoxazole therapy for ocular toxoplasmosis. Ophthalmology 99:920–925, 1992.
10. Silveira C, Belfort R Jr, Burnier M Jr, Nussenblatt R: Acquired toxoplasmosis infection as the cause of toxoplasmic retinochoroiditis in families. Am J Ophthalmol 106:362–364, 1988.
11. Tabbara KF: Ocular toxoplasmosis: Toxoplasmic retinochoroiditis. Int Ophthalmol Clin 35:15–29, 1995.
12. Tamesis RR, Foster CS: Toxoplasmosis. In Albert DM, Jakobiec FA (eds): Principles and Practice of Ophthalmology: Clinical Practice. Philadelphia, W.B. Saunders, 1994, pp 929–934.
13. Tamesis RR, Foster CS: Ocular syphilis. Ophthalmology 97:1281–1287, 1990.
14. Weiss MJ, Velazquez N, Hofeldt AJ: Serologic tests in the diagnosis of presumed toxoplasmic retinochoroiditis. Am J Ophthalmol 109:407–411, 1990.
15. Zaidman GW: The ocular manifestations of Lyme disease. Int Ophthalmol Clin 33:9–22, 1993.

42. MASQUERADE SYNDROMES

Vinay N. Desai, M.D., and Jay S. Duker, M.D.

1. Define a masquerade syndrome.

The term **masquerade syndrome** refers to ophthalmic disorders that are not primarily inflammatory but present clinically as either anterior or posterior uveitis. These entities may be mistaken for primary uveitis, leading to inappropriate treatment and possible ocular morbidity and systemic mortality.

2. Name the most common syndromes that masquerade as uveitis of the anterior and posterior segments.

Masquerade Syndromes

SEGMENT	AGE IN YEARS	SIGNS OF INFLAMMATION	DIAGNOSTIC STUDIES*
Anterior segment			
Retinoblastoma	< 15	Flare, cells, pseudohypopyon	Aqueous tap for LDH levels and cytology
Leukemia	< 15	Flare, cells, heterochromia	Bone marrow, peripheral blood smear, aqueous cytology
Intraocular foreign body	Any age	Flare, cells	X-ray, ultrasound
Malignant melanoma	Any age	Flare, cells	Fluorescein, ultrasound
Juvenile xantho-granuloma	< 15	Flare, cells, hyphema	Examination of skin, iris biopsy
Peripheral retinal detachment	Any age	Flare, cells	Ophthalmoscopy
Posterior segment			
Retinitis pigmentosa	Any age	Cells in vitreous	ERG, EOG, visual fields
Reticulum cell sarcoma	15+	Vitreous exudate, retinal hemorrhage or exudates, retinal pigment epithelium infiltrates	Cytology study of aqueous and vitreous
Lymphoma	15+	Retinal hemorrhage exudates, vitreous cells	Node biopsy, bone marrow, physical examination
Retinoblastoma	< 15	Vitreous cells, retinal exudates	Ultrasound, aqueous tap
Malignant melanoma	15+	Vitreous cells	Fluorescein, ultrasound
Multiple sclerosis	15+	Periphlebitis	Neurologic examination

LDH = lactic dehydrogenase, ERG = electroretinogram, EOG = electrooculogram.
From American Academy of Ophthalmology: Ophthalmology Basic and Clinical Science Course, Sect. 6. San Francisco, American Academy of Ophthalmology, 1997.

3. Describe the clinical features of retinoblastoma.

Retinoblastoma is the most common primary intraocular malignancy in children, usually presenting before the age of two. The most common presenting signs of retinoblastoma are leukocoria (white pupillary reflex) and strabismus. Occasionally, necrosis of the tumor may produce significant inflammation in the anterior or posterior segment. Tumor cells may become layered in the anterior chamber, producing a "pseudohypopyon." Retinoblastoma cells may gain access to the vitreous, where they appear as vitreous seeds, simulating inflammatory vitritis. Other examples of true posterior uveitis that present with significant inflammation include toxoplasmosis, toxocariasis, cysticercosis, and pars planitis. Ultrasonography may help to differentiate retinoblastoma from these entities. Calcification may be seen within the retinoblastoma tumor but not in the other diseases.

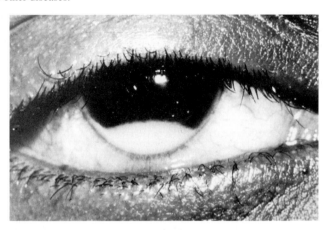

Pseudohypopyon due to seeding of retinoblastoma cells in the anterior chamber. (From Shields JA, Shields CL: Intraocular Tumors—A Text and Atlas. Philadelphia, W.B. Saunders, 1992, p 310, with permission.)

4. Which clinical entity may present with chronic intraocular inflammation, refractory to corticosteroids, in a patient over the age of 50?

Primary intraocular lymphoma, or reticulum cell sarcoma, as it was formerly called, may present in this fashion. Most patients present with bilateral involvement associated with vitreous cells, anterior chamber reaction, and retinal and choroidal infiltrates. The retinal infiltrates may be patchy and associated with hemorrhage and exudate. However, a dense vitritis may be the only presenting sign. Most patients eventually develop some form of central nervous system (CNS) involvement. CT or MRI imaging may demonstrate CNS tumors. In almost all cases a vitreous aspirate establishes the diagnosis. Current treatment includes ocular and CNS irradiation combined with intrathecal chemotherapy.

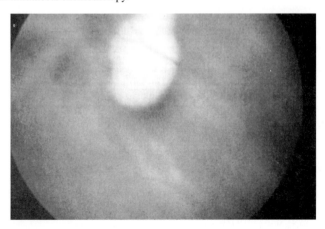

Yellow-white chorioretinal infiltrate in intraocular lymphoma. (From Shields JA, Shields CL: Intraocular Tumors—A Text and Atlas. Philadelphia, W.B. Saunders, 1992, p 499, with permission.)

5. Which ocular tissue is most commonly affected clinically by leukemia?

The retina is the most commonly affected ocular tissue clinically. Retinal involvement includes vascular dilation, tortuosity, retinal hemorrhages, cotton-wool spots, and peripheral retinal neovascularization. The retinal hemorrhages may have white centers consisting of leukemic cells or platelet–fibrin aggregates (Roth spots). In contrast, the choroid is the most commonly involved tissue histopathologically. However, choroidal involvement is rarely detected clinically but may produce serous retinal detachment. Fluorescein angiography of such detachments demonstrates multiple areas of hyperfluorescence at the level of the retinal pigment epithelium (RPE) similar to that found in the Vogt-Koyanagi-Harada syndrome. Leukemic involvement of the anterior segment may present with conjunctival mass, iris heterochromia, anterior chamber cell and flare, pseudohypopyon, spontaneous hyphema, and elevated intraocular pressure. Optic nerve infiltration and orbital involvement are common.

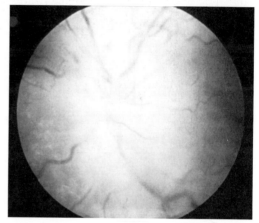

Leukemic infiltration of the optic nerve head, retina, and choroid in an 8-year-old child. (From Shields JA, Shields CL: Intraocular Tumors—A Text and Atlas. Philadelphia, W.B. Saunders, 1992, p 506, with permission.)

6. Through which mechanism can a malignant melanoma produce inflammatory signs?

Necrotic tumors may elicit an intense inflammatory response associated with seeding of tumor cells into the vitreous cavity and anterior segment. Occasionally, melanophages or tumor cells containing melanin produce a brown pseudohypopyon. Blockage of the trabecular meshwork by tumor cells may result in elevated intraocular pressure (melanomalytic glaucoma). Necrosis of the tumor may result in spontaneous vitreous hemorrhage. Other clinical findings include iris heterochromia and serous retinal detachment with shifting subretinal fluid. Ultrasound examination and fluorescein angiography help to establish the diagnosis.

7. Which condition may produce spontaneous hyphema in a child?

Juvenile xanthogranuloma is a systemic condition consisting of one or more benign tumors. Ocular involvement may present with recurrent anterior chamber reaction and spontaneous hyphema (see figure, next page). The xanthogranuloma has small fleshy tumors on the iris. Diagnosis is made with iris biopsy or by finding similar lesions on the skin. If the patient develops recurrent hyphema and secondary glaucoma, treatment with topical and systemic corticosteroids is advised.

8. Describe several other entities that may simulate anterior or posterior uveitis.

1. **Long-standing peripheral retinal detachment** may produce a severe anterior chamber reaction and posterior synechiae. Careful ophthalmoscopy and ultrasonography help to detect the retinal detachment.

2. **Retained intraocular foreign bodies** associated with trauma may cause persistent anterior and posterior segment inflammation. Examination with computed tomography or ultrasonography should demonstrate the abnormality.

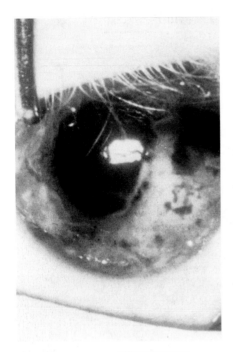

Large solitary juvenile xanthogranuloma that had given rise to a spontaneous hyphema in a 7-month old child. (From Shields JA, Shields CL: Intraocular Tumors—T Text and Atlas. Philadelphia, W.G. Saunders, 1992, p 296, with permission.)

3. Patients with **multiple sclerosis** may present with peripheral uveitis consisting of cells in the vitreous cavity and periphlebitis. Occasionally, patients with multiple sclerosis present with a granulomatous anterior uveitis.

4. **Retinitis pigmentosa** may present with vitreous cell and posterior subcapsular cataract. However, pigment deposition in the retina in clumps giving a "bone spicule" pattern, attenuated retinal vessels, mottling and atrophy of the RPE, and waxy pallor of the optic nerve help to distinguish this disease from other true inflammatory disorders. The diagnosis can be confirmed with an extinguished electroretinogram and electrooculogram and ring scotoma on visual field testing.

BIBLIOGRAPHY

1. Char DH: Clinical Ocular Oncology. New York, Churchill Livingstone, 1989.
2. Char DH, Ljung BM, Miller T, et al: Primary intraocular lymphoma (ocular reticulum cell sarcoma): Diagnosis and management. Ophthalmology 95:625–630, 1988.
3. Clements DB: Juvenile xanthogranuloma treated with local steroids. Br J Ophthalmol 50:663–665, 1966.
4. Fraser DJ Jr, Font RL: Ocular inflammation and hemorrhage as initial manifestations of uveal malignant melanoma: Incidence and prognosis. Arch Ophthalmol 97:1311–1314, 1979.
5. Heckenlively JR (ed): Retinitis Pigmentosa. Philadelphia, J.B. Lippincott, 1988.
6. Kincaid MC, Green WR: Ocular and orbital involvement in leukemia. Surv Ophthalmol 27:211–232, 1983.
7. Lim JI, Tessler HH, Goodwin JA: Anterior granulomatous uveitis in patients with multiple sclerosis. Ophthalmology 98:142–145, 1991.
8. Rao NA, Forster DJ, Spalton DJ: Masquerade syndromes and AIDS. In Podos SM, Yanoff M (eds): Textbook of Ophthalmology, 1992, pp 9.1–9.8.
9. Shields JA, Augsburger JJ: Current approaches to the diagnosis and management of retinoblastoma. Surv Ophthalmol 25:347–372, 1981.
10. Shields JA, Shields CL: Intraocular Tumors—A Text and Atlas. Philadelphia, W.B. Saunders, 1992.
11. Zimmerman LE: Ocular lesions of juvenile xanthogranuloma. Nevoxanthoendothelioma. Trans Am Acad Ophthalmol Otolaryngol 69:412–439, 1965.

43. OCULAR MANIFESTATIONS OF AIDS

Tamara R. Vrabec, M.D., and Vincent F. Baldassano, M.D.

1. Who is at greatest risk for developing AIDS-related eye disease?

Patients with severely reduced CD4+ T-lymphocyte counts are most likely to develop AIDS-related eye disease.

2. What is the most common ocular manifestation of AIDS?

Retinal microvasculopathy that manifests clinically as cotton-wool spots (CWS). Most patients are asymptomatic. CWSs are more common as the CD4+ T-lymphocyte count declines, reaching a prevalence of 45% in patients with counts < 50 cells/ml.

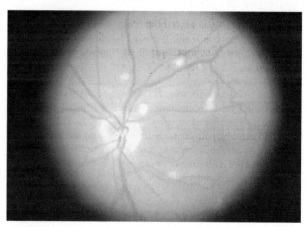

Cotton-wool spots are infarcts of the nerve fiber layer. Unlike early infiltrates of CMV retinitis, they do not enlarge, do not have associated hemorrhage, and may resolve in several weeks.

3. What is the most common ocular opportunistic infection in AIDS?

Cytomegalovirus (CMV) is by far the most common cause of opportunistic ocular infection and most frequently results in necrotizing retinitis. Other less common ocular opportunistic infectious agents in patients with AIDS include herpes zoster, toxoplasmosis, and cryptococcus.

4. What is the incidence of CMV retinitis?

Among patients whose CD4+ count is less than 50 cells/ml, 20% per year develop CMV retinitis.

5. Describe the early symptoms of CMV retinitis.

Floaters and loss of visual field (tunnel vision or blind spots) may be early symptoms of CMV retinitis.

6. How does CMV retinitis present clinically?

Classic ophthalmologic findings include white areas of retinal necrosis with associated hemorrhage and minimal vitreous inflammation (see figure, next page).

7. What drugs are most commonly used to treat CMV retinitis? How do they work?

Ganciclovir, foscarnet, and cidofovir are antiviral medications used to treat CMV retinitis. They work by inhibiting viral DNA polymerase. It is important to note that all are virostatic, not virocidal.

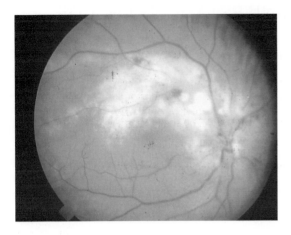

CMV retinitis is characterized by areas of retinal infiltrate with associated hemorrhage. Note optic nerve involvement. (See Fig. 14, Color Plates.)

8. For how long should treatment be continued in CMV retinitis?

For the remainder of the patient's life because of the virostatic nature of the medications and the suppressed immune system of the host. Lifetime maintenance therapy with antiviral medications is required to control the retinitis.

9. What is the treatment strategy for CMV retinitis?

Treatment of CMV retinitis includes an initial 2 weeks of intravenous or intraocular induction therapy with either ganciclovir or foscarnet followed by intravenous, oral, or intraocular maintenance therapy. Cidofovir is administered once weekly for induction and then every other week for maintenance. Despite maintenance therapy, the retinitis will relapse in most patients (mean period to relapse varies from 2–8 months, depending on the drug and/or route of delivery), and the interval to relapse shortens as the duration of treatment extends. When relapse occurs, reinduction (2–3 weeks of high-dose IV medication or multiple intraocular injections) is indicated. If resistance occurs (no clinical response to 8 weeks of reinduction), change in medication or route of delivery is indicated. Combination therapy with ganciclovir and foscarnet is more effective than high-dose single-drug therapy for recurring CMV retinitis; however, only 23% of patients can tolerate treatment because of toxicity (57%) or inconvenience (20%).

10. Name the main toxicity of ganciclovir.

The main toxicity of ganciclovir is bone marrow toxicity with neutropenia and/or thrombocytopenia. Neutropenia may be limited by concurrent use of granulocyte colony-stimulating factor (GCSF). Intraocular ganciclovir implant releases medication to the intraocular space only and therefore causes no systemic toxicity.

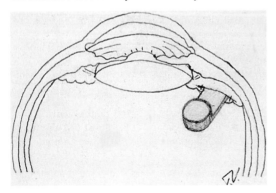

The intraocular ganciclovir implant is sutured to the sclera and extends into the vitreous cavity. The drug delivery system slowly releases ganciclovir over 8 months. It may be replaced when the drug supply is exhausted. Although it is not associated with the systemic toxicity seen with oral or intravenous therapy, the implant provides no prophylaxis against systemic CMV or CMV retinitis in the fellow eye.

11. Name the toxicities of foscarnet and cidofovir.

The main toxicity of foscarnet is renal toxicity, which occurs in about 30% of patients. Other toxicities include electrolyte imbalance, anemia, and, less commonly, neutropenia. The principal toxicity associated with cidofovir is nephrotoxicity.

12. What is HAART and how is it affecting the treatment of CMV retinitis?

HAART (highly active antiretroviral therapy) uses a combination of protease inhibitors plus other antiretroviral agents. HAART has resulted in significant and sustained increases in CD4 counts and remission of CMV retinitis following discontinuation of maintenance treatment.

13. What is progressive outer retinal necrosis (PORN)?

PORN is an extremely aggressive form of retinitis in the AIDS population. Caused by herpes zoster virus, it is temporally associated with herpes zoster skin lesions, which may or may not be in the periocular region. Blindness develops in > 80% of patients due to either relentless progression of infection despite therapy or secondary retinal detachment. Dilated fundus examination and periodic follow-up to screen for outer retinal necrosis are indicated for patients with AIDS who develop herpes zoster retinitis.

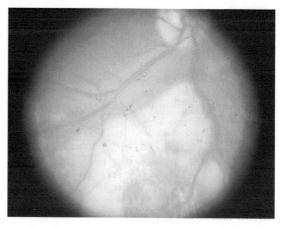

Progressive outer retinal necrosis typically affects the outer retina with sparing of retinal vessels. Note the areas of perivascular clearing and absence of associated hemorrhage.

14. Why do retinal detachments develop in cases of infectious retinitis? How often do they occur?

Retinal infections may cause multiple necrotic retinal holes that over time lead to retinal detachment. Retinal detachments occur in 34% of patients with CMV retinitis and 50% of patients with PORN.

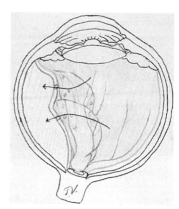

CMV-related retinal detachment is caused by multiple necrotic retinal holes that develop in areas of infectious retinitis. Liquid vitreous passes through the holes into the potential space beneath the retina and results in retinal detachment.

15. How are most AIDS-related retinal detachments repaired?

Lasers may be used to demarcate or wall off small peripheral retinal detachments, especially in patients who are not well enough to tolerate surgery. Because detachments are the result of multiple tiny necrotic holes, standard repair with scleral buckle is not effective, and vitrectomy with silicone oil injection is often required. The silicone oil replaces the vitreous and tamponades the multiple holes to prevent redetachment.

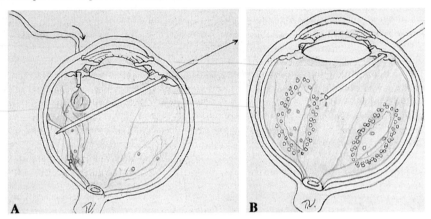

Surgical repair of CMV-related retinal detchment. *A,* Fluid is aspirated from the subretinal space as silicone oil is simultaneously injected into the vitreous cavity. *B,* Endolaser is applied to surround areas of necrotic retina. The silicone oil replaces the vitreous and acts as a permanent tamponade that prevents fluid from reaccumulating in the subretinal space.

16. Explain how ocular syphilis presents in patients with AIDS.

Ocular findings are variable and may range from iritis to necrotizing retinitis that mimics CMV retinitis. Syphilis is not an opportunistic infection by definition, because most patients who develop it have $CD4^+$ T-cell counts > 250 cell/ml. Concurrent CNS syphilis is present in 85% of HIV-positive patients with ocular syphilis. Hence, evaluation of cerebrospinal fluid is mandated for all HIV-positive patients with ocular syphilis. Syphilis may be seronegative (negative rapid plasmin reagin test despite active infection) in the HIV-positive population. Regardless of clinical findings, syphilis in patients with AIDS should be treated as tertiary disease with a 10-day course of intravenous antibiotics.

17. How should optic neuritis in patients with AIDS be diagnosed and managed?

Retrobulbar optic neuritis is an idiopathic inflammatory optic neuropathy often associated with demyelinating disease in young patients. The appearance of the optic disc (intraocular portion of the optic nerve) is normal despite visual loss. Idiopathic inflammatory retrobulbar optic neuritis must be considered a diagnosis of exclusion in patients with AIDS, and intravenous steroids should not be used until infection is ruled out.

18. What diagnoses should be considered in cases of retrobulbar optic neuritis in patients with AIDS?

Cryptococcal infection and syphilis. Cryptococci may cause acute, severe optic neuropathy from direct invasion of the optic nerve. Visual prognosis is often poor despite treatment. Work-up for optic neuropathy also should include review of medications. Ethambutol, an antimycobacterial drug commonly used in HIV-positive patients, may cause toxic optic neuropathy. Optic neuropathy related to direct HIV infection of the optic nerve is controversial.

19. What is papillitis?

Papillitis is direct infection of the optic disc, the visible intraocular portion of the optic nerve. The optic nerve appears white and necrotic, and vision is severely compromised. CMV may cause papillitis, often in association with adjacent retinitis. Vision may respond to treatment with antiviral medications.

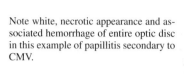

Note white, necrotic appearance and associated hemorrhage of entire optic disc in this example of papillitis secondary to CMV.

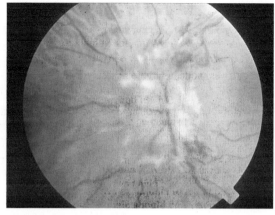

20. What are the causes of papilledema in patients with AIDS?

Papilledema is defined as disc swelling secondary to increased intracranial pressure. Early optic nerve dysfunction is minimal, and vision is usually preserved. The most likely causes in patients with AIDS include CNS infection (cryptococcus, toxoplasmosis) or malignancy (lymphoma).

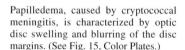

Papilledema, caused by cryptococcal meningitis, is characterized by optic disc swelling and blurring of the disc margins. (See Fig. 15, Color Plates.)

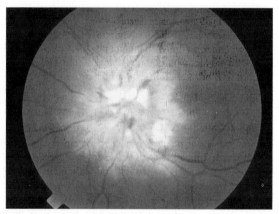

21. What is the most common malignancy in the periocular region of patients with AIDS?

Kaposi's sarcoma is the most common periocular malignancy (see figure, next page). This aggressive tumor of endothelial call origins affects 35% of bisexual HIV-positive males and is viscerally disseminated in 70% of cases. Ocular findings are observed in 20% of patients with visceral disease. Skin lesions are more common than conjunctival lesions. Orbital tumors are rare.

22. How should ocular Kaposi's sarcoma be managed?

Treatment is indicated only in patients with cosmetic or functional (i.e., eyelid does not close because of tumor) problems. Because most patients are treated for systemic disease initially, local ocular treatment is reserved until systemic treatment has been completed. If lesions persist, conjunctival lesions may be excised, and skin lesions may be treated with cryotherapy (flat lesions) or external beam radiation (nodular lesions).

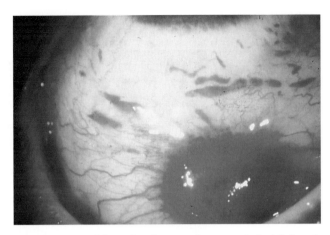

Kaposi's sarcoma of the conjunctiva most often occurs in the inferior cul-de-sac. Flat lesions may be easily mistaken for subconjunctival hemor-rhage. (Courtesy of Drs. Carol and Jerry Shields, Philadelphia.) (See Fig. 16, Color Plates.)

23. What other periocular malignancies may develop?

Squamous cell carcinoma of the conjunctiva has been reported with increasing frequency in patients with AIDS. The lesions may mimic papillomas or be more characteristic masses with as-sociated leukoplakia. Young patients with conjunctival squamous cell carcinoma should be tested for HIV.

24. Which medications may be associated with ocular toxicity?

Rifabutin, when used in combination with clarithromycin and fluconazole, has been reported to cause severe hypopyon iritis and, in rare instances, sterile endophthalmitis. Ethambutol may cause optic neuropathy.

BIBLIOGRAPHY

 1. Arevalo JF, Gonzales C, et al: Intravitreous and plasma concentrations of ganciclovir and foscarnet after intravenous therapy in patients with AIDS and cytomegalovirus retinitis. J Infect Dis 172:951–956, 1995.
 2. Deeks SG, Smith M, Holodniy M, Kahn JO: HIV-1 protease inhibitors. A review for clinicians. JAMA 227:145–153, 1997.
 3. Dugel PU, Gill PS, Frangieh GT, et al: Ocular adnexal Kaposi's sarcoma in AIDS. Am J Ophthalmol 110:500–503, 1990.
 4. Dugel PU, Gill PS, Frangieh GT, et al: Treatment of ocular adnexal Kaposi's sarcoma in AIDS. Ophthalmology 99:1127–1132, 1992.
 5. Engstrom RE Jr, Holland GN, Margolis TP, et al: Progressive outer retinal necrosis syndrome. Ophthalmology 101:1488–1452, 1994.
 6. Freeman WR, Chen A, Henderly DE, et al: Prevalence and significance of acquired immunodeficiency-related retinal microvasculopathy. Am J Ophthalmol 107:229–235, 1989.
 7. Holland GN, Sidikaro Y, Krieger AE, et al: Treatment of cytomegalovirus retinopathy with ganciclovir. Ophthalmology 94:815–823, 1987.
 8. Jabs DA, Enger C, Bartlett JG: Cytomegalovirus retinitis and acquired immunodeficiency syndrome. Arch Ophthalmol 107:75–80, 1989.
 9. Karp CL, Scott IU, Chang TS, Pflugfelder SC: Conjunctival intrapeithelial neoplasia. A possible marker for HIV infection? Arch Ophthalmol 114:257–261, 1996.
10. Lim JI, Enger C, Haller JA, et al: Improved visual results after surgical repair of cytomegalovirus-related retinal detachments. Ophthalmology 101:264–269, 1994.
11. Martin DF, et al: Treatment of CMV retinitis with a sustained release intraocular implant. A randomized, controlled clinical trial. Arch Ophthalmol 112:1530–1539, 1994.

12. Passo MS, Rosenbaum JT: Ocular syphilis in patients with human immunodeficency virus infection. Am J Ophthalmol 106:1–6, 1988.

13. Saran BR, Maguire AM, Nichols C, et al: Hypopyon uveitis in patients with AIDS treated for systemic *Mycobacterium avium* complex infection with rifabutin. Arch Ophthalmol 112:1159–1165, 1994.

14. Spector SA, Busch DF, Follansbee S, et al: Pharmacokinetic, safety, and antiviral profiles of oral ganciclovir in persons infected with the human immune deficiency virus: A phase I/II study. J Infect Dis 171:1431–1437, 1995.

15. Stenson SM, Freidberg DN: AIDS and the Eye. New Orleans, Contact Lens Association of Ophthalmologists, 1995.

16. Studies of Ocular Complications of AIDS Research Group: Mortality in patients with the acquired immunodeficiency syndrome treated with either foscarnet or ganciclovir for cytomegalovirus retinitis. N Engl J Med 326:213–220, 1992.

IX. Retina

44. TOXIC RETINOPATHIES

Philip G. Hykin, FRCS, FRCOphth

1. Describe the clinical features of chloroquine retinopathy.

Patients notice paracentral scotomas, nyctalopia, color vision defects, and blurred vision. In the early stages of toxicity, mild mottling of the perifoveal retinal pigment epithelium is seen in conjunction with a reduced foveal reflex. Peripheral pigmentary changes often occur at this stage but may be overlooked. Macular pigmentary changes progress to a classic bull's eye maculopathy. In the later stages, generalized retinal pigmentary changes occur with vascular attenuation and optic disc pallor.

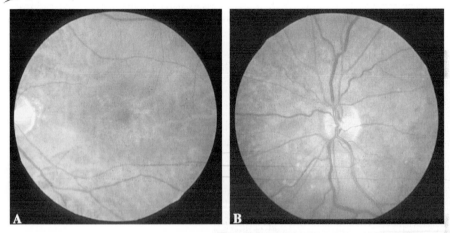

Bull's eye maculopathy of chloroquine retinopathy (*A*). Advanced chloroquine maculopathy (*B*).

2. What doses of chloroquine and hydroxychloroquine cause retinopathy?

Retinopathy is extremely unlikely with a total dose < 100 gm of chloroquine or < 300 gm of hydroxychloroquine and rare with a total dose < 300 gm or 700 gm, respectively. Perhaps more importantly retinopathy is unlikely with a daily dose < 4.4 mg/kg/day of chloroquine or < 7.7 mg/kg/day of hydroxychloroquine. A daily dose > 8 mg/kg/day of hydroxychloroquine produces retinopathy in 40% of cases.

3. How should patients taking chloroquine and hydroxychloroquine be monitored?

Before commencing hydroxychloroquine therapy, a baseline assessment should include a detailed clinical examination with special attention to pigmentary changes in the macular area. Threshold static perimetry with a red light in scotopic conditions may elicit parafoveal scotomata indicative of retinal damage before clinical or fluorescein angiographic evidence of retinal damage. Abnormalities may be found in electroretinography (ERG), electrooculography (EOG), and dark adaptation tests, but they generally indicate more widespread retinal damage. Further review is recommended yearly, until the total dose approaches 700 gm, when more regular review may be necessary, or until symptoms develop.

4. What management is advised for chloroquine retinopathy?

If retinal toxicity is present, hydroxychloroquine or chloroquine should be stopped immediately. Clinical improvement may be noted, but typically progression continues because of the slow excretion of the drugs. Studies in laboratory animals suggest that NH_4Cl and dimercapol increase renal excretion of chloroquine, but they have not been proved effective in the clinical setting.

5. Is the pathogenesis of chloroquine and hydroxychloroquine retinopathy understood?

The earliest histopathologic changes of chloroquine retinopathy include membranous cytoplasmic bodies in ganglion cells and degenerative changes in the outer segments of photoreceptors. However, chloroquine has a selective affinity for melanin, and it has been suggested that this affinity reduces the ability of melanin to combine with free radicals and protect visual cells from light and radiation toxicity. Other authors believe that direct damage to photoreceptors occurs.

6. How may thioridazine affect the retina?

Thioridazine (Mellaril) may cause complaints of nyctalopia, dyschromatopsia, and poor vision. The earliest retinal changes are a fine mottling or granularity to the retinal pigment epithelium posterior to the equator, which may progress to marked pigmentary atrophy and hypertrophic pigment plaques. Vascular attenuation and optic atrophy may follow. Toxicity is said to be uncommon with daily doses < 800 mg/day but may develop rapidly with doses over 1200 mg/day.

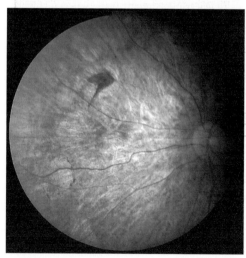

Marked retinal pigment epithelial loss and clumping due to thioridazine toxicity.

7. What other phenothiazines cause retinopathy?

Retinal toxicity has been reported with other phenothiazines, including chlorpromazine. However, these compounds are less likely to cause retinopathy, probably because they lack the piperdylethyl side group of thioridazine. It is thought that 1200–2400 gm/day of chlorpromazine for at least 12 months is required before toxicity occurs.

8. How may quinine sulfate cause retinopathy?

Quinine sulfate is used for nocturnal cramps and malaria prophylaxis. It may cause retinal toxicity after a single large ingestion (4 gm). The therapeutic window is narrow with some patients taking a daily dose of 2 gm. Patients develop blurred vision, nyctalopia, nausea, tinnitus, dysacusis, and even coma within 2–4 hours of ingestion. The acute findings include dilated pupils, loss of retinal transparency due to ganglion cell toxicity, and dilated retinal vessels. As the acute phase resolves, vessel attenuation and optic disc pallor result. Visual acuity improves after the acute phase.

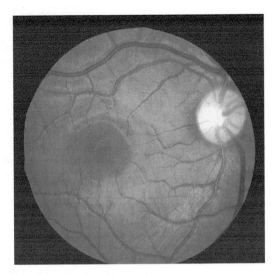

Mild loss of retinal transparency due to quinine sulfate toxicity.

9. What are the similarities and differences in electrophysiologic tests between chloroquine and phenothiazine retinopathy?

The ERG in chloroquine toxicity may show an enlarged A wave and depressed B wave, whereas it is generally depressed in phenothiazine toxicity. The EOG is decreased in both, but only progressive disease is significant in chloroquine retinopathy because some decrease is common shortly after starting chloroquine therapy. Dark adaptation may remain normal in chloroquine toxicity even in late cases, whereas adaptation is delayed in phenothiazine toxicity.

10. What is unusual about cystoid macula edema due to nicotinic acid?

Nicotinic acid is used in conjunction with dietary restriction of fats for the treatment of hyperlipidemia in doses of 1–3 gm/day. Although typical cystoid macula edema is seen clinically, fluorescein angiography shows no late leakage, suggesting that the edema is due to intracellular edema in Müller cells.

11. Name the substances that may cause crystalline retinopathy.

1. Tamoxifen
2. Canthoxanthine
3. Talc (often seen with intravenous drug abuse)
4. Drugs that cause secondary oxalosis
   • Methoxyfluorane anesthesia
   • Ethylene glycol
   • Salicylate ingestion in the presence of renal failure

12. What is the mechanism of retinopathy caused by talc?

Talc is used as a filler in methylphenidate hydrochloride (Ritalin) pills that drug addicts may crush and inject intravenously. Initially the talc particles embolize the lungs but after prolonged abuse ($\geq$ 12,000 pills) pulmonary arteriovenous shunts allow talc into the systemic circulation. Emboli to the retinal arterioles may lead to marked peripheral and posterior closure (see figures, next page), resulting in retinal neovascularization, vitreous hemorrhage, and ischemic maculopathy.

13. How should talc retinopathy be managed?

Immediate cessation of Ritalin abuse is essential. If neovascularization and vitreous hemorrhage are present, peripheral panretinal photocoagulation should be considered. There is no effective treatment for ischemic maculopathy.

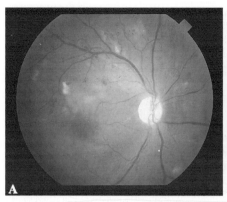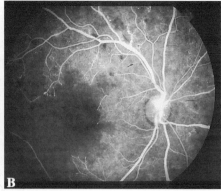

Talc retinopathy, showing fine perifoveal talc particles (*A*) and extensive resultant posterior pole retinal vascular closure on fluorescein angiography (*B*).

14. What is xanthopsia? Which drug may cause it?

Xanthopsia is the unusual symptom of yellow vision. Along with hemeralopia (reduced visual acuity in the presence of increased background illumination), blurred vision, poor color vision, and paracentral scotomas, it is due to digitalis toxicity.

15. What are the clinical features of tamoxifen retinopathy? How much drug is necessary to cause symptoms?

Patients are typically asymptomatic, although significantly reduced visual acuity has been reported. Small crystals are seen deposited in the inner retina in the macular area. Punctate retinal pigment epithelial changes and cystoid macular edema may occur. Toxicity has been reported in patients taking between 20–320 mg/day.

16. Is silver known to cause retinopathy?

Argyrosis is a discoloration of the skin caused by silver. It typically occurs in radiographers and in patients who use silver nitrate mouthwashes for recurrent streptococcal sore throat. Silver is probably deposited at the level of Bruch's membrane/choriocapillaris and in red light blocks choroidal vessel fluorescence. Fluorescein angiography demonstrates a dark choroid.

17. Can intraocular injection of antibiotics cause retinopathy?

Inadvertent intraocular injection of gentamicin may result in the rapid onset of retinal whitening in the macular area. Optic atrophy and retinal pigment epithelial changes develop later. The visual prognosis is poor, and neovascular glaucoma may develop. Macular infarction has been reported after intravitreal injection of 400 μg, although 200 μg is probably safe. Similar problems may occur with tobramycin and other aminoglycosides.

18. In what circumstances can oxygen therapy be toxic to the retina?

Retrolental fibroplasia was the name originally given to extensive neovascularization and retinal detachment in premature infants who had been given postnatal oxygen therapy. It is now believed that the retinal changes are primarily due to immaturity, which may arrest normal developmental retinal neovascularization, and that a further insult to the retina, such as postnatal oxygen therapy or systemic sepsis, may precipitate retinopathy of prematurity.

19. What is interferon retinopathy?

Interferon may cause retinal changes that include cotton-wool spots, retinal hemorrhages, macula edema, capillary nonperfusion, and vascular occlusions. The mechanism may be immune complex deposition in the retinal vasculature followed by leukocyte infiltration and vascular closure. Interferon alpha may aggravate autoimmune thyroiditis and polyarthropathy in 10% of cases by stimulating antibody production.

20. What effects may iron overload have on the retina?

A retained iron intraocular foreign body may lead to darkening of the iris, orange deposits in the anterior subcapsular region of the lens, anterior and posterior vitritis, pigmentary retinopathy, and progressive loss of field. The intraocular foreign body should be removed as soon as possible.

21. Retinal thromboembolic events are caused by what drugs?

Oral contraceptives have been associated with central, branch, and cilioretinal artery occlusions and central retinal vein occlusion. Considerable controversy surrounds the role of oral contraceptives in causing these events, but stopping the oral contraceptive pill seems advisable. Talc retinal emboli are discussed in question 12, and periorbital steroid injection with inadvertent arterial penetration may result in extensive embolization of the retinal circulation.

22. What chelating agents may cause maculopathy?

Desferrioxamine, a chelating agent used to treat iron overload, particularly in thalassemia major, may cause blurred vision, nyctalopia, and ring scotomata. The fundus may show bilateral widespread retinal pigment epithelial derangement.

BIBLIOGRAPHY

1. Cohen SV, Quertel G, Egasse D, et al: The dark choroid in systemic aggrosis. Retina 13:312–316, 1993.
2. Gass JDM: Toxic diseases affecting the pigment epithelium and retina. In Gass JDM (ed): Stereoscopic Atlas of Macular Diseases, 4th ed. St. Louis, Mosby, 1997.
3. Swartz M: Other diseases: Drug toxicity, metabolic and nutritional conditions. In Ryan SJ (ed): Retina, 2nd ed. St. Louis, Mosby, 1994.
4. Weiner A, Sandberg MA, Raudie AR, et al: Hydroxychloroquine retinopathy. Am J Ophthalmol 106:286–292, 1988.

45. COATS' DISEASE

William Tasman, M.D.

1. What is Coats' disease?

Exudation and retinal telangiectasia are hallmarks of the disorder, which is named for the British ophthalmologist who first described this condition in 1908. It comes on painlessly and may be slow and insidious in its development. In many instances, Coats' disease is not discovered until it is well advanced.

2. List the clinical characteristics of Coats' disease.

1. Occurs most frequently in young males
2. Usually unilateral
3. Not familial and not known to be associated with any systemic disease
4. Characteristic retinal vascular lesions are telangiectatic-like "light bulb" aneurysms that are associated with capillary drop-out and sometimes vascular sheathing, usually in the fundus periphery (see figures *B* and *F*, page 281)
5. Exudation, a prominent feature, has a predilection to accumulate in the posterior pole of the fundus (see figure *A*, page 281); it contains cholesterol.
6. May lead to retinal detachment, cataract, glaucoma, and phthisis bulbae.

3. What is the incidence in women?

Although some researchers have questioned whether Coats' disease actually occurs in women, 8 to 10% of cases occur in women.

4. What is the most common age at which Coats' disease becomes apparent?

Between 8 and 10 years of age. However, it can be noted in infancy and often is much more severe when noted early in life.

5. What percentage of cases are unilateral vs. bilateral?

About 80 to 90% of the cases are unilateral. When bilateral cases do develop, there is usually asymmetry, with one eye being much more involved than the other.

6. Are the retinal vascular changes easy to detect?

Usually if the patient is cooperative, it is not hard to diagnose the peripheral retinal telangiectasia. In younger patients, however, these changes can be subtle. Under anesthesia, it is possible to perform fluorescein angiography, which usually helps to confirm the diagnosis.

7. How does this condition differ from Leber's miliary aneurysms?

Leber described retinal miliary aneurysms within a couple of years of Coats. He suggested that the conditions were one and the same, and that is the generally accepted thinking at the present time.

8. Do we know the etiology of Coats' disease?

The precise etiology for Coats' disease has not been determined. Some studies suggest that the retinal changes are not predominantly inflammatory in nature. We have few additional insights into the underlying cause, and at this point one would have to say that the etiology remains obscure.

9. Are there any conditions with which Coats' disease can be confused?

When there is exudation in the macula and peripheral retinal telangiectasia, but no retinal detachment, the disease can frequently be competently diagnosed. In advanced stages, there are a number of conditions that Coats' disease may simulate, most notably the malignant intraocular tumor in infancy and childhood, retinoblastoma. It has been estimated that approximately 3.9%

of eyes originally diagnosed as harboring retinoblastoma were subsequently discovered to have Coats' disease.

10. Are there other conditions beside retinoblastoma that can simulate Coats' diseases?

Angiomatosis retinae (von Hippel-Lindau syndrome), one of the phakomatoses, can cause exudation in the macula. This condition is autosomally dominantly inherited and has visceral and central nervous system hemangioblastomas as part of the syndrome. In addition, visceral cysts and tumors, including renal cell carcinoma, may occur. Early in its onset, the fundus picture is different from Coats' disease in that angiomatosis retinae will demonstrate a dilated and tortuous afferent arteriole and an efferent draining venule entering and leaving a reddish balloon-like mass, usually in the fundus periphery. Other conditions to be considered in the diagnosis are hyperplastic primary vitreous, which is usually unilateral and which occurs in a microphthalmic eye. Retinopathy of prematurity may present with a retinal detachment, but usually there is a history of significant prematurity in patients affected with this disorder.

11. Other than fluorescein angiography, what may be helpful in confirming the diagnosis?

Ultrasonography may help to differentiate between Coats' disease and retinoblastoma by detecting the presence or absence of subretinal calcifications. Calcification is found in retinoblastoma, but it is extremely rare in Coats' disease.

12. Is it advisable to obtain a CT?

CT is perhaps the single most valuable test because of its ability to delineate intraocular morphology, to qualify retinal densities, and to detect associated orbital or intracranial abnormalities. However, this does expose a young patient to low levels of radiation if studies are repeated periodically.

13. Can aspiration of subretinal exudates aid in diagnosis?

The key diagnostic findings in the analysis of subretinal aspirates are the presence of cholesterol crystals and pigment-laden macrophages and the absence of tumor cells. Reserve this technique for patients in whom retinoblastoma has been ruled out by all other noninvasive means, because tumor seeding can occur.

14. How is Coats' disease managed?

It is desirable to treat the condition before exudate accumulates in the macular area. Treatment is directed at the peripheral telangiectatic vascular abnormalities. Photocoagulation can be used to eliminate these abnormal vessels. In patients with exudation under the peripheral vascular telangiectasia, cryotherapy may be preferable (see figure D, next page). Elimination of the defective vessels prevents further leakage and is followed by resorption of the exudate.

15. How long does it take for the exudate to disappear?

Resorption of the exudate may take up to a year or more before it is completely gone.

16. Is more than one treatment necessary?

If more than two quadrants have retinal telangiectasia, two to three treatments may be required.

17. Once the abnormal vessels are gone, is the patient considered cured?

Recurrence, which is usually heralded by the reappearance of exudate and is almost always associated with new vascular abnormalities, can occur even many years later. It is recommended that patients be followed up at 6-month intervals.

18. Can this condition be managed once the retina has detached?

The drainage of subretinal exudative fluid and the placement of a scleral buckle may, in some cases, help to reattach the retina. Less commonly, vitrectomy may be performed, and internal drainage of fluid and cholesterol may be accomplished through a retinotomy. At the same time, it is necessary to treat the abnormal vessels by photocoagulation or cryotherapy. The vision in these eyes, however, is usually quite limited, and sometimes, despite reattachment of the retina, there is no light perception.

19. If left untreated, what is the outcome?

Untreated Coats' disease does not invariably lead to intractable glaucoma. However, retinal detachment and neovascular glaucoma are the ultimate complications that may lead to loss of the globe.

20. When should an eye with Coats' disease be enucleated?

When retinoblastoma cannot be ruled out or when neovascular glaucoma is present in blind, painful eyes.

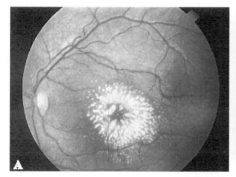
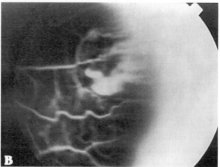

A, Exudate in the posterior pole of a 9-month-old infant girl prior to treatment. *B,* Peripheral retinal telangiectasia seen on fluorescein angiography in the temporal periphery of patient shown in part *A.*

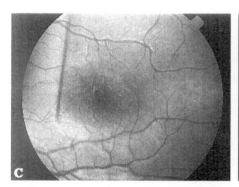
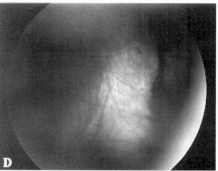

C, Two years after treatment, the exudate has absorbed. *D,* Area of cryotherapy peripherally 2 years later.

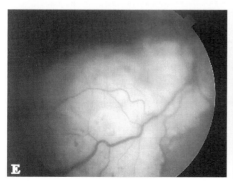
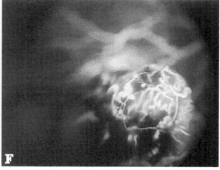

E, Exudation in the posterior pole of a 16-year-old patient with Coats' disease. *F,* Peripheral telangiectasia seen on fluorescein angiography in the temporal fundus periphery of the patient shown in part *E.*

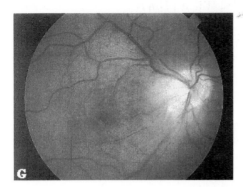

G, Two years after treatment, the exudate in the posterior pole has absorbed.

BIBLIOGRAPHY

1. Coats G: Forms of retinal disease with massive exudation. R Lond Ophthalmol Hosp Rep 17:440–525, 1908.
2. Coats G: Über retinitis exsudativa (retinitis haemorrhagica externa). Albrecht von Graefes Arch Klin Exp Ophthalmol 18:275–327, 1912.
3. Egerer I, Tasman W, Tomer TL: Coats' disease. Arch Ophthalmol 92:109–112, 1974.
4. Haik BG, Saint Louis L, Smith ME, et al: Computed tomography of the nonrhegmatogenous retinal detachment in the pediatric patient. Ophthalmology 92:1133–1142, 1985.
5. Howard GM, Ellsworth RM: Differential diagnosis of retinoblastoma: A statistical survey of 500 children: I. Relative frequency of the lesions which simulate retinoblastoma. Am J Ophthalmol 60:610–617, 1965.
6. Leber T: Über eine durch Vorkommen multipler Miliaraneurysmen charakterisierte Form von Retinaldegeneration. Arch Ophthalmol 81:1–14, 1912.
7. Ridley ME, Shields JA, Brown GC, et al: Coats' disease: Evaluation of management. Ophthalmology 898:1381–1387, 1982.
8. Tarkkanen A, Laatikainen L: Coats' disease: Clinical, angiographic, histopathological findings and clinical management. Br J Ophthalmol 67:766–776, 1983.

46. FUNDUS TRAUMA

Jeffrey P. Blice, M.D.

1. What are the mechanisms of injury to the fundus in blunt trauma?

Blunt trauma to the sclera can produce a direct effect on the underlying choroid and retina. In addition, a concussive effect from force transmitted through the vitreous may be seen away from the initial point of impact. The sudden deformation of the globe may cause stretching of the retina and retinal pigment epithelium (RPE) and traction on the vitreous base. The shearing forces generated by this traction may tear the retina in the area of the vitreous base or result in avulsion of the vitreous base.

2. What clinical entity is caused by the contrecoup mechanism?

Indirect damage from the concussive effect of an injury tends to occur at the interfaces of tissue with greatest differences in density, most commonly the lens–vitreous interface and posterior vitreoretinal interface. The transmitted force may cause fragmentation of photoreceptor outer segments and damage to the receptor cell bodies. Clinically, these areas appear as opacified retina and are termed **commotio retinae**. Although the retinal whitening is only temporary, resolving over 3–4 weeks, permanent damage may occur. Loss of vision depends on the amount and location of early photoreceptor loss. The RPE underlying an area of commotio may develop a granular hyperpigmentation or atrophic appearance and lead to decreased vision. The eponym associated with this entity is Berlin's edema; however, there is no true intra- or extracellular edema and no fluoroscein leakage is seen.

3. Name the five types of retinal breaks seen in fundus trauma.
1. Retinal dialyses
2. Horseshoe tears
3. Operculated holes
4. Macular holes
5. Necrotic dissolution of the retina

4. Where are retinal dialyses most commonly seen?

Retinal dialyses are usually located in the superonasal or inferotemporal quadrants. Trauma is more clearly related to the superonasal than inferotemporal dialyses. Dialyses may be associated with avulsion of the vitreous base. Because they can lead to retinal detachment, a careful depressed exam of all patients with a history of blunt trauma is essential. Prophylactic treatment of all dialyses with cryopexy or laser photocoagulation is recommended in the hope of decreasing the likelihood of future retinal detachments.

5. When do retinal detachments occur with dialyses?

Retinal detachments present at variable intervals after injury; however, the dialysis is usually detectable early or immediately at the time of injury. Approximately 10% of dialysis-related detachments present immediately, 30% within 1 month, 50% within 8 months and 80% within 2 years. Most trauma victims are young with a formed vitreous that tamponades a break or dialysis, but as the vitreous eventually liquefies, fluid passes through retinal breaks causing detachments. The nature of the vitreous in such cases may explain the delay in presentation of the detachments.

6. Besides retinal dialyses, do other trauma-related breaks need to be treated prophylactically?

Horseshoe tears and operculated holes in the setting of acute trauma are usually treated by cryopexy or laser photocoagulation. Macular holes require pars plana vitrectomy with gas exchange if closure of the hole is attempted; however, macular holes usually do not progress to retinal detachments. Surgery is not performed for the purposes of prophylactic closure. Direct injury with necrosis of the retina is usually associated with underlying choroidal injury so that a chorioretinal adhesion may be formed spontaneously. However, any accumulation of subretinal fluid or persistent traction on damaged retina makes prophylactic treatment reasonable.

7. What is the prognosis for repair of a retinal detachment associated with a dialysis?

Dialysis-related detachments are usually smooth, thin, and transparent. Intrarenal cysts are common, and one-half have demarcation lines. In addition, proliferative vitreoretinopathy is rare. The characteristics of the detachment are suggestive of its chronic nature and insidious onset; however, the prognosis for repair with conventional scleral buckling techniques is good.

8. Describe the clinical features of a choroidal rupture.

The retina is relatively elastic, and the sclera is mechanically strong. Bruch's membrane, the structure between the retinal pigment epithelium and choriocapillaris, is neither elastic nor strong. Consequently, it is susceptible to the stretching forces exerted on the globe in blunt trauma. Bruch's membrane usually tears along with the choriocapillaris and RPE. Choroidal ruptures may be found at the point of contact with the globe or in the posterior pole as a result of indirect forces. Clinically, choroidal rupture appears as a single area or multiple areas of subretinal hemorrhage, usually concentric and temporal to the optic nerve. The hemorrhage may dissect into the vitreous. As the blood resolves, a crescent-shaped or linear white area is seen where the rupture occurred. With time, surrounding RPE hyperplasia or atrophy may be seen.

9. Are there any long-term complications of choroidal ruptures?

The visual consequences of a choroidal rupture depend on its location with respect to the fovea. A patient with a choroidal rupture near the fovea may have good vision; however, the break in Bruch's membrane predisposes the patient to the development of a choroidal neovascular membrane, which may threaten vision long after the initial injury. Therefore, patients at risk should be followed regularly and advised of the potential complication.

10. Can orbital adnexal trauma result in fundus abnormalities?

High-velocity missile injuries may cause an indirect concussive injury to the globe, resulting in retinal breaks and ruptures in Bruch's membrane that resemble a claw. A fibroglial scar with pigment proliferation forms, but retinal detachment is rare, possibly because a firm adhesion develops, acting as a retinopexy. Chorioretinitis sclopetaria is the name given to this clinical entity.

11. What are the signs of a scleral rupture?

When a laceration or obvious deformation of the globe is not visible, other findings raise the index of suspicion that an injury may be more serious than initially thought. The presence of an afferent pupillary defect (APD), poor motility, marked chemosis, and vitreous hemorrhage raise the suspicion of an open globe. Other findings that may be helpful include a deeper than normal anterior chamber and a low intraocular pressure; however, in an eye with a posterior rupture and incarcerated uvea the intraocular pressure may be normal.

12. Why is the initial exam of a severely traumatized eye important?

A poor outcome is associated with initially poor visual acuity, presence of an APD, large wounds (> 10 mm) or wounds extending posterior to the rectus muscles, and vitreous hemorrhage. The first person to evaluate the traumatized eye may have the only opportunity to assess the best visual acuity. The delay often associated with referral to other institutions or dealing with life-threatening complications may result in diffusion of vitreous hemorrhage and corneal or other anterior segment abnormalities that preclude an adequate view of the posterior segment. The first look may be the only look at a traumatized eye.

13. Where is the most likely place for a globe to rupture?

The globe may rupture anywhere, depending on the nature of the injury. However, the globe most often ruptures at the limbus, beneath the recti muscles, or at a surgical scar. The sclera is thinnest and therefore weakest behind the insertions of the recti muscles. The site of a previous cataract extraction or glaucoma procedure is weaker than normal sclera.

14. Outline the goals of managing a ruptured globe.

1. Identify the extent of the injury. Perform a 360° peritomy, inspecting all quadrants. If necessary, disinsert a muscle to determine the extent of a laceration.

2. Rule out a retained foreign body. In any case of projectile injury, sharp lacerations, uncertain history, or questionable mechanism of injury, consider a CT to detect a foreign body.

3. Close the wound, and limit reconstruction as much as possible. Close the sclera with a relatively large suture (e.g., 8-0 or 9-0 Nylon), and reposit any protruding uvea. If vitreous is protruding, cut it flush with the choroidal tissues, using fine scissors and a cellulose sponge or automated vitreous cutter.

4. Guard against infection. Prophylactic IV antibiotic treatment should include an aminoglycoside in combination with a cephalosporin or vancomycin. Clindamycin may be added if coverage for *Bacillus* sp. is desired.

5. Protect the remaining eye. Place a shield over the fellow eye during the repair procedure to prevent accidental injury. Counsel the patient at the earliest opportunity about the need for protective eyewear to prevent future injury.

15. Discuss the role of CT and MRI in the detection of intraocular foreign bodies.

The best method of detection of intraocular foreign bodies is indirect ophthalmoscopy. If a view of the posterior segment is impossible, CT is the next best alternative. A CT scan is excellent for the detection of metallic foreign bodies but also detects glass or even plastic foreign bodies in some instances. When an organic foreign body is suspected, MRI offers the advantage of better soft tissue discrimination and is an excellent supplement to CT. However, any suspicion of a metallic foreign body prevents the use of MRI. Ultrasonography also supplements the information provided by a CT, possibly detecting a radiolucent foreign body as well as providing information about the status of the retina and vitreous. Plain films of the orbit are still useful for the detection of a foreign body if a CT scanner is not available; however, the ability to localize and detect nonmetallic foreign bodies is more limited.

16. Do all intraocular foreign bodies need to be removed immediately? Which ones require early vitrectomy for removal?

All foreign bodies do not require immediate removal. The decision to remove a foreign body at the time of initial repair is complex and depends somewhat on the preferences of the surgeon and the specific situation. However, in a patient with acute traumatic endophthalmitis or a known toxic or reactive foreign body, vitrectomy at the time of initial repair or soon after is a reasonable option.

17. Which metals are toxic to the eye?

The toxicity of a metal is related to the reduction-oxidation potential (redox potential). Metals such as copper and iron have a low redox potential and tend to dissociate into their respective ionic forms, making them more toxic. Pure forms are more reactive than alloys. The ocular toxicity from an iron foreign body is called siderosis. When copper is the offending agent, the condition is named chalcosis. Other metals, such as gold, platinum, silver, and aluminum, are relatively inert. Nonmetallic substances such as glass, plastic, porcelain, and rubber are also relatively inert and pose no threat of toxicity on the basis of their chemical composition.

18. List the clinical findings in siderosis bulbi.

Iron tends to be deposited in epithelial tissues. Hyperchromic heterochromia of the involved iris and a mid-dilated, minimally reactive pupil are seen. Brownish dots are visible in the lens from iron deposition in the lens epithelium, along with generalized yellowing of the lens from involvement of the cortex. The retinal effects of iron toxicity can be detected and followed by electroretinography (ERG). Pure iron particles may cause a flat ERG in 100 days. Clinically, a pigmentary degeneration with sclerosis of vessels, retinal thinning, and, later, atrophy develops in the periphery and progresses posteriorly. If not removed initially, the potential toxic effects of a foreign body can be monitored by clinical exam and serial ERG. However, siderosis generally causes progressive gradual visual loss unless the foreign body is removed.

19. Do all copper foreign bodies cause chalcosis?

Foreign bodies less than 85% pure copper cause chalcosis; greater than 85% pure copper foreign bodies cause sterile endophthalmitis. Copper ions are deposited in basement membranes. In the cornea Descemet's membrane may be affected, causing a Kaiser Fleischer ring, a brownish discoloration of the peripheral cornea. The iris may be sluggishly reactive to light and have a greenish color. Deposition of copper in the anterior capsule results in a "sunflower" cataract, and the vitreous may become opacified. ERG findings are similar but may improve if the foreign body is removed.

20. Posttraumatic endophthalmitis is caused most commonly by what organisms?

The most common organism associated with endophthalmitis in the setting of acute trauma is *Staphylococcus aureus*. Skin flora are the most likely source of contamination of a traumatic ocular wound. Infections due to *Bacillus cereus*, although much less common (estimates range from 8–25%), are important because of the severity and damage caused by the infection. In any ocular injury contaminated by soil, the possibility of infection with *B. cereus* needs to be considered and the regimen of prophylactic antibiotics adjusted accordingly.

21. Outline the role of prophylactic antibiotics.

Posttraumatic endophthalmitis is a relatively rare complication of penetrating ocular trauma, occurring in only 7% of cases; however, the potential for devastation to the eye warrants prophylactic treatment. In cases of obvious endophthalmitis, a grossly contaminated wound, or contaminated foreign body, initial intravitreal antibiotic injection should be considered. Postoperatively, all ruptured or lacerated globes should be treated with prophylactic topical and systemic antibiotics for 3–5 days. Although the Endophthalmitis Vitrectomy Study (EVS) showed no benefit to systemic antibiotic treatment in postoperative endophthalmitis, the issue of prophylaxis in trauma was not addressed.

22. What regimen of antibiotics is used to treat posttraumatic endophthalmitis?

The choice of intravitreal injections is directed at covering a broad spectrum of organisms. Although a number of combinations are possible, a regimen with coverage for typical pathogens is vancomycin, 1 mg/0.1 cc, or clindamycin, 1 mg/0.1 cc, in combination with amikacin, 0.2–0.4 mg/0.1 cc, or gentamicin, 0.1 mg/0.1 cc. Frequent topical treatment with a fortified aminoglycoside and vancomycin should be initiated postoperatively in addition to systemic antibiotics for 3–5 days.

23. Does injury to one eye place the other eye at risk for visual loss?

Granulomatous inflammation may affect both the noninjured and injured eye weeks to years after a penetrating injury. Sympathetic ophthalmia (SO) is a bilateral granulomatous uveitis manifested by anterior segment inflammation and multiple yellow-white lesions in the peripheral fundus. Complications include cataract, glaucoma, optic atrophy, exudative retinal detachments, and subretinal fibrosis. Exposure of the immune system to a previously immunologically isolated antigen in the uvea probably triggers the response. Eighty percent of cases develop within 3 months of injury, and 90% develop within 1 year. Cases of SO have occurred after ocular surgery. Therapy is directed at immunosuppression with steroids, cyclosporin, and/or cytotoxic agents. Most patients retain 20/60 vision or better at 10-year follow-up, but complications limit vision in many patients.

24. How can the uninjured eye be protected from the long-term sequelae of penetrating ocular injury?

The incidence of SO is extremely rare (< 0.5% of penetrating trauma). The only known way to prevent the disease absolutely is enucleation of the injured eye 10–14 days after the injury.

With modern repair techniques, the potential for vision in severely injured eyes has improved; therefore, enucleation as prophylactic treatment for SO should be reserved only **for eyes confirmed to have no visual potential**. Removal of the inciting eye after inflammation has developed may improve the final acuity of the noninjured eye, but the inciting eye may eventually retain the best visual acuity. Enucleation as a treatment is reserved for inciting eyes with **no visual potential**.

25. Can trauma elsewhere in the body cause fundus abnormalities?

Cotton-wool spots, usually in the peripapillary distribution, retinal hemorrhages, and optic disc edema have been described after severe head injury or compressive chest trauma. Purtscher's retinopathy, the name given to this entity, is a result of microvascular occlusion presumed to be embolic in nature; however, the true pathogenesis is unknown. A similar appearance in other conditions, such as acute pancreatitis, collagen vascular disease, renal dialysis, and eclampsia, suggests a systemic process with secondary retinal capillary occlusion. The fundus manifestations in severe trauma may be related to the generally poor condition of patients who sustained such trauma rather than the trauma itself. Vitreous, preretinal, and retinal hemorrhages may be seen in birth trauma; however, if seen in the absence of such trauma or other causes (leukemia or bleeding diathesis), nonaccidental trauma should be suspected. Ocular manifestations are present in 40% of abused children, and the ophthalmologist is first to recognize the abuse in 6% of cases. Suspicious injuries need to be reported to protect children from further abuse.

BIBLIOGRAPHY

1. Cox MS, Schepens CL, Freeman HM: Retinal detachment due to ocular contusion. Arch Ophthalmol 76:678–685, 1966.
2. Delori F, Pomerantzeff O, Cox MS: Deformation of the globe under high-speed impact: Its relation to contusion injuries. Invest Ophthalmol 8:290–301, 1969.
3. Tasman W: Peripheral retinal changes following blunt trauma. Trans Am Ophthalmol Soc 70:190–198, 1972.
4. Federman JL, Gouras P: Retina and vitreous. In Podos SM, Yanoff M (eds): Textbook of Ophthalmology, vol 9. St. Louis, Mosby, 1994, pp 15.1–15.12.
5. Kelley JS, Dhaliwal RS: Traumatic choroidopathies. In Ryan SJ (ed): Retina, vol 2. St. Louis, Mosby, 1994, pp 1783–1796.

47. AGE-RELATED MACULAR DEGENERATION

Joseph I. Maguire, M.D., F.A.C.S.

1. What is age-related macular degeneration?

Age-related macular degeneration (ARMD) is the leading cause of significant, irreversible central visual loss in the Western world. It is characterized by age-dependent alterations of the sensory retina, retinal pigment epithelium and choriocapillaris complex in the central retina (macula). The macula is defined clinically by the area roughly within the major temporal vascular arcades and serves our sharp, discriminating vision. Incidence of disease is age-dependent, and prevalence steadily increases past the age of 55. Recent attempts have been made to develop a common international classification, but most clinicians still divide ARMD into exudative or wet and nonexudative or dry forms.

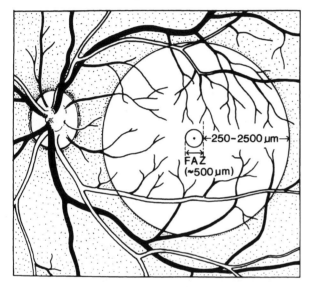

The clinical macula describes that area of retina encompassed by the temporal arcade vessels.

2. Who gets ARMD?

Anyone can. The greatest statistical association of macular degeneration is increasing age. All long-term epidemiologic studies indicate an increasing prevalence of exudative and nonexudative macular changes, as well as visual loss, with increasing age. Most reports point to a greater incidence of exudative disease in women over men. In addition, skin pigmentation also seems to play an important role, at least in exudative disease. African-Americans have a significantly smaller incidence of choroidal neovascularization compared with Caucasians.

3. What etiologic factors are involved in the development of ARMD?

The cause of ARMD is unknown. In addition to increasing age, female gender, heredity, white race, smoking, nutrition, scleral rigidity, photic exposure, and hypertension have been implicated as additional risk factors.

4. What are the clinical signs of ARMD?

1. Drusen
2. Pigmentary alterations

   3. Exudative changes
      • Hemorrhage
      • Hard exudate
      • Subretinal and subretinal pigment epithelial and intraretinal fluid
   4. Atrophy
      • Incipient
      • Geographic

5. What are the symptoms of ARMD?
   1. Visual blurring
   2. Central scotomas
   3. Metamorphopsia

Metamorphopsia is visual distortion. Images may appear smaller (micropsia) or larger (macropsia) than they really are. Patients frequently comment that straight lines such as door jams, tile patterns, phone poles, or other straight-edge surfaces appear curved. Special graphs called Amsler grids—which test the central 20° of vision—are effective home-testing devices for eyes at higher risk for development of exudative age-related macular degeneration.

6. What is dry or nonexudative ARMD?

Nonexudative ARMD is characterized by drusen, pigmentary changes, and atrophy. Drusen are the most common and earliest finding in dry age-related macular degeneration. Drusen represent metabolic byproducts of retinal pigment epithelial cell metabolism. They vary in shape, size, and color. Hard drusen are small, discrete, yellow-to-white nodules, whereas soft drusen tend to be larger and more amorphous. Soft drusen may coalesce with neighboring drusen and are frequently associated with overlying pigmentary changes either from photoreceptor dysfunction or retinal pigment epithelial demise. Progressive retinal pigment epithelial disruption eventually causes loss of overlying sensory retina and underlying choriocapillaris. Such developments result in localized atrophic regions that extend and coalesce around the fovea and eventually involve the fovea itself.

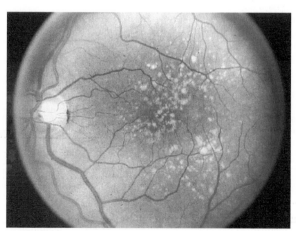

Drusen are the byproduct of retinal metabolism and manifest as focal yellow-white deposits deep to the retinal pigment epithelium. They serve as a marker of nonexudative age-related macular degeneration.

7. What is wet or exudative ARMD?

Exudative ARMD is characterized by the development of vascular changes and/or fluid under the sensory retina and retinal pigment epithelium. Choroidal neovascular membranes and pigment epithelial detachments progressing to endstage disciform macular scarring are the classic presentations of wet age-related macular degeneration. Ophthalmoscopically choroidal neovascular membranes are slate-to-green subretinal lesions associated with hard exudate, hemorrhage, or fluid. These vessels originate from the normal choriocapillaris and enter the subretinal space through defects in Bruch's membrane—a collagenous layer separating the choroidal circulation from the retina. Pigment epithelial detachments are dome-shaped clear, turbid, or blood-filled elevations of the retinal pigment epithelium; they may or may not be associated with choroidal neovascular ingrowth.

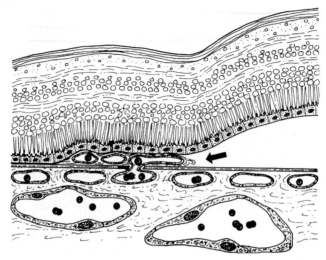

Choroidal neovascular membranes gain access to the subretinal space via defects in Bruch's membrane (arrow). Once there, these vessels may cause bleeding and disciform scar formation, resulting in overlying retinal dysfunction.

8. How does ARMD cause visual loss?

ARMD ultimately leads to visual loss via permanent alterations in the sensory retina, retinal pigment epithelium, and choroid within the macula. These changes may arise from the development of disciform scarring secondary to choroidal neovascularization or atrophy in which areas of retina cease to exist.

9. What is fluorescein angiography?

Fluorescein angiography is a photographic test used in the diagnosis and treatment of ARMD. Fluorescein dye is injected via an antecubital vein while simultaneous photographs of the macula are taken with a fundus camera. Fluorescein dye demonstrates fluorescence when stimulated with visible light in the blue frequency range. This property, along with anatomic constraints in the retinal and choroidal circulations, allows the identification and localization of abnormal vascular processes, such as choroidal neovascularization, that are found frequently in ARMD.

10. What is indocyanine green videoangiography?

Indocyanine green (ICG) videoangiography is a photographic technique stylistically related to fluorescein angiography. The major difference is the use of ICG dye, which has a peak absorption and emission in the infrared range, whereas the spectral qualities of fluorescein dye are in the visible light range. The advantage of ICG angiography is that it allows visualization through pigment and thin blood. It consequently gives a much better view of the choroid and occult choroidal neovascularization. Current reports show that areas of choroidal neovascularization are localized in an additional 25–35% of eyes using ICG and fluorescein compared with fluorescein angiography alone.

11. What is the difference between occult and classic choroidal neovascularization?

Classic choroidal neovascularization (top figure) is clinically well defined with a gray-to-green hue. Fluorescein angiography demonstrates a well-defined hyperfluorescent lesion with a cartwheel configuration that increases in intensity over the course of the study.

Occult neovascularization (bottom figure) usually demonstrates a poorly defined stippled pigmented appearance with associated retinal thickening. It is not well localized with fluorescein angiography, exhibiting a diffuse punctate hyperfluorescence.

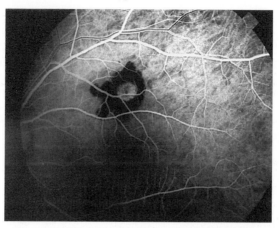

Angiographically, classic choroidal neovascular membranes appear as focal hyperfluorescent lesions deep to the retina. This example shows a corona of hypofluorescence which is associated hemorrhage.

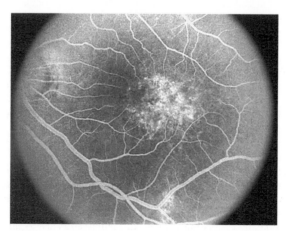

Unfortunately, the majority of choroidal neovascularization is nondiscrete or occult in character. This presentation is often not fully localized with fluorescein angiography. It has a punctate hyperfluorescent pattern with nondiscrete borders.

12. What is the only proven treatment for ARMD?

The only statistically proven effective therapy for ARMD is laser photocoagulation. Its proven use is limited to selected eyes with exudative disease.

13. What is the Macular Photocoagulation Study (MPS)?

The MPS is a multicenter study sponsored by the National Institutes of Health to evaluate the utility of laser in the treatment of extrafoveal exudative ARMD, ocular histoplasmosis, and idiopathic choroidal neovascular membranes. Over time it has also investigated the benefits of laser in juxtafoveal and subfoveal neovascularization, as established in its guidelines.

14. How does laser treatment affect exudative ARMD?

Laser treatment theoretically works by causing a thermal burn and coagulating abnormal vasculature. However, local environmental effects, such as retinal pigment epithelial stimulation and increased oxygenation, also may play crucial roles.

15. What percentage of patients with exudative ARMD can be effectively treated with laser photocoagulation?

Using Macular Photocoagulation Study guidelines, no more than 25% of current patients with ARMD are candidates for laser photocoagulation. Since over one-third of eyes that are treatable have subfoveal lesions and over 50% of successfully treated lesions recur within 3 years, the capacity of laser in the treatment and preservation of vision becomes even more limited.

16. Why is the treatment of exudative ARMD with laser frequently frustrating?

Laser treatment of exudative ARMD is vexing for two main reasons:

1. A majority of patients cannot be offered laser therapy which will preserve central vision because of the foveal position of the vessels or their nondiscrete nature.

2. Even successfully treated eyes have a recurrence rate of greater than 50% within 3 years.

17. What is the role of nutrition in the treatment and prophylaxis of ARMD?

Currently, the role of nutrition in the treatment and prophylaxis of ARMD is unknown. Multiple short-term studies are conflicting or inconclusive in their efforts to establish a therapeutic link. Theoretically, the intake of certain vitamins and trace elements, involved through association with certain enzymes in free radical scavenging, may play a role in modulating the aging process.

18. What is the role of medical management in the treatment of ARMD?

Currently, medical management involves investigative work into compounds with antiangiogenic properties, including alpha-interferon and thalidomide. These agents have caused the successful regression of neovascular changes in selected vascular neoplasms and animal models of neovascularization.

19. What is photodynamic therapy? How does it differ from laser photocoagulation?

Photodynamic therapy (PDT) is an investigative treatment for exudative ARMD. It employs a light-activated drug that is activated by low-power light in a specific wavelength. When injected intravenously, the agent travels in the blood system to the eye, where it is sensitized by an external nonthermal light source. This process causes free radical formation with localized damage to choroidal neovascular processes but spares overlying neurosensory retina, whereas laser causes full-thickness burns of retina and choroid. Because so many exudative features of ARMD are foveal, PDT hopefully eliminates choroidal neovascular changes while preserving overlying retina.

20. Name additional treatment strategies currently under investigation for ARMD.

Additional treatment strategies currently under investigation in ARMD include:

1. Radiation therapy
   - External beam
   - Radioactive plaque therapy
   - External probe application
2. Submacular surgery
   - Removal of choroidal neovascular membranes
   - Removal of submacular hemorrhage
3. Laser treatment for drusen in nonexudative disease

21. What is the role of surgery in removing choroidal neovascular membranes in ARMD?

The benefits of submacular surgery for choroidal neovascular membrane removal have not been established. Selected cases with preretinal pigment epithelial membranes have been reported in ARMD, but they are limited in number. The Submacular Surgery Trial (SST) is currently evaluating in randomized fashion the benefits of submacular surgery vs. laser photocoagulation in subfoveal choroidal neovascularization associated with ARMD.

22. What are low vision aids?

Low vision support involves the use of devices that maximize an eye's visual function through magnification, lighting, and training aimed at allowing patients to take advantage of near peripheral vision. Such aids take many forms, including special spectacles, magnifiers, closed circuit television devices, digitally enhanced cameras, and overhead viewers. People often can read print and carry out important functions not possible without such support. In people with untreatable bilateral visual loss, evaluation for low vision support is critical.

BIBLIOGRAPHY

1. Chakravarthy U, Houston RF, Archer DB: Treatment of age-related subfoveal neovascular membranes by teletherapy: A pilot study. Br J Ophthalmol 77:265–273, 1993.
2. D'Amato RJ, Adamis AP: Angiogenesis inhibition in age-related macular degeneration. Ophthalmology 102:1261–1262, 1995.
3. Eye Disease Case–Control Study Group: Antioxidant status and neovascular age-related macular degeneration. Arch Ophthalmol 111:104–109, 1993.
4. The Framingham Study: VI. Macular degeneration. Surv Ophthalmol 24:428–435, 1980.
5. The International ARM Epidemiological Study Group: An international classification and grading system for age-related maculopathy and age-related macular degeneration. Surv Ophthalmol 39:367–374, 1995.
6. Gass JDM: Drusen and disciform macular detachment and degeneration. Arch Ophthalmol 90:206–217, 1973.
7. Macular Photocoagulation Study Group: Argon laser photocoagulation for neovascular maculopathy: Three year results from randomized clinical trials. Arch Ophthalmol 104:694–701, 1986.
8. Moisseiev J, Alhalel A, Masuri R, Treister G: The impact of the Macular Photocoagulation Study results on the treatment of exudative age-related macular degeneration. Arch Ophthalmol 113:185–189, 1995.
9. Pieramici DJ, Bressler NM, Bressler SB, Schachat AP: Choroidal neovascularization in black patients. Arch Ophthalmol 112:1043–1046, 1994.
10. Thomas MA, Grand MG, Williams DF, et al: Surgical management of subfoveal choroidal neovascularization. Ophthalmology 99:952–968, 1992.
11. Yannuzzi LA, Slakter JS, Sorenson JA, et al: Digital indocyanine green videoangiography and choroidal neovascularization. Retina 12:191–223, 1992.
12. Young R: Pathophysiology of age-related macular degeneration. Surv Ophthalmol 31:291–306, 1987.

48. RETINOPATHY OF PREMATURITY

J. Arch McNamara, M.D.

1. What is retinopathy of prematurity?

Retinopathy of prematurity (ROP) is a vasoproliferative retinal disease that affects infants born prematurely. It has two phases. In the acute phase, normal vascular development goes awry with the development of abnormal vessels that proliferate, occasionally with associated fibrous proliferation. In the chronic or late proliferation phase, retinal detachment, macular ectopia, and severe visual loss may occur. More than 90% of cases of acute ROP go on to spontaneous regression.

2. Who gets retinopathy of prematurity?

Infants weighing less than 1,500 grams at birth and those born at a gestational age of 32 weeks or less are at risk for developing ROP. The disease is more likely to affect the smallest and most premature of infants. The incidence of acute ROP in infants weighing less than 1 kilogram at birth is 3 times greater than that of infants weighing between 1 and 1½ kilograms. Infants born at 23–27 weeks' gestation have a particularly high chance of developing ROP.

3. Who should be screened for retinopathy of prematurity?

Guidelines published by the American College of Obstetrics and Gynecology and the American Academy of Pediatrics recommend that all infants weighing less than 1,250 grams at birth and those that require oxygen in excess of room air during the first 7 days of life should be examined. Infants at particularly high risk are those who weigh less than 1,000 grams at birth and those born at less than 27 weeks' gestation. The first exam should take place at 4–6 weeks after birth. The frequency of follow-up examinations is based on the retinal status at the time of the first exam. Exams should be done every 1–2 weeks either until there is complete retinal vascularization or until two successive 2-week examinations show stage 2 ROP in zone III (more on staging below). Infants should then be examined every 4–6 weeks until the retina is fully vascularized. If there is prethreshold disease (see below), examinations should be done every week until threshold disease occurs (at which point treatment should be offered) or until the disease regresses.

4. How is retinopathy of prematurity classified?

The International Classification of Retinopathy of Prematurity (ICROP) is the system used for describing the findings in ROP. ICROP defines the location of disease in the retina and the extent of involvement of the developing vasculature. It also specifies the stage of involvement with levels of severity ranging from 1 (least affected) to 5 (severe disease).

For the purpose of defining location, the retina is divided into three zones with the optic nerve as the center since vascularization starts from the optic nerve and progresses peripherally (see figure, top of next page, left). Zone I consists of a circle, the radius of which subtends an angle of 30° and extends from the disc to twice the distance from the disc to the center of the macula (twice the disc-to-fovea distance in all directions from the optic disc). Zone II extends from the edge of zone I peripherally to a point tangential to the nasal ora serrata and around to an area near the temporal anatomic equator. Zone III is the residual temporal crescent of retina anterior to zone II.

Staging pertains to the degree of abnormal vascular response observed. Staging for the eye as a whole receives the stage of the most severe manifestation present. Stage I (demarcation line) is defined as a thin but definite structure that separates avascular retina anteriorly from the vascularized retina posteriorly. Abnormal branching of vessels can be seen leading up to the line. It is flat and white and is in the plane of the retina. Stage 2 (ridge) is present when the line of stage 1

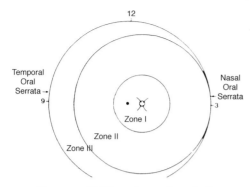

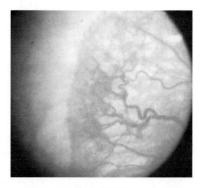

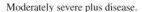
The zones of ROP are shown schematically.   Stage 3 ROP.

has height and width and occupies a volume extending out of the plane of the retina. The ridge may be pink or white. Vessels may leave the plane of the retina to enter it. Small tufts of new vessels may be seen on the surface of the retina posterior to the ridge. These vessels do not constitute fibrovascular growth. Stage 3 (ridge with extraretinal fibrovascular proliferation) is present when fibrovascular proliferation is added to the ridge of stage 2 (see figure, above right). Stage 4 ROP exists when there is subtotal retinal detachment. Retinal detachments in ROP are concave, tractional retinal detachments. Stage 4A ROP is a subtotal retinal detachment that does not involve the central macula. Typically, it is present in the temporal region of zones II and III. Stage 4B ROP is a subtotal retinal detachment that involves the central macula. Lastly, stage 5 ROP is a total retinal detachment. These retinal detachments are funnel-shaped but may have an open or closed configuration in their anterior and posterior areas. The old term for ROP, retrolental fibroplasia, was coined because of the most severe form of retinal detachment in which the retina is totally detached and drawn up into a fibrous mass behind the lens.

5. What is "plus disease"?

Plus disease is indicative of progressive vascular incompetence and is a strong risk factor for development of more severe ROP. Anteriorly, plus disease manifests itself as iris vascular engorgement and pupillary rigidity. Posteriorly, plus disease appears as retinal venous dilation and arterial tortuosity in the posterior pole. It is graded as mild, moderate, or severe (see figure). When plus disease is present in the posterior pole, a plus sign (+) is added to the number stage of the disease, e.g., stage 3+.

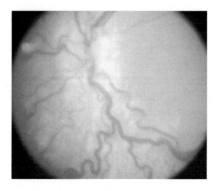

Moderately severe plus disease.

6. When should acute retinopathy of prematurity be treated?

Since ROP can lead to blindness from retinal detachment, treatment to prevent progression to retinal detachment is indicated. However, 90% of infants who develop acute ROP undergo spontaneous regression. Treatment should therefore only be performed for those infants who have a high risk of developing retinal detachment. The Cryotherapy for Retinopathy of Prematurity (Cryo-ROP) Study set out to determine whether or not treatment for ROP would prevent poor outcomes. For the purposes of that study, a level of disease (called "threshold disease") was chosen at which 50% of infants were predicted to go blind without treatment. This prediction was appropriate for the Cryo-ROP Study and remains the level of clinical disease at which treatment is recommended.

Threshold disease is defined as the presence of at least five contiguous or eight cumulative 30° sectors (clock hours) of stage 3 ROP in zone I or II, in the presence of plus disease (see figure). Zone I ROP can progress rapidly to a disastrous outcome, and, therefore, treatment at a lesser level of disease may be appropriate in this posterior zone. Thus, "prethreshold" ROP is defined as zone I, any stage; zone II, stage 2 with plus disease; or zone II with extraretinal fibrovascular proliferation less than threshold. When ROP reaches prethreshold, examinations should be performed weekly.

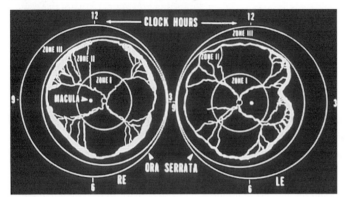

The Cryo-ROP definition of threshold disease is shown schematically.

7. How do you treat acute ROP?

Cryotherapy has been the standard of care for treating acute ROP. More recently, multiple studies have reported on the efficacy of treating ROP with laser photocoagulation delivered by the indirect ophthalmoscope. "Indirect laser" has become the most common form of treatment for acute ROP.

Indirect laser can be delivered in the intensive care nursery without having to take the infant to the operating room. An "isolation room" in the nursery is a desirable location because it allows for others to be shielded from the laser energy. Intravenous sedation is administered at the discretion of the neonatologist, who should be immediately available to manage any possible systemic complications. The pupils are dilated and a lid speculum is inserted. Diode or argon laser is then applied to the entire peripheral avascular zone using a laser indirect ophthalmoscope. The peripheral retina is brought into view with the aid of a pediatric scleral depressor, such as the Flynn depressor. The laser spot desired is a dull white or gray spot, and the spots are placed approximately 1–1½ lesion-widths apart (see figure). With the IRIS Medical, Inc. (Mountain View, CA), diode

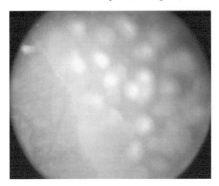

Appearance of the peripheral fundus immediately after laser treatment.

laser, it is advisable to start with a power of 200 milliwatts and a duration of 200 milliseconds. Critical focus on the retina is essential. If the desired lesion is not obtained, the power should be increased in 50 milliwatt increments until the desired result is obtained.

8. How is cryotherapy applied?

Cryotherapy is still preferred by some ophthalmologists for managing acute ROP. As for laser treatment, intravenous sedation can be administered at the discretion of the neonatologist. Some ophthalmologists prefer general anesthesia because of the greater stress on the infant and the greater risk of cardiopulmonary complications with cryotherapy than with laser photocoagulation. The pupils are dilated and a lid speculum is inserted. Cryotherapy is applied to the entire peripheral avascular zone using a hand-held cryo-pencil. The peripheral retina is brought into view using the cryo-pencil as a scleral depressor. A white freeze spot seen for 1–2 seconds is the desired endpoint. The lesions are placed contiguously.

9. Does posterior ROP respond to treatment?

Zone I and posterior zone II disease have a worse prognosis than more anterior ROP. In the Cryo-ROP Study, the beneficial effect of treatment for zone I threshold ROP was limited to a reduction in unfavorable anatomic outcome rate from 92% to 75% at 3 months follow-up. Studies have shown that 100% of eyes with any amount of extraretinal fibrovascular proliferation in zone I and approximately 70% of eyes with vascularization limited to zone I or posterior zone II and stage 1 or stage 2 ROP will progress to threshold disease. Investigations have shown that laser photocoagulation for posterior disease can limit the likelihood of an unfavorable anatomic outcome to approximately 20%.

10. What is the expected result following laser for ROP?

Various reports have quoted a regression rate of approximately 90% following laser photocoagulation for threshold ROP. If regression is to occur, plus disease is usually less on the first week's follow-up visit. There may not be much change in the extraretinal fibrovascular proliferation (ERFP). By 2 weeks, one should start to see a reduction in the ERFP.

11. When should you consider re-treatment for ROP?

Laser photocoagulation for threshold ROP is successful at inducing regression of the acute disease in approximately 90% of cases. Occasionally (approximately 10% of the time) supplemental treatment after the initial session is necessary to induce regression. Re-treatment should be considered if there is worse disease (worse plus disease and increased extraretinal fibrovascular proliferation) at the 1-week visit or persistently active disease (extraretinal fibrovascular proliferation with plus disease) and the presence of "skip lesions" (areas of apparently missed treatment) or widely spaced laser lesions at the 2-week visit. Additional treatment should be applied to previously untreated areas rather than treating over old laser spots. In a similar fashion, supplemental cryotherapy can be applied to "skip areas" if there has not been an adequate response to initial cryotherapy treatment.

12. What can be done for more advanced stages of ROP?

Stage 4B and progressive stage 4A retinal detachments may be managed with scleral buckling surgery. There is an approximated 60% rate of retinal reattachment with approximately 35% of those infants with attached retinae having useful vision. Vitrectomy surgery may be tried for more advanced stage 5 ROP. However, the anatomic and visual success rates are extremely poor.

13. What are some of the late complications of ROP?

The late complications of ROP include myopia, retinal pigmentation, dragging of the retina (see figure, top of next page), lattice-like vitreoretinal degeneration, retinal holes, retinal detachment, and angle closure glaucoma. Obviously, these children need long-term follow-up by both a retina specialist and a pediatric ophthalmologist. Amblyopia and strabismus are also common.

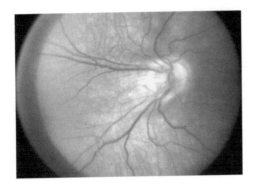

Moderate temporal dragging of the macula due to regressed ROP.

14. What is the differential diagnosis for ROP?

The differential differs depending on the extent of the disease. In less severe ROP, conditions that lead to peripheral retinal vascular changes and retinal dragging should be considered. In more severe disease, the differential diagnosis of a white pupillary reflex must be considered.

Differential Diagnosis of Retinopathy of Prematurity

LESS SEVERE DISEASE	MORE SEVERE DISEASE
Familial exudative vitreoretinopathy	Congenital cataract
Incontinentia pigmenti (Bloch-Sulzberger syndrome)	Persistent hyperplastic primary vitreous (PHPV)
	Retinoblastoma
X-linked retinoschisis	Ocular toxocariasis
	Intermediate uveitis
	Coats' disease
	Advanced X-linked retinoschisis
	Vitreous hemorrhage

BIBLIOGRAPHY

1. Capone AJ, Diaz-Rohena R, Sternberg PJ, et al: Diode laser photocoagulation for zone I threshold retinopathy of prematurity. Am J Ophthalmol 116:444–450, 1993.
2. Cryotherapy for Retinopathy of Prematurity Cooperative Group: Multicenter trial of cryotherapy for retinopathy of prematurity: Preliminary results. Arch Ophthalmol 106:471–479, 1988.
3. Cryotherapy for Retinopathy of Prematurity Cooperative Group: Multicenter trial of cryotherapy for retinopathy of prematurity: Three-month outcome. Arch Ophthalmol 108:195–204, 1990.
4. Cryotherapy for Retinopathy of Prematurity Cooperative Group: Multicenter trial of cryotherapy for retinopathy of prematurity: One-year outcome—structure and function. Arch Ophthalmol 108:1408–1416, 1990.
5. Cryotherapy for Retinopathy of Prematurity Cooperative Group: Multicenter trial of cryotherapy for retinopathy of prematurity: 3-1/2 year outcome—structure and function. Arch Ophthalmol 111:339–344, 1993.
6. Cryotherapy for Retinopathy of Prematurity Cooperative Group: The natural ocular outcome of premature birth and retinopathy: Status at one year. Arch Ophthalmol 112:903–912, 1994.
7. Cryotherapy for Retinopathy of Prematurity Cooperative Group: Multicenter trial of cryotherapy for retinopathy of prematurity: Snellen visual acuity and structural outcome at 5-1/2 years after randomization. Arch Ophthalmol 114:417–424, 1996.
8. Fleming T, Runge P, Charles S: Diode laser photocoagulation for prethreshold, posterior retinopathy of prematurity. Am J Ophthalmol 114:589–592, 1992.
9. Flynn J, Tasman W: Retinopathy of Prematurity: A Clinician's Guide. New York, Springer-Verlag, 1992.
10. Goggin M, O'Keefe M: Diode laser for retinopathy of prematurity: Early outcome. Br J Ophthalmol 77:559–562, 1993.

11. Iverson D, Trese M, Orgel I, Williams G: Laser photocoagulation for threshold retinopathy of prematurity. Arch Ophthalmol 108:1342–1343, 1991.
12. Landers M, Toth C, Semple H, Morse L: Treatment of retinopathy of prematurity with argon laser photocoagulation. Arch Ophthalmol 110:44–47, 1992.
13. McNamara J, Tasman W: retinopathy of prematurity. Ophthalmol Clin North Am 3:413–427, 1990.
14. McNamara J, Tasman W, Brown G, Federman J: Laser photocoagulation for stage 3+ retinopathy of prematurity. Ophthalmology 98:576–580, 1991.
15. McNamara J, Tasman W, Vander J, Brown G: Diode laser photocoagulation for retinopathy of prematurity: Preliminary results. Arch Ophthalmol 110:1714–1716, 1992.
16. McNamara J: Laser treatment for retinopathy of prematurity. Curr Opin Ophthalmol 4:76–80, 1993.
17. Quinn G, Dobson V, Barr C, et al: Visual acuity in infants after vitrectomy for severe retinopathy of prematurity. Ophthalmology 98:5–13, 1991.
18. Quinn G, Dobson V, Barr C, et al: Visual acuity of eyes after vitrectomy for ROP: Follow-up at 5-1/2 years. Ophthalmology 103:595–600, 1996.
19. Schaffer D, Palmer E, Plotsky D, et al: Prognostic factors in the natural course of retinopathy of prematurity. Ophthalmology 100:230–236, 1993.
20. Seiberth V, Linderkamp O, Vardarli I, et al: Diode laser photocoagulation for stage 3+ retinopathy of prematurity. Graefes Arch Clin Exp Ophthalmol 233:489–493, 1995.
21. The Committee for the Classification of Retinopathy of Prematurity: An international classification of retinopathy of prematurity. Arch Ophthalmol 102:1130–1134, 1984.
22. The International Committee for the Classification of the Late Stages of Retinopathy of Prematurity: An international classification of retinopathy of prematurity. Part II: The classification of retinal detachment. Arch Ophthalmol 105:906–912, 1987.
23. Vander J, Handa J, McNamara J, et al: Early laser photocoagulation for posterior retinopathy of prematurity: A randomized controlled clinical trial. Ophthalmology 104:1731–1734, 1997.

49. DIABETIC RETINOPATHY

James F. Vander, M.D.

1. Name the three types of diabetic retinopathy and their characteristic clinical features.

1. **Background diabetic retinopathy.** The typical fundus features are related to loss of capillary integrity—specifically, microaneurysms, dot and blot hemorrhages, hard yellow exudate, and macular edema.

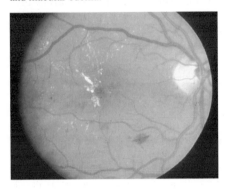

Background diabetic retinopathy with exudate, hemorrhages, and edema. (See Fig. 17, Color Plates.)

2. **Preproliferative diabetic retinopathy.** Typical features are related to early signs of retinal capillary occlusion. Findings include those associated with background diabetic retinopathy as well as extensive cottonwool spots, extensive intraretinal hemorrhages, venous beading, and intraretinal microvascular abnormalities (IRMA).

3. **Proliferative diabetic retinopathy.** Typical features are related to the consequences of extensive retinal capillary nonperfusion. Fundus findings include those of preproliferative diabetic retinopathy as well as the development of neovascularization of the disc (NVD), neovascularization elsewhere in the retina (NVE), preretinal and/or vitreous hemorrhage, and vitreoretinal traction with traction retinal detachment.

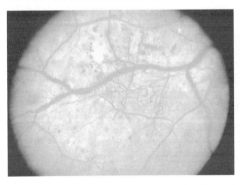

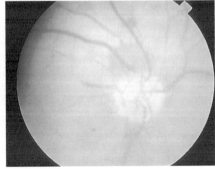

Preproliferative retinopathy with venous beading and IRMA.

Neovascularization of the disc in proliferative retinopathy.

2. What is the most common cause of vision loss in diabetic retinopathy?
Macular edema.

3. Who is at risk for the development of diabetic retinopathy?

All patients with diabetes mellitus are at risk for diabetic retinopathy. Relative risk factors include the following:

1. Duration of diabetes. The longer diabetes has been present, the greater the risk of some manifestation of diabetic retinopathy. After 10–15 years over 75% of patients show some signs of retinopathy.

2. Age. Diabetic retinopathy is uncommon before puberty even in patients who were diagnosed shortly after birth. Background diabetic retinopathy appears sooner in patients diagnosed with diabetes after the age of 40 years. This may be related to duration of disease before diagnosis.

3. Diabetic control. The Diabetic Control and Complications Trial (DCCT) clearly demonstrated a correlation between poor long-term glucose control and subsequent development of diabetic retinopathy as well as other complications of diabetes.

4. Renal disease. Proteinuria is a particularly good marker for the development of diabetic retinopathy. This association may not be causal, but a patient with renal dysfunction should be followed more closely.

5. Systemic hypertension. Again the causal nature of the relationship is not certain.

6. Pregnancy. Diabetic retinopathy may progress rapidly in patients who are pregnant. Patients with preexisting retinopathy are at particular risk.

4. What is the significance of the hemoglobin A_1C? What is its correlation with the development of diabetic retinopathy?

Hemoglobin A_1C measures serum glycosolated hemoglobin, which is an indicator for the average level of serum glucose for the preceding 3 months. Thus, it provides a report card of the adequacy of glucose control for the preceding 3 months without identifying peaks, valleys, or timing of glucose fluctuation. The hemoglobin A_1C has been found to correlate most closely with the development of diabetic retinopathy. Nondiabetic patients typically have a level of 6 or less. The DCCT demonstrated that hemoglobin A_1C less than 8 was associated with a significantly reduced risk of retinopathy when compared with a value greater than 8.

5. What is the recommendation for screening in patients with diabetes?

Patients with juvenile insulin-dependent diabetes should have a dilated ophthalmologic examination 5 years after diagnosis. Patients with type II, adult-onset diabetes should be examined at diagnosis. All diabetic patients should have an annual dilated funduscopic examination; more frequent examinations depend on the findings.

6. What are the fluorescein angiographic features of each of the three types of diabetic retinopathy?

1. **Background retinopathy.** The large retinal vessels seem to fill normally. Pinpoint areas of early hyperfluorescence correspond to microaneurysms, whereas dot and blot hemorrhages show hypofluorescence. Microaneurysms leak in the later frames with blurring of margins and diffusion of fluorescein dye, whereas hemorrhages remain hypofluorescent throughout the study. Telangiectasis also shows early hyperfluorescence with late leakage of fluorescein dye. Hard yellow exudate generally does not appear on a fluorescein angiogram unless it is extremely thick, in which case it reveals hypofluorescence. Macular edema usually is apparent as fluorescein leaks into the retina as the angiogram progresses. (See figures, next page, top left and top right.)

2. **Preproliferative retinopathy.** In addition to the features of background diabetic retinopathy, patients show evidence of retinal capillary loss. Cottonwool spots are usually hypofluorescent, sometimes with late hyperfluorescence along the margins. Areas of capillary dropout appear as smooth, hypofluorescent "ground-glass" patches, often with staining at the margins in the later frames of the angiogram. IRMA fills in the arterial phase of the angiogram and does not leak significantly in the later frames (see figure, next page, bottom left).

3. **Proliferative retinopathy.** Extensive retinal capillary loss is seen early in the angiogram with diffuse leakage at the edges of the ischemic areas in the later frames. NVD and NVE show

intense early hyperfluorescence with marked leakage developing rapidly (see figure, below, bottom right).

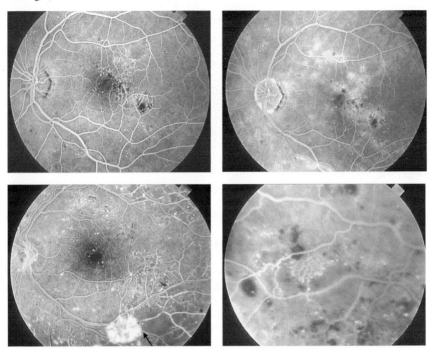

Top left, Early phase fluorescein angiogram shows pinpoint hyperfluorescence corresponding to micro-aneurysms.

Top right, Later phase shows leakage with diffusion of dye and blurring of the microaneurysms.

Bottom left, Neovascularization (NVE) (arrow) is markedly hyperfluorescent early and develops at the border of perfused and nonperfused retina.

Bottom right, IRMA does not leak on fluorescein angiography.

7. What is the definition of clinically significant macular edema (CSME)?

CSME, as defined in the Early Treatment Diabetic Retinopathy study (ETDRS), is present in patients with any one of the following:

1. Retinal thickening within 500 microns of the center of the fovea

2. Hard yellow exudate within 500 microns of the center of the fovea with adjacent retinal thickening (see figure, next page, left)

3. At least one disc area of retinal thickening, any part of which is within 1 disc diameter of the center of the fovea

CSME describes the fundus features as seen on stereoscopic high-magnification viewing of the macula. Visual acuity is not relevant; a patient with 20/20 vision may still have CSME. The fluorescein angiographic appearance is not relevant for the definition of CSME. Monocular viewing of the macula with a direct ophthalmoscope or a solitary color photograph is not adequate for diagnosing CSME, nor is the low-magnification view provided by the indirect ophthalmoscope.

8. What are the results of the ETDRS concerning treatment of diabetic macular edema?

The ETDRS showed that macular laser treatment for patients with CSME reduced the risk of doubling of the visual angle (for example, 20/40 worsening to 20/80) from 24% to 12% over a 3-year period. This benefit was detected over all levels of visual acuity. Significant visual improvement is uncommon after macular laser treatment. The goal is to prevent worsened vision in the future. Treatment is directed at areas of diffuse leakage by using a grid pattern and areas of focal leakage by treatment of the leaking abnormality. Resolution of macular edema may take several months and retreatment is occasionally necessary (figure at right).

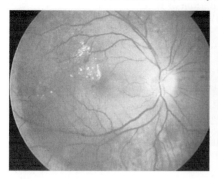 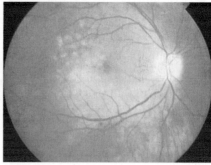

Left, Clinically significant macular edema with thickening and exudate within 500 microns of the center of the fovea.

Right, Four months after focal laser, the edema and exudate are gone.

9. What other findings did the ETDRS report?

The ETDRS also was designed to determine whether aspirin use was helpful or harmful in patients with diabetic retinopathy; the study concluded that it was neither. The study also assessed the role of early panretinal laser treatment for proliferative disease (see below).

10. What is the definition of high-risk characteristics (HRC)?

HRC was used by the Diabetic Retinopathy Study (DRS) to describe patients at a high risk of severe vision loss from proliferative diabetic retinopathy. The study found that patients with (1) NVE and vitreous hemorrhage, (2) mild NVD and vitreous hemorrhage, and (3) moderate or severe NVD with or without vitreous hemorrhage are at high risk for severe vision loss over the ensuing 3 years. Initiation of full-scatter panretinal photocoagulation (PRP) greatly reduced the risk of severe vision loss in patients with HRC. Subsequently, the EDTRS found that for patients with preproliferative retinopathy and/or early proliferative retinopathy without HRC, there was no clear-cut benefit to initiation of full-scatter PRP. So long as careful follow-up can be assured, PRP may be safely withheld in such cases.

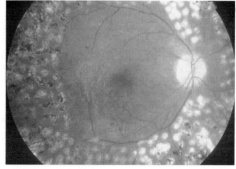

Panretinal photocoagulation (PRP) several months after treatment. (See Fig. 18, Color Plates.)

11. What are the side effects of PRP?

PRP does not improve vision but is performed to prevent the blinding complication of proliferative retinopathy. Loss of peripheral vision and night vision are the major concerns. Loss of central vision also may result from exacerbation of macular edema. Thus, if possible, macular focal laser should be performed before PRP when both are indicated. Other complications include impaired accommodation, papillary dilation, and inadvertent macular burns.

12. Do all patients treated with PRP show resolution of HRC?

No. As many as one-third of patients do not show resolution of NVD or NVE, and in some cases there will be no apparent regression.

13. What is the role of supplemental PRP?

The DRS evaluated the placement of 2,000 spots of PRP. For patients who do not show regression of high-risk characteristics or who have persistent vitreous hemorrhage, it is not clear whether additional PRP improves the long-term visual prognosis. Patients have been reported with 7,000 or more spots of PRP, and in some cases recurrent vitreous hemorrhage persists.

14. What are the indications for fluorescein angiography in diabetic retinopathy?

Fluorescein angiography is not part of the definition of either clinically significant macular edema for patients with background retinopathy or high-risk characteristics for patients with proliferative disease. The indications for treatment are based on clinical rather than angiographic features. Nevertheless, fluorescein angiography is important, particularly for patients with diabetic maculopathy. Most patients considered for treatment of macular edema should have a fluorescein angiogram to determine the focal and diffuse areas of leakage and thus to guide the treating physician during placement of the laser. Areas of capillary nonperfusion also are treated with a grid pattern, which can be determined angiographically. The proximity of focal areas of leakage to the foveal avascular zone (FAZ) also can be demonstrated on fluorescein angiography. Treatment too close to the FAZ carries a higher risk of vision loss and therefore should be done with caution. In patients with unexplained vision loss, the cause may be macular ischemia, which is nicely demonstrated on fluorescein angiography. Finally, patients with a vitreous hemorrhage of uncertain etiology may benefit from a fluorescein angiogram. In patients with significant media opacity, a fluorescein angiogram may demonstrate retinal neovascularization that was not apparent clinically.

15. What is the differential diagnosis of diabetic retinopathy?

The differential diagnosis includes branch or central retinal vein obstruction, ocular ischemic syndrome, radiation retinopathy, hypertensive retinopathy, and miscellaneous proliferative retinopathies such as sarcoidosis, sickle cell hemoglobinopathy, and other less common causes. In patients with typical macular features of background retinopathy, such as microaneurysms and macular edema, but no evidence of diabetes mellitus, the disease usually is categorized as idiopathic juxtafoveal telangiectasia.

16. What is the significance of neovascularization of iris (NVI) in diabetes?

NVI is an ominous sign of severe proliferative diabetic retinopathy and generally requires urgent treatment. Neovascularization of the iris may progress to occlude the trabecular meshwork in a relatively short period, leading to severe neovascular glaucoma. This dreaded complication of proliferative disease usually can be avoided if heavy PRP can be placed before the angle has become occluded.

17. What are the indications for vitrectomy in diabetic retinopathy?

1. **Vitreous hemorrhage.** Vitreous hemorrhage obscuring the visual axis causes severe vision loss. Although it generally clears spontaneously, for patients with more extensive hemorrhage vitrectomy may be indicated. The Diabetic Retinopathy Vitrectomy Study (DRVS) studied eyes with vitreous hemorrhage reducing vision to 5/200 or worse. The study demonstrated a strong benefit for patients with type I diabetes, perhaps related to extensive fibrovascular proliferation. Guidelines are variable, but most surgeons wait at least 3 months for patients to clear spontaneously unless occupational or personal needs demand early intervention or extensive untreated

fibrovascular proliferation is known to be present. The development of iris neovascularization also may prompt earlier vitrectomy.

2. **Traction retinal detachment.** Most surgeons agree that traction retinal detachment involving the macula is an indication for diabetic vitrectomy. If the vitreoretinal traction can be relieved within weeks or a few months of onset, visual results are excellent. Long-standing traction retinal detachments generally do not respond favorably in terms of visual recovery. Progressive extramacular traction retinal detachment moving toward the fovea is occasionally an indication for surgery, although this indication is controversial.

3. **Combined traction–rhegmatogenous retinal detachment.** The development of combined retinal detachment with an open retinal break is an indication for vitrectomy. Such detachments are notoriously difficult to fix and usually are taken to surgery shortly after diagnosis.

4. **Refractory macular edema.** Patients with a taut posterior hyaloid face producing chronic macular edema that is not responsive to focal laser therapy can undergo surgery, sometimes with significant visual improvement. It is believed that the chronic traction of the vitreous face on the macula produces persistent leakage and that the edema can resolve only after traction is released.

18. What are the complications of vitrectomy for diabetes?

1. **Progression of cataract.** Progressive nuclear sclerotic or posterior subcapular cataracts occur frequently after vitrectomy. The risk of secondary neovascular glaucoma may be higher in patients in whom the lens is removed intraoperatively.

2. **Nonhealing corneal epithelial defects.** The cornea may swell, and the surface may break down during vitrectomy. Diabetic patients are prone to poor healing of corneal epithelial defects.

3. **Retinal detachment.** Retinal detachment may be related to a peripheral tear near one of the sclerotomy sites or posteriorly as a result of persistent or recurrent vitreoretinal traction.

4, **Vitreous hemorrhage.** Some degree of vitreous hemorrhage is frequently present postoperatively. It generally clears quickly.

BIBLIOGRAPHY

1. Benson WE, Brown GC, Tasman W: Diabetes and Its Ocular Complications. Philadelphia, W.B. Saunders, 1988.
2. Diabetic Control and Complications Trial Research Group: The effect of intensive diabetes treatment on the progression of diabetic retinopathy in insulin dependent diabetes mellitus. Arch Ophthalmol 113:36–51, 1995.
3. Diabetic Retinopathy Study Research Group: Photocoagulation treatment of proliferative diabetic retinopathy. Clinical application of Diabetic Retinopathy Study (DRS) findings, DRS report number 8. Ophthalmology 88:583–600, 1981.
4. Diabetic Retinopathy Vitrectomy Study Research Group: Early vitrectomy for severe vitreous hemorrhage in diabetic retinopathy: Two year results of a randomized trial. Diabetic Retinopathy Vitrectomy Study report 2. Arch Ophthalmol 103:1644–1652, 1985.
5. Early Treatment for Diabetic Retinopathy Study Research Group: Photocoagulation for diabetic macular edema: Early Treatment for Diabetic Retinopathy Study report number 1. Arch Ophthalmol 103:1796–1806, 1985.

50. RETINAL ARTERIAL OBSTRUCTION

Jay S. Duker, M.D.

1. What types of retinal arterial obstructions can occur?

Retinal arterial obstructions are generally divided into branch retinal arterial obstructions and central retinal arterial obstructions depending on the precise site of obstruction. A branch retinal arterial obstruction (BRAO) occurs when the site of blockage is distal to the lamina cribrosa of the optic nerve—in other words, within the visible vasculature of the retina. A BRAO can involve as large an area as three-quarters of the retina, or as small an area as just a few microns. A central retinal artery obstruction (CRAO) occurs when the blockage is within the optic nerve substance itself. The site of obstruction is therefore not generally visible on ophthalmoscopy in a CRAO. In a CRAO most, if not all, of the retina is affected.

Obstructions more proximal to the central retinal artery, in the ophthalmic artery, or even in the internal carotid artery can cause visual loss as well. Ophthalmic arterial obstructions can be difficult to differentiate from CRAO on a clinical basis.

2. What causes a retinal artery to become blocked?

The typical causes differ for CRAO and BRAO. Because the site of obstruction is not visible on clinical examination and, in general, the central retinal artery is too small to image with most techniques, the precise cause of most CRAOs cannot be definitely determined. It is currently believed that most CRAO are caused by thrombus formation. Localized intimal damage in the form of atherosclerosis probably incites the thrombus in most cases. In about 20% of cases, an embolus is visible in the central retinal artery or one of its branches, suggesting an embolic cause (see figure). Extrinsic mechanical compression due to orbital or optic nerve tumor, hemorrhage, or inflammation is a rare cause. Inflammation in the form of vasculitis, optic neuritis, or even orbital disease (e.g., mucormyocosis) can cause a CRAO as well. Trauma with direct damage to the optic nerve or blood vessels can lead to CRAO. In addition, system coagulopathies can also be associated with both CRAO and BRAO.

Over 90% of BRAOs are the result of emboli. Cholesterol, calcium, fibrin, and platelets have all been implicated individually or together. Emboli are usually visible in the retinal arterial tree. In an older individual, the most common source of emboli is the ipsilateral carotid artery. In a

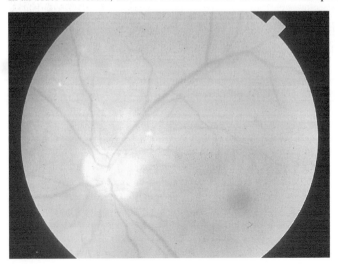

A CRAO caused by emboli. Note the refractile particles in the central retinal artery in the center of the optic disc as well as in two branch retinal arteries superior to the optic disc.

younger person, it is more likely to be cardiac in origin. Rarely, intraocular inflammations such as toxoplasmosis or herpes retinitis (the acute retinal necrosis syndrome) can lead to BRAO.

3. Describe typical symptoms of a retinal arterial obstruction.

The hallmark symptom of an acute retinal arterial obstruction is abrupt, painless loss of sight in the visual field that corresponds to the territory of the obstructed artery. In a CRAO this would be most, if not all, of the visual field. In some patients, an artery derived from the choroidal circulation, called a cilioretinal artery, may perfuse a small amount of the central retina. The cilioretinal artery, which is present in up to 20% of individuals, remains patent when the site of obstruction is the central retinal artery. Some of the visual field corresponding to the territory of the patent cilioretinal vessel can be spared in select individuals. Cilioretinal artery sparing can rarely leave a patient with 20/20 (normal) central vision, albeit with a very constricted visual field (see figure).

Occasionally, patients report stuttering visual loss or episodes of amaurosis fugax prior to arterial obstruction. Pain is not generally a part of retinal arterial obstruction unless some other underlying disease is present (e.g., giant cell arteritis, ocular ischemia).

In a BRAO, the visual field loss can vary from up to three-quarters of the visual field to as little as a few degrees, depending on the territory of the obstructed vessel. Often, the central vision will be 20/20, as the macular area can be spared.

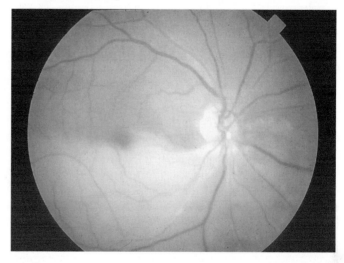

Typical inferior hemispheric BRAO. The visual acuity was 20/20, but there was a marked superior visual field defect.

4. What do you see on examination when a retinal arterial obstruction has occurred?

The decreased blood flow results in ischemic whitening of the retina in the territory of the obstructed artery (see figure, next page). Because the retinal vasculature only supplies circulation to the inner retina (the outer retina gets its circulation from the choroid), the ischemia is limited to the inner retina. The retinal whitening is most pronounced in the posterior pole where the nerve fiber layer of the inner retina is thickest.

In an arterial obstruction, the retinal arteries distal to the blockage appear thin and attenuated. The blood column may be interrupted in both the distal arteries and the corresponding draining veins. This phenomenon has been labeled "box-carring." Splinter retinal hemorrhages on the disc are common. Embolic material may be visible in the central retinal artery where it exits the disc or in one of the branches of the central retinal artery. In most instances, a cherry-red spot will be visible in the macular area.

The most common sites of obstruction in a BRAO are the retinal arterial bifurcations. Because there are more bifurcations and more retinal vessels in the temporal retina, temporal BRAOs are more common than nasal BRAOs.

In a CRAO, the visual acuity is usually quite poor. The patient typically can only discern motion or, perhaps, count fingers at several feet. Many episodes of BRAO result in only peripheral visual loss with intact central acuity.

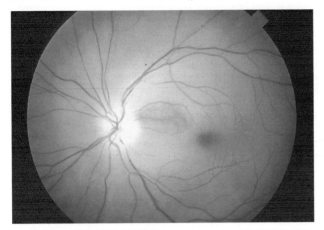

Typical appearance of a CRAO. Note the ischemic retinal whitening with a cherry-red spot. There is a patent cilioretinal artery present just temporal to the optic nerve producing a small area of unaffected, normal-appearing retina. (See Fig. 19, Color Plates.)

5. What is a cherry-red spot?

A cherry-red spot represents a pathologic appearance of the macula, the center of the retina. There are two main causes: ischemia and abnormal depositions. A cherry-red spot occurs in CRAO because of the retinal whitening of the surrounding nerve fiber layer. The fovea itself has no nerve fibers, so its appearance does not change from normal. The retinal whitening surrounding the normal reddish tint of the macular area produces the cherry-red spot.

6. What other conditions result in a cherry-red spot of the retina and how can you differentiate these from an arterial obstruction?

Besides CRAO, a cherry-red spot can occur in conditions of abnormal deposition into the cells of the retinal nerve fiber layer. The classic example is Tay-Sachs disease, a sphingolipidosis. A cherry-red spot has been reported in other sphingolipidoses as well, such as Farber syndrome, Sandoff disease, Niemann-Pick, Goldberg syndrome, Gaucher disease, and gangliosidase GM1-type 2. A cherry-red spot has also been reported in Hurler syndrome (MPS I-H), B-galactosidase deficiency (MPS-VII), Hallevorden-Spatz Disease, and Batten-Mayou-Vogt-Spielmeyer disease.

Ischemic cherry-red spot can be differentiated from these other entities by the history of visual loss, concurrent systemic disease, age of the patient, and the appearance of the surrounding retinal blood vessels and retina.

7. Is there any ancillary testing that can be done to confirm the diagnosis?

In most cases, CRAO and BRAO can be accurately diagnosed clinically by an experienced observer. In cases in which the diagnosis is in doubt, an intravenous fluorescein angiogram can be performed. This will show a significant diminution in dye flow through the obstructed vessels. A color Doppler ultrasound evaluation of the orbital circulation can also be used to determine the degree of obstruction and to differentiate an ophthalmic artery obstruction from CRAO.

8. Which systemic diseases are associated with retinal arterial obstruction?

Although many systemic diseases are associated with retinal arterial obstruction, over 50% of all affected patients will manifest no apparent cause for their retinal disease. The most common association is ipsilateral carotid artery disease, which is present in about one-third of affected patients. About 10% of arterial obstructions are associated with giant cell arteritis. This is a critical association to be aware of because visual loss can occur rapidly in the fellow eye in these patients, and prompt administration of intravenous corticosteroids may prevent the contralateral visual loss.

In both CRAO and BRAO, all patients should be evaluated for embolic sources from the carotid artery system and the heart using carotid noninvasive testing and echocardiogram. In some instances, esophageal echocardiography is necessary to detect embolic sources. Holter monitoring to detect a cardiac arrhythmia may be appropriate in select patients.

9. Do you always have to test for giant cell arteritis?

It is of paramount importance that giant cell arteritis be ruled out in all patients over the age of 50 with a CRAO. A stat erythrocyte sedimentation rate should be performed and, if it is high, or if there is clinical suspicion of giant cell arteritis, then a biopsy should be considered.

BRAO associated with giant cell arteritis is exceedingly uncommon.

10. Which patients are at risk to get a retinal arterial obstruction?

Patients who have suffered an arterial obstruction in one eye are at more risk for developing an obstruction in the contralateral eye. The risk of bilaterality is about 10%. Patients with known carotid artery disease, diseased heart valves, or cardiac arrythmias are also at increased risk. In addition, conditions that result in abnormal rheologic parameters such as pancreatitis, lupus, pregnancy, and amniotic fluid emboli can result in artery obstructions as well.

11. Can any prophylactic treatment be given?

With the exception of corticosteroid treatment for giant cell arteritis, prophylaxis against arterial obstructions is not generally given. The utility of anticoagulation to prevent retinal arterial obstructions in the setting of known carotid disease is not definitively proven. Extrapolation from studies showing a benefit of the risk of subsequent stroke in this situation suggests that anticoagulation is useful to lower the risk of arterial obstruction as well. The same conclusion may be extrapolated from the studies proving a benefit for carotid endarterectomy for appropriate patients with carotid arterial disease.

12. What is the incidence of bilateral retinal arterial obstructions?

Ten percent.

13. Is there any proven treatment for retinal arterial obstruction?

There is no proven treatment for either CRAO or BRAO. Some investigators feel that none of the treatments currently recommended do any good. Because the inner retina is highly sensitive to loss of perfusion, intervention is rarely, if ever, attempted in anyone with an obstruction more than 72 hours old.

Proposed therapies for retinal arterial obstructions are as follows:
1. Dislodging emboli to a more distal location
2. Dissolving thrombi
3. Increasing oxygenation to the retina
4. Protecting surviving retinal cells from ischemic damage

The traditional approach to CRAO includes paracentesis, ocular massage, and medications to lower intraocular pressure. All three of these interventions are an attempt to dislodge any embolus that may be present. A paracentesis is the removal of a small amount of aqueous humor via a small needle (30 gauge or 27 gauge). This can be done in an office setting. Although generally simple and safe, it has rarely been reported to cause endophthalmitis.

Increasing oxygenation to the retina is attempted by having patients inhale a mixture of 95% oxygen and 5% carbon dioxide (carbogen) for 10 minutes out of every 2 hours for 24 to 48 hours after the blockage. The purpose of the carbon dioxide is to counteract the normal retinal arterial vasoconstriction that occurs when pure oxygen is inhaled. This theoretically increases the oxygenation to the ischemic inner retina; however, there is no clinical evidence that any beneficial effect is achieved. Carbogen should not be employed in any individual with chronic obstructive pulmonary disease.

More recently, both systemic (via intravenous infusion) and local (directly into the ophthalmic artery via an arterial catheter) infusions of clot-dissolving medications (streptokinase, tissue plasminogen activator, urokinase, heparin) have been given for retinal arterial obstruction. Although the initial reports are encouraging, these therapies are not without risk and should be reserved for obstructions less than 48 hours old. These medications should be given only by experienced personnel under close supervision. Because branch retinal arterial obstructions do not usually affect central vision, such invasive procedures probably should not be attempted in these cases.

At the present time, there are no means to "rescue" ischemic retinal tissue. This is an area of active research and, in the future, this may be possible.

14. Why is the retina so sensitive to arterial inflow problems?

The retina is a highly metabolic organ and is therefore sensitive to ischemia. The central retinal artery is an end-artery with no true normal anastomosis. As part of the central nervous system, the retina is unable to regenerate if damaged.

15. How do you tell a retinal arterial obstruction from a retinal venous obstruction?

Simple—white versus red. The hallmark of retinal arterial obstructions is ischemic retinal whitening. The hallmark of retinal venous obstruction is retinal hemorrhage in the territory of the obstructed vessel. In addition, the retinal veins will appear dilated and tortuous as opposed to thin and attenuated.

Warning: Rarely, a patient may present with a combined obstruction. Obstructions of a branch retinal artery or the central retinal artery in conjunction with a central retinal venous obstruction have been reported. This produces a combined fundus picture (i.e., whitening from ischemia with red from retinal hemorrhage).

16. Is acute obstruction of a retinal artery an emergency?

CRAO is considered a true ophthalmic emergency, even though there is no proven treatment. Because the retina is highly sensitive to ischemia, if treatment is contemplated it should be initiated as quickly as possible. Although animal studies indicate that more than 90 minutes of ischemia produce irreversible retinal cell death, clinical experience suggests that some eyes can tolerate ischemia for up to 72 hours and still recover.

If a potentially risky intervention such as anticoagulation is contemplated, the visual loss should be no more than 48 hours old to maximize the possibility of recovery and the overall risk/benefit ratio. Optimal timing for anticoagulation is within 6 to 8 hours of visual loss.

17. What does the retina look like months or years after an arterial obstruction?

The retinal vessels look attenuated and the optic disc is often pale owing to the loss of the retinal nerve fiber layer. Because the retina itself is transparent and the underlying retinal pigment epithelium and choroid are unaffected by a pure CRAO or BRAO, the retina itself looks normal.

18. Are there any other late complications after retinal arterial obstructions?

In about 15% of eyes following CRAO, neovascularization of the iris occurs. It is usually seen within 3 months of the CRAO and can result in a severe type of glaucoma (elevated intraocular pressure) called neovascular glaucoma. If neovascularization of the iris is detected, a laser treatment to the ischemic retina, panretinal photocoagulation (PRP), is usually performed. Neovascularization is extremely rare after BRAO.

BIBLIOGRAPHY

1. Arruga J, Sanders MD: Ophthalmologic findings in 70 patients with evidence of retinal embolism. Ophthalmology 89:1336–1347, 1982.
2. Atebara NH, Brown GC, Cater J: Efficacy of anterior chamber paracentesis and carbogen in treating acute nonarteritic central retinal artery obstruction. Ophthalmology 102:2029–2035, 1995.
3. Brown GC, Magargal LE: Central retinal artery obstruction and visual acuity. Ophthalmology 89:14–19, 1982.

4. Brown GC, Magargal LE, Sergott R: Acute obstruction of the retinal and choroidal circulations. Ophthalmology 93:1373–1382, 1986.
5. Duker JS, Brown GC: Recovery following acute obstruction of the retinal and choroidal circulations. Retina 8:257–260, 1988.
6. Duker JS, Sivalingham A, Brown GC, Reber R: A prospective study of acute central retinal artery obstruction. Arch Ophthalmol 109:339–342, 1991.
7. Greven CM, Slusher MM, Weaver RG: Retinal arterial occlusions in young adults. Am J Ophthalmol 120:776–783, 1995.
8. Hayreh SS, Podhajsky P: Ocular neovascularization with retinal vascular occlusion. II. Occurrence in central and branch retinal artery obstruction. Arch Ophthalmol 100:1585–1596, 1982.
9. Schmidt D, Schumaker M, Wakhloo AK: Microcatheter urokinase infusion in central retinal artery occlusion. Am J Ophthalmol 113:429–434, 1992.

51. RETINAL VENOUS OCCLUSIVE DISEASE

Vernon K. W. Wong, M.D.

BRANCH RETINAL VEIN OCCLUSION

1. What are the symptoms of a branch vein occlusion (BRVO)?

Patients may notice an acute, painless loss of vision if there is macular edema, ischemic maculopathy, or intraretinal hemorrhage involving the fovea. BRVOs that occur in the nasal quadrants may be asymptomatic. Longstanding BRVOs can present with floaters or an abrupt decrease in vision from vitreous hemorrhage.[4,10,11]

2. What are the clinical signs of a BRVO?

Ophthalmoscopy can reveal intraretinal hemorrhages in a segmental pattern, cotton-wool spots, and macular edema in a recent BRVO. In a chronic BRVO, optociliary collateral vessels (very tortuous, dilated vessels) macular retinal pigment epithelium changes, and neovascularization of the retina or disc can develop.[4,10,11]

3. Are there any systemic associations in patients with a BRVO?

Hypertension is a risk factor for a BRVO. About 10% of patients with a BRVO will develop a retinal vein occlusion in the fellow eye.[4,11]

4. Where do BRVOs most commonly occur?

In the superotemporal quadrant.

5. Are there different types of BRVOs?

BRVOs can be broken down into ischemic and nonischemic types. A nonischemic BRVO is defined as less than 5 disc areas of retinal capillary nonperfusion, as documented by fluorescein angiography. An ischemic BRVO is defined as greater than 5 disc areas of retinal capillary nonperfusion, as documented by fluorescein angiography.[4,11]

6. What are the complications of a BRVO?

Patients with a nonischemic BRVO can lose vision secondary to macular edema. Patients with an ischemic BRVO can lose vision from macular edema, ischemic maculopathy, vitreous hemorrhage (VH), traction retinal detachment (TRD), or rhegmatogenous retinal detachment (RRD). If ischemia occurs in the macula, a patient may complain of central vision loss, and ophthalmoscopy may not reveal macular edema. A fluorescein angiogram will demonstrate an enlarged and irregular foveal avascular zone. About 40% of patients with ischemic BRVOs develop neovascularization of the retina (NVE) or disc (NVD). In approximately 60% of the patients who develop neovascularization, traction from the vitreous may cause these new vessels to bleed, leading to VH and decreased vision. Rarely, traction on the new vessels may lead to a TRD or a retinal tear that progresses to a RRD.[3,4,10,11]

7. What is the treatment for an uncomplicated BRVO?

Patients with a nonischemic BRVO without macular edema can be followed clinically for the development of macular edema and for progression into an ischemic BRVO and its complications, including ischemic maculopathy, NVE, NVD, VH, TRD, and RRD.[4,10,11]

8. Is there any treatment for a patient with a BRVO and macular edema?

The Branch Vein Occlusion Study was a multicenter, randomized, controlled clinical trial designed to answer whether argon laser photocoagulation was useful in improving visual acuity in eyes with a BRVO and macular edema that reduced vision to 20/40 or worse. The study found that 65% of eyes treated with argon laser photocoagulation compared with 37% of the control eyes gained two or more lines of vision, a difference that was statistically significant. The study investigators recommend argon laser photocoagulation for patients with a BRVO of at least 3 months in duration and vision 20/40 or worse secondary to macular edema.[1]

9. Is there any treatment for a patient with an ischemic BRVO?

The Branch Vein Occlusion Study was also designed to answer whether peripheral scatter argon laser photocoagulation could prevent the development of retinal neovascularization and prevent vitreous hemorrhage in patients who had already developed neovascularization. It was found that significantly less neovascularization developed in patients treated with laser than in control patients. In patients with neovascularization that was treated, the development of vitreous hemorrhage was significantly less than in the control patients. Although the Branch Vein Occlusion Study was not designed to determine whether peripheral scatter laser treatment should be applied before rather than after the development of neovascularization, data accumulated in the study suggested that there was minimal risk for severe vision loss if laser treatment was performed after the development of neovascularization. The study investigators recommend peripheral scatter argon laser photocoagulation for patients with a BRVO at the time that neovascularization develops.[3]

CENTRAL RETINAL VEIN OCCLUSION

10. What are the symptoms of a central retinal vein occlusion (CRVO)?

Patients may complain of sudden, painless loss of vision. Occasionally, patients may complain of a painful, red eye because they have developed neovascular glaucoma secondary to an ischemic CRVO.[4,8,11]

11. What are the clinical signs of a CRVO?

In an acute CRVO, ophthalmoscopy reveals intraretinal hemorrhages in all four quadrants and a dilated, tortuous retinal venous system. The disc may be swollen, and there may be cotton wool spots and cystoid macular edema. Patients with an ischemic CRVO can develop anterior segment or posterior segment neovascularization, which manifests as new vessels on the iris, angle, disc, or retina. In longstanding CRVOs, patients may have optociliary venous collaterals, cystoid macular edema, macular retinal pigment epithelium changes, and retinal venous collaterals.[4,8,11]

12. What are the risk factors for a central retinal vein occlusion (CRVO)?

Hypertension, diabetes mellitus, hyperviscosity syndromes, and increased intraocular pressure are risk factors for a CRVO.

13. Are there different types of CRVOs?

CRVOs can be broken down into ischemic and nonischemic types. A nonischemic CRVO is defined as less than 10 disc areas of capillary nonperfusion on fluorescein angiography, whereas an ischemic CRVO is defined as greater than 10 disc areas of capillary nonperfusion on fluorescein angiography. Clinically, patients with an ischemic CRVO have poor vision, an afferent pupillary defect, and extensive intraretinal hemorrhages.[4,6]

14. What are the complications of a CRVO?

Patients with a nonischemic CRVO can lose vision secondary to macular edema. Patients with an ischemic CRVO can lose vision from macular edema, ischemic maculopathy, neovascular glaucoma (NVG), vitreous hemorrhage (VH), traction retinal detachment (TRD), or rhegmatogenous retinal detachment (RRD). If ischemia occurs in the macula, a patient may complain of central vision loss, and ophthalmoscopy may not reveal macular edema. A fluorescein angiogram will demonstrate an enlarged and irregular foveal avascular zone. The most feared complication of an ischemic CRVO is anterior segment neovascularization, which can lead to NVG. About 15% of patients with ischemic CRVOs develop neovascularization of the retina or disc (NVE, NVD). Traction from the vitreous may cause these new vessels to bleed, leading to VH and decreased vision. Rarely, traction on the new vessels may lead to a TRD or a retinal tear that progresses to a RRD.[4,5,8,11]

15. What is the treatment for an uncomplicated CRVO?

Patients with a nonischemic CRVO without macular edema can be followed clinically for the development of macular edema and for progression into an ischemic CRVO and its complications, including ischemic maculopathy, NVG, VH, TRD, and RRD .[4,6,8,11]

16. Is there any treatment for a patient with a CRVO and macular edema?

The Central Vein Occlusion Study was a multicenter, randomized, controlled clinical trial designed to answer whether argon laser photocoagulation was useful in improving visual acuity in eyes with a CRVO and macular edema that reduced vision to 20/50 or worse. Patients were randomized to macular grid photocoagulation or no treatment. There was no difference between the visual acuity in treated and untreated eyes. The study investigators do not recommend macular grid photocoagulation for patients that met the study entry criteria.[7]

17. What is the recommended treatment for a patient with an ischemic CRVO?

The Central Vein Occlusion Study was also designed to answer whether panretinal argon laser photocoagulation could prevent the development of anterior segment neovascularization and neovascular glaucoma. Patients with ischemic CRVOs defined as greater than 10 disc areas of capillary nonperfusion, as documented by fluorescein angiography, were randomized to prophylactic panretinal argon laser photocoagulation or treatment only at the time of development of anterior segment neovascularization. Although prophylactic laser decreased the incidence of anterior segment neovascularization, laser at the time of development of anterior segment neovascularization was effective in preventing neovascular glaucoma. The study investigators recommend careful follow-up of patients with an ischemic CRVO and panretinal photocoagulation at the time a patient develops 2 clock hours of iris neovascularization or any angle neovascularization.[5,9]

BIBLIOGRAPHY

1. Branch Vein Occlusion Study Group: Argon laser photocoagulation for macular edema in branch vein occlusion. Am J Ophthalmol 98:271–282, 1984.
2. Branch Vein Occlusion Study Group: Argon laser photocoagulation for macular edema in branch vein occlusion (letter). Am J Ophthalmol 99:218–219, 1985.
3. Branch Vein Occlusion Study Group: Argon laser scatter photocoagulation for prevention of neovascularization and vitreous hemorrhage in branch vein occlusion. Arch Ophthalmol 104:34–41, 1996.
4. Brown GC: Retinal vascular disease. In Tasman W, Jaeger EA (eds): The Wills Eye Hospital Atlas of Clinical Ophthalmology. Philadelphia, Lippincott-Raven, 1996, pp 168–173.
5. Central Vein Occlusion Study Group: A randomized clinical trial of early panretinal photocoagulation for ischemic central vein occlusion: The Central Vein Occlusion Study Group N report. Ophthalmology 102:1434–1444, 1995.
6. Central Vein Occlusion Study Group: Baseline and early natural history report: The central vein occlusion study. Arch Ophthalmol 111:1087–1095, 1993.
7. Central Vein Occlusion Study Group: Evaluation of grid pattern photocoagulation for macular edema in central vein occlusion: The central vein occlusion study group M report. Ophthalmology 102:1425–1433, 1995.
8. Clarkson JC: Central retinal vein occlusion. In Ryan SJ (ed): Retina, 2nd ed. St. Louis, CV Mosby, 1994, pp 1379–1386.
9. Clarkson JG, Coscas G, Finkelstein D, et al: The CVOS group M and N reports (letter). Ophthalmology 103:350–354, 1996.
10. Finkelstein D: Retinal branch vein occlusion. In Ryan SJ (ed): Retina, 2nd ed. St. Louis, CV Mosby, 1994, pp 1386–1392.
11. Gass JDM: Stereoscopic Atlas of Macular Disease Diagnosis and Treatment, 4th ed. St. Louis, CV Mosby, 1997, pp 546–563.

52. RETINAL DETACHMENT

Michael J. Borne, M.D.

1. What is retinal detachment?

Retinal detachment is separation of the neurosensory retina from the underlying retinal pigment epithelium with accumulation of fluid in the potential space between the two layers. The types of retinal detachment include rhegmatogenous, traction, and exudative.

- In **rhegmatogenous retinal detachments**, a break in the retina allows fluid from the vitreous cavity access to the potential space between the retina and retinal pigment epithelium.
- **Traction retinal detachment** occurs when epiretinal tissue forms and contracts, pulling the retina away from the pigment epithelial layer. Occasionally the severe traction caused by epiretinal membranes may cause a tear in the retina, creating a combination rhegmatogenous-traction detachment.
- **Exudative retinal detachments** are produced by retinal and choroidal conditions that damage the blood-retina barrier and allow fluid to accumulate in the subretinal space (the potential space between the retina and retinal pigment epithelium).

2. What are the major characteristics of each type of retinal detachment?

1. **Rhegmatogenous retinal detachments** typically have a corrugated appearance caused by intraretinal edema (see figure). Obviously, they are associated with a retinal break, although in a small percentage of cases the break is not easily identifiable. Decreased intraocular pressure, pigmented cells in the vitreous cavity, and vitreous hemorrhage are also associated with rhegmatogenous detachments. Fixed folds and other signs of proliferative vitreoretinopathy strongly suggest a rhegmatogenous detachment.

2. **Traction retinal detachments** are characterized by a smooth and stiff-appearing retinal surface. In most cases, the epiretinal membranes causing the traction may be observed ophthalmoscopically. The detachment is usually concave toward the front of the eye. The most common location of the tractional membranes is in the postequatorial region; the traction detachment rarely extends to the ora serrata.

3. **Exudative retinal detachments** are characterized by shifting subretinal fluid. The subretinal fluid accumulates according to gravitational forces and detaches the retina in the area where it accumulates. Thus, the fluid is noted to shift when the patient is viewed in a upright compared with a supine position. The surface of the retina is usually smooth in exudative detachments, compared with the corrugated appearance of a rhegmatogenous detachment. Occasionally the retina may be seen directly behind the lens in exudative detachments. This rarely occurs in rhegmatogenous detachments, unless severe vitreoretinal traction is present.

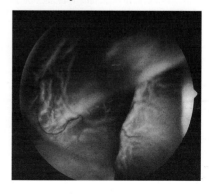

Bullous rhegmatogenous retinal detachment with mobile, corrugated appearance. (See Fig. 20, Color Plates.)

3. What are the major causes of exudative retinal detachments?

The major causes of exudative retinal detachments are intraocular tumors, intraocular inflammatory diseases, and congenital abnormalities. Intraocular neoplasms, such as choroidal melanomas, choroidal hemangiomas, and metastatic choroidal tumors, are most likely to produce serous retinal detachments. Intraocular inflammation, such as posterior scleritis, Harada's disease, severe posterior uveitis, and central serous choroidretinopathy, occasionally produce shifting subretinal fluid. The most common congenital abnormalities known to produce exudative retinal detachment are optic pits, nanophthalmos, and the morning glory disc syndrome.

4. How does the retina remain attached?

The retinal photoreceptors and retinal pigment epithelial (RPE) cells are oriented with the apices of each cell in apposition. An interphotoreceptor matrix between the cells forms a "glue" that helps to maintain cellular apposition. It also has been postulated that the RPE functions as a cellular pump to remove ions and water from the interphotoreceptor matrix, providing a "suction force" that helps to keep the retina attached.

5. What are the major predisposing factors for rhegmatogenous retinal detachments?

The main predisposing factors for rhegmatogenous detachments are previous cataract surgery, lattice degeneration, and myopia. The incidence of rhegmatogenous retinal detachment after cataract surgery is approximately 2 in 1000. The incidence becomes much higher after complicated cataract surgery, including posterior capsule rupture, vitreous loss, and retained lens fragments. Some studies have shown an incidence of rhegmatogenous detachments after complicated cataract surgery as high as 15%. Currently, approximately one-half of all primary rhegmatogenous detachments occur in patients with a history of cataract surgery.

Lattice degeneration is a peripheral retinal degeneration characterized by thinning of the retina with liquefaction of the overlying vitreous, which results in a high risk for retinal tears and breaks. Lattice degeneration is found in 6–7% of the population and is often bilateral. Lattice degeneration is the direct cause of primary rhegmatogenous retinal detachment in about 25% of eyes.

High myopes have a high risk of retinal detachment for several reasons. First, the incidence of lattice degeneration is higher in myopes. Second, myopes tend to have a higher rate of posterior vitreous detachment. Of greater importance, myopic eyes have a higher rate of retinal breaks due to the thin peripheral retina. The rate of retinal breaks tends to be higher with increasing myopia.

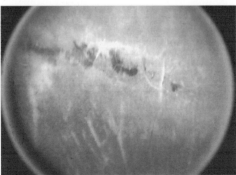

Lattice degeneration

6. What are the signs and symptoms of a retinal break?

Flashes and floaters are the classic symptoms. Pigmented cells or blood in the vitreous strongly suggests the possibility of a retinal break.

7. What are the types of retinal breaks?

1. **Horseshoe tear** (see figure). A flap of retina created by vitreous traction gives the appearance of a horseshoe. The open end of the horseshoe is anterior. A retinal vessel may bridge the gap of the tear. The risk of subsequent retinal detachment is high, especially with acute tears.

2. **Operculated tear.** When a piece of retina is completely torn away by vitreous traction, the fragment is seen floating over the retinal defect. The risk of retinal detachment is lower than with a horseshoe tear.

3. **Atrophic hole.** A round hole without evidence of retinal traction is often associated with lattice degeneration. The risk of retinal detachment is low.

4. **Dialysis.** A disinsertion of the retina at the ora serrata is most common in the inferotemporal quadrant. The second most common site is superonasal. A frequent cause is trauma.

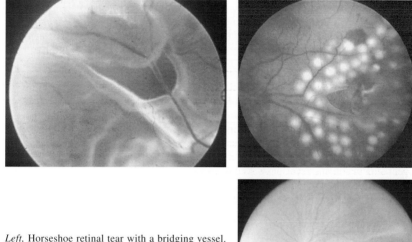

Left, Horseshoe retinal tear with a bridging vessel. (See Fig. 21, Color Plates.) *Top right,* Horseshoe retinal tear after laser photocoagulation. *Bottom right,* Retinal detachment resulting from inferotemporal dialysis.

8. What are the options for repair of retinal detachment?

First, consideration of the type of retinal detachment is important before identifying the modality of treatment. Exudative retinal detachments are approached entirely differently from rhegmatogenous or traction detachments. Exudative detachments are repaired by treating the primary cause of the fluid extravasation into the subretinal space. For example, retinal detachment associated with choroidal melanoma is addressed by treatment of the tumor with radiation, thermotherapy, or resection. Exudative retinal detachments related to intraocular inflammatory conditions are generally treated by aggressive antiinflammatory regimens. Rarely does an exudative detachment require primary surgical repair.

On the other hand, treatment of rhegmatogenous and traction retinal detachment is primarily surgical. Traction retinal detachments caused by diabetes or proliferative vitreoretinopathy require relief of all traction membranes before the retina will remain reattached.

Small, localized rhegmatogenous detachments are usually treated by cryotherapy or barrier laser photocoagulation. Rarely, an asymptomatic localized detachment may be treated with close observation only. If significant vitreous traction is present on the retinal tear, especially if the tear is superior in location, or if a large amount of subretinal fluid is found, more definitive treatment is usually indicated. Options include pneumatic retinopexy, Lincoff balloon, scleral buckling, and pars plana vitrectomy. Scleral buckling surgery is the time-honored approach and has been applied routinely since the 1950s. Pars plana vitrectomy was first performed in the late 1960s and has become the operation of choice for some surgeons. Pneumatic retinopexy has gained popularity since the early 1980s.

9. Which patients are the best candidates for pneumatic retinopexy?

Pneumatic retinopexy involves injection of an inert gas or sterile air into the vitreous cavity; strict positioning is required to place the gas bubble in contact with the retinal break. If the break is closed with the surface tension from the gas bubble, the retinal pigment epithelium can pump the subretinal fluid back into the choroid and allow retinal reattachment. The break is sealed either with cryotherapy at the time of gas injection or with laser photocoagulation after the retina is flattened. The ideal candidates are patients with a detachment caused by a single retinal break in the superior 8 clock hours or multiple breaks if all of the tears are within 1–2 clock hours of each other. Obviously, the patient must not have a systemic disease or mechanical problem that precludes the positioning requirements. Phakic patients tend to do slightly better than patients with a history of cataract surgery.

10. Which patients are poor candidates for pneumatic retinopexy?

Patients with retinal detachment due to multiple tears in several locations are poor candidates for pneumatic retinopexy. In addition, patients with a detachment due to a single tear but with tears in other areas of attached retina are poor candidates for pneumatic retinopexy. Proliferative vitreoretinopathy, especially if fixed folds are present, lessens the chances for reattachment with pneumatic retinopexy. And, as stated above, patients with rheumatoid arthritis or other systemic conditions who are unable to obey the strict postoperative positioning requirements are poor candidates.

11. What are the advantages of scleral buckling and pars plana vitrectomy?

Both scleral buckling and pars plana vitrectomy reduce vitreous traction mechanically. Scleral buckling involves the surgical placement of a silicone band or sponge, either sewn to the sclera as an exoplant or implanted in the sclera after a partial-thickness scleral bed is surgically created (see figure). Scleral buckles provide smooth, broad relief of vitreous traction. Subretinal fluid may be drained at the time of placement of the scleral buckle with an external sclerostomy and intraocular gas may be injected into the vitreous cavity as an adjunct to aid in retinal reattachment. Scleral buckles are especially effective in anterior retinal breaks, which typically are present after cataract surgery. Another advantage of scleral buckling is the opportunity to repair the retinal detachment from a purely external approach with no intraocular invasion.

With vitrectomy, it is possible to relieve vitreous traction directly with the vitrectomy cutter. This technique is especially useful in cases with very posterior breaks. Vitrectomy is advantageous in cases of retinal detachment with vitreous hemorrhage or vitreous opacities that obscure a view of the retinal breaks. Vitrectomy also allows the surgeon to remove epiretinal membranes when proliferative vitreoretinopathy is present. When vitrectomy is performed, the vitreous cavity must be filled with gas to reattach the retina. The presence of intravitreal gas hastens the development of cataract in phakic patients.

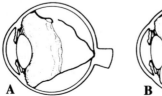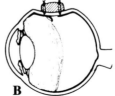

Placement of a scleral buckle.

12. What are the major risks and complications with scleral buckling and pars plana vitrectomy?

Risks of infection and hemorrhage are found with any invasive ocular procedure. The risk of a scleral buckle infection is less than 3%. Other risks and complications from scleral buckles include angle closure glaucoma, acute glaucoma from intraocular gas injection, intraocular hemorrhage from perforation during drainage of subretinal fluid, and anterior segment ischemia and necrosis. The surgically placed buckles may cause extrusion or intrusion over time, and, if the buckle is placed under an extraocular muscle, strabismus may result. Vitrectomy involves the risks of endophthalmitis, iatrogenic retinal breaks, retinal or vitreous incarceration in the sclerostomy sites, and glaucoma from the use of intraocular gases.

13. What intraoperative findings should be confirmed at the time of scleral buckle placement?

The most important intraoperative decisions at the time of scleral buckling procedures are to find and treat all retinal tears and to place the scleral buckle in a position to support all retinal breaks. After the buckle has been temporarily placed, the surgeon should confirm that the tears are flat on the buckle. If the tears are not flat, the placement of the buckle should be checked with scleral depression. If the buckle is in the appropriate position but fluid still exists between the retina and the buckle, the decision to drain subretinal fluid or to inject an intravitreal gas bubble should be made. If the detachment is primarily inferior in location, most surgeons prefer to have the retina completely attached before leaving the operating room. Superior detachments may flatten with gas injection and postoperative positioning; the decision for subretinal fluid drainage adds potential complications.

14. What three factors should be confirmed with indirect ophthalmoscopy at the conclusion of scleral buckling surgery?

Apposition of the scleral buckle to the retinal breaks, absence of complications at the drainage site, and absence of central retinal artery pulsations should be confirmed before final closure. If pulsations are present, the intraocular pressure is high enough to cause an obstruction. The pressure should be lowered.

15. How should cases of rhegmatogenous retinal detachment be approached if pars plana vitrectomy is the chosen treatment?

The placement of the infusion cannula must be carefully confirmed to avoid flushing fluid or air into the subretinal space. Vitreous traction on all retinal breaks should be relieved if possible. Care must be taken to avoid damaging retinal blood vessels if they are coursing across the retinal tears. The infusion pressure should be kept low, and instruments should be passed through the sclerostomy sites infrequently to avoid retinal incarceration. A complete posterior vitreous detachment should be created if possible. Sclerostomy sites should be checked carefully at the end of the case to evaluate for iatrogenic retinal breaks. All retinal tears should be treated completely with laser or cryotherapy. Finally, the intraocular pressure must be measured if intraocular gas is used.

16. Which gases may be used inside the eye? In what concentrations?

The inert gases sulfur hexafluoride (SF_6) and perfluoropropane (C_3F_8), along with sterile air, are the most commonly used intraocular gases. Nonexpansile mixtures are composed of approximately 20% sulfur hexafluoride and 14% perfluoropropane. These are the most commonly used mixtures when the vitreous cavity is filled with gas, as in vitrectomy. Pure 100% gas injection allows a larger bubble to form with a smaller volume of injection. This technique is advantageous in patients with pneumatic retinopexy and scleral buckles. Typically, sulfur hexafluoride expands to 2 or 3 times its initial volume, and perfluoropropane expands to about 4 times its initial volume. Thus, injection of 0.4 cc of each gas produces a 20–40% intravitreal gas bubble when they are injected as a pure concentration.

17. What are the primary causes of failure of initial retinal detachment repair?

Except for cases of severe proliferative vitreoretinopathy (PVR) in which epiretinal membranes cause traction retinal detachments (see figure), failures of retinal detachment repair are caused by an open retinal break. With pneumatic retinopexy, the most common reasons for failure include poor patient compliance with positioning requirements, inadequate identification of all retinal breaks, and development of new retinal tears from vitreous traction related to intravitreal gas. After scleral buckling surgery, failure to flatten the retina or to keep it attached results most often from undetected retinal breaks, continued vitreous traction with new, extended, or reopened retinal breaks, or a a misplaced scleral buckle. Inadequate photocoagulation or cryotherapy, continued vitreous traction, and new or missed breaks are the most common reasons for failure after pars plana vitrectomy. Ten percent of retinal placements have evidence of PVR. However, only 10–25% of these progress to require treatment for detachment.

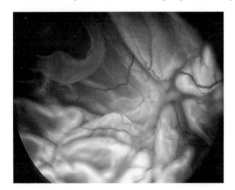

Severe proliferative vitreoretinopathy with total retinal detachment. (See Fig. 22, Color Plates.)

18. What are the major objectives in repair of traction retinal detachment?

When traction retinal detachments are due to proliferative diabetic retinopathy, one of the major aims is relief of all anteroposterior traction (see figure). A complete posterior vitreous separation must be created to remove or segment all retinal traction. Segmentation of diabetic tractional membranes is effective if no anterior traction remains. Delamination of traction membranes is accomplished by carefully identifying the plane between epiretinal tissue and the retina and lysing all adhesions. In advanced PVR, retinal traction may be so severe that the retina must be cut to relieve all retinal traction. In cases with such severe traction, especially when a retinotomy must be created, silicone oil is often useful as a long-acting tamponade. The silicone oil is usually removed after 3–6 months but may be left in place longer if the retina appears unstable.

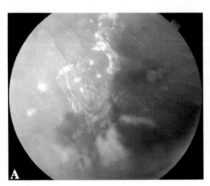 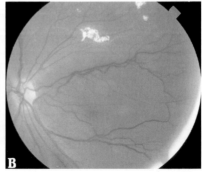

A, Proliferative diabetic retinopathy causing localized tractional retinal detachment. (See Fig. 23, Color Plates.)
B, Reattachment of retina after membrane peeling.

19. Describe the classification system for proliferative vitreoretinopathy.

The Retina Society published a classification system for PVR in 1983 which was updated in 1991. The three grades—A, B, and C—describe increasing severity of the disease. Posterior or anterior location of the proliferations has been emphasized, along with the number of clock hours involved. Five contraction types also have been described. Focal, diffuse, subretinal, circumferential, and anterior displacement are descriptive terms to quantify the type of contraction.

BIBLIOGRAPHY

1. Benson WE: Retinal Detachment: Diagnosis and Management, 2nd ed. Philadelphia, J.B. Lippincott, 1988.
2. Davis MD: Natural history of retinal breaks without detachment. Arch Ophthalmol 92:183–194, 1974.
3. Hilton GF, McLean EB, Chuang EL: Retinal Detachment: Ophthalmology Monograph Series. San Francisco, American Academy of Ophthalmology, 1989.
4. Machemer R, Aaberg TM, Freeman HM, et al: An updated classification of retinal detachment with proliferative vitreoretinopathy. Am J Ophthalmol 112:159–165, 1991.
5. Prophylactic therapy of retinal breaks. Surv Ophthalmol 22:41–47, 1977.

53. RETINOBLASTOMA

Carol L. Shields, M.D.

1. What is retinoblastoma?

Retinoblastoma is the most common eye cancer in children. It is believed to arise from primitive retinoblasts.

2. How common is retinoblastoma?

Retinoblastoma occurs with a frequency of about 1 in 14,000 live births. Approximately 250 to 300 children in the United States each year are diagnosed with retinoblastoma.

3. What causes retinoblastoma?

There are no determined causes for the cancer. Advanced paternal age and excess cancer in relatives have been found to be associated with retinoblastoma.

4. On what chromosome is the genetic mutation associated with retinoblastoma?

The genetic mutation associated with retinoblastoma is found on chromosome 13 in the region 13q14. It is believed that this single locus exists for all forms of retinoblastoma. The esterase D gene is closely linked to this site.

5. What syndrome is associated with retinoblastoma?

The 13q deletion syndrome is associated with retinoblastoma. The characteristic findings include microcephaly, broad prominent nasal bridge, hypertelorism, microphthalmos, epicanthus, ptosis, protruding upper incisors, micrognathia, short neck with lateral folds, large low-set ears, facial asymmetry, imperforate anus, genital malformations, perineal fistula, hypoplastic or absent thumbs, toe abnormalities, and psychomotor and mental delay.

6. What is the laterality of retinoblastoma?

Retinoblastoma is unilateral in approximately 67% of cases and bilateral in 33% of cases.

7. What are the most common presenting findings of retinoblastoma?

In the United States, leukocoria is the presenting feature in nearly 50% of cases and strabismus in 20%. Other less common presenting features include poor vision, red eye, glaucoma, and orbital cellulitis.

8. What are the most common lesions simulating retinoblastoma?

Of all patients referred to an ocular oncology center with the diagnosis of possible retinoblastoma, about 50% prove to have retinoblastoma and 50% are found to have pseudo-retinoblastoma. The most common pseudoretinoblastomas include persistent hyperplastic primary vitreous in 28% of patients. Coats' disease in 16%, and ocular toxocariasis in 16%.

9. At what age does retinoblastoma typically present?

Retinoblastoma is diagnosed at an average age of 18 months. Blilateral cases are recognized at an average of 12 months and unilateral cases at 23 months. In 8% of cases, the tumor is first diagnosed after age 5 years.

10. What is trilateral retinoblastoma?

Trilateral retinoblastoma is the association of bilateral retinoblastoma with midline brain tumors, especially pinealoblastoma. Trilateral disease represents 3% of all retinoblastoma cases and typically occurs before the age of 5 years.

11. What second cancers are associated with retinoblastoma?

The most common second cancers associated with retinoblastoma include osteosarcoma (especially of the femur), cutaneous melanoma, and other sarcomas. The peak incidence for second cancers is age 13 years, but these tumors can occur at anytime during the patient's life. Second cancers are believed to be related to germline mutation of chromosome 13.

12. How often do eyes with retinoblastoma present with glaucoma?

From a clinical standpoint, 17% of eyes with retinoblastoma have glaucoma, most often neovascular or angle closure glaucoma. From a pathology standpoint, glaucoma is present in 40% of eyes that come to enucleation.

13. How often does retinoblastoma invade the optic nerve?

Optic nerve invasion by retinoblastoma occurs in 29% of eyes that come to enucleation. Usually it occurs in the prelaminar area. Risks for optic nerve invasion by retinoblastoma include a large exophytic tumor measuring greater than 15 mm and secondary glaucoma.

14. What is the survival rate with retinoblastoma?

In the United States in the 1990s, 90–95% of the children with retinoblastoma survive. Risks for metastatic disease include substantial optic nerve, choroidal, or orbital invasion by the tumor.

15. What are the growth patterns of retinoblastoma?

The growth patterns are endophytic and exophytic. Endophytic retinoblastoma arises from the inner retina and seeds the vitreous. Exophytic retinoblastoma arises from outer retinal layers and causes a solid retinal detachment. A variant of endophytic retinoblastoma is the diffuse infiltrating retinoblastoma. These patterns impart no difference to the patient's life prognosis.

16. What is the differential diagnosis of endophytic retinoblastoma?

The differential diagnosis of endophytic retinoblastoma includes various inflammatory or infectious processes of the eye in children such as toxocariasis, endophthalmitis, or advanced uveitis.

17. What is the differential diagnosis of exophytic retinoblastoma?

The differential diagnosis of exophytic retinoblastoma includes Coats' disease, retinal capillary hemangioma, and other causes of rhegmatogenous or nonrhegmatogenous retinal detachment in children.

18. Can retinoblastoma spontaneously regress?

Yes, about 3% of all cases of retinoblastoma are classified as spontaneously regressed. These tumors nevertheless carry the risk for recurrence and the same genetic implications as other retinoblastoma.

19. What are the pathology features of a well-differentiated retinoblastoma?

Flexner-Wintersteiner rosettes and fleurettes represent well-differentiated retinoblastoma.

20. List the options for management of an eye with intraocular retinoblastoma.

Enucleation	Thermotherapy
External beam radiotherapy	Chemothermotherapy
Plaque radiotherapy	Cryotherapy
Laser photocoagulation	Chemoreduction

21. What are the conservative options for management of a small retinoblastoma (> 3 mm) posterior to the equator of the eye? (See figure, next page.)

Laser photocoagulation, thermotherapy, chemothermotherapy, and plaque radiotherapy are the most conservative options. Cryotherapy is generally limited to small tumors anterior to the equator of the eye.

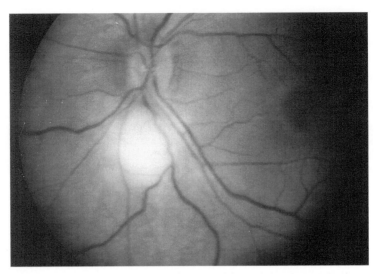

Small retinoblastoma adjacent to the optic nerve that is suitable for conservative treatment with laser photo-coagulation, thermotherapy, chemotherapy, or plaque radiotherapy.

22. What are the conservative options for management of a small retinoblastoma (< 3 mm) anterior to the equator of the eye?

Cryotherapy, laser photocoagulation, and plaque radiotherapy are the most conservative options. It is difficult to deliver appropriate thermotherapy or chemothermotherapy to the peripheral retina.

23. What are the risks of external beam radiotherapy to the patient?

External beam radiotherapy can cause short-term and long-term effects. The short-term effects include dry eye, cilia loss, and cutaneous erythema. The long-term effects include persistent dry eye, cataract, retinopathy, papillopathy, orbital fat atrophy, maldevelopment of the orbital bones, and, importantly, second cancers in the radiation field.

24. What are the chances that a child with bilateral retinoblastoma will have a future baby with retinoblastoma?

The quoted risk is 40%.

Chance of Having A Baby with Retinoblastoma

	PARENTS*	AFFECTED CHILD	NORMAL SIBLING
A. No Family History			
Bilateral retinoblastoma	6%	40%	1%
Unilateral retinoblastoma	1%	8%	1%
B. Positive Family History			
Bilateral retinoblastoma	40%	40%	7%
Unilateral retinoblastoma	40%	40%	7%

* Chance of having another baby with retinoblastoma.

25. What is the most often used classification scheme for retinoblastoma?

The Reese Ellsworth classification scheme was devised in the 1950s to predict survival of the eye with retinoblastoma, not survival of the patient. At that time, external beam radiotherapy was the only widely available conservative modality to save the eye.

Reese Ellsworth Classification System

Group 1: Very Favorable
A. Solitary tumor less than 4 disc diameters (DD) in size, at or behind the equator
B. Multiple tumors, none over 4 DD in size, all at or behind the equator

Group 2: Favorable
A. Solitary tumor 4–10 DD in size, at or behind the equator
B. Multiple tumors, 4–10 DD in size, behind the equator

Group 3: Doubtful
A. Any tumor anterior to the equator
B. Solitary tumor, larger than 10 DD, behind the equator

Group 4: Unfavorable
A. Multiple tumors, some larger than 10 DD in size
B. Any lesion extending anteriorly to the ora serrata

Group 5: Very Unfavorable
A. Massive tumors involving over half the retina
B. Vitreous seeding

---

26. How does retinoblastoma appear on ultrasound?

On ultrasound, retinoblastoma appears as a mass originating from the retina with acoustic solidity and high internal reflectivity. Foci of calcium can be seen as dense echoes.

27. How does retinoblastoma appear on computed tomography?

On computed tomography, retinoblastoma appears as a solid mass within the globe with foci of bone density, representing calcium. Often retinal detachment can be detected.

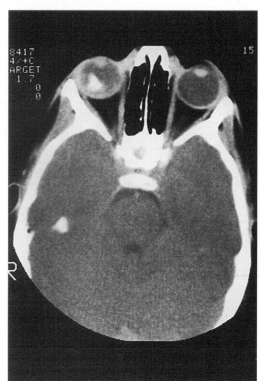

Computed tomography of eye with retinoblastoma showing the calcified mass within the right globe.

28. How does retinoblastoma appear on magnetic resonance imaging?

On magnetic resonance imaging, retinoblastoma shows a hyperintense signal to the vitreous on T1-weighted images and a hypointense signal on T2. Contrast enhancement can be seen. The foci of calcium remain hypointense on both T1 and T2 without enhancement. Areas of necrosis appear similar to calcium except that they show enhancement.

BIBLIOGRAPHY

1. Murphree AL, Munier FL: Retinoblastoma. In Ryan SJ (ed): Retina. St. Louis, Mosby, 1994, pp 571–626.
2. Shields CL, Shields JA, De Potter P: Newer treatment modalities for retinoblastoma. Curr Opin Ophthalmol 7:20–26, 1996.
3. Shields JA (ed): Update on Malignant Ocular Tumors. International Ophthalmology Clinics, Boston, Little, Brown, 1993.
4. Shields JA, Shields CL: Intraocular Tumors: A Text and Atlas. Philadelphia, W.B. Saunders, 1992, pp 305–392.
5. Shields JA, Shields CL: Surgical management of retinoblastoma. In Tasman WS, Jaeger EA (eds): Duane's Clinical Ophthalmology. Foundations of Clinical Ophthalmology, vol 6. Philadelphia, J.B. Lippincott, 1996, pp 1–13.

54. PIGMENTED LESIONS OF THE OCULAR FUNDUS

Jerry A. Shields, M.D.

1. What is the main differential diagnosis of a relatively flat pigmented fundus lesion?
- Choroidal nevus (see figure)
- Congenital hypertrophy of the retinal pigment epithelium (CHRPE) (see figure)

2. What ophthalmoscope features help to differentiate choroidal nevus and CHRPE?
Choroidal nevus is generally a slate gray lesion with a slightly ill-defined border. Drusen may be present on the surface of the lesion. CHRPE is usually black, has a sharply demarcated border, and may have depigmented lacunae through which the underlying choroid can be visualized.

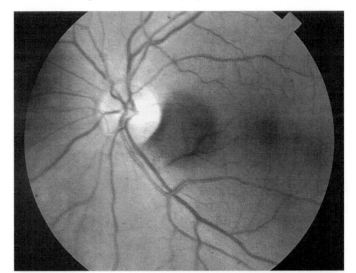

Typical choroidal nevus adjacent to the optic disc.

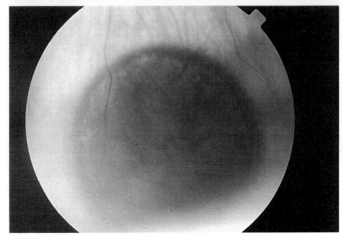

Congenital hypertrophy of the retinal pigment epithelium.

3. What is the difference in the natural course of a choroidal nevus and CHRPE?

Although both lesions are benign and usually stationary, CHRPE has no malignant potential. In contrast, choroidal nevus occasionally evolves into malignant melanoma.

4. What is the main differential diagnosis of an elevated pigmented fundus lesion?
- Choroidal melanoma
- Subretinal hemorrhage
- Tumor of the retinal pigment epithelium

5. What ophthalmoscopic features help to differentiate a choroidal melanoma from a subretinal hemorrhage?

In general, a choroidal melanoma is a rather homogeneous brown-to-black lesion with smooth surface. Subretinal hemorrhage in the macular area (age-related macular degeneration) or in the peripheral fundus (peripheral disciform degeneration) initially has a reddish-blue color; as it undergoes resolution, it has a more heterogeneous color with areas of fresh red blood and older yellow blood.

6. What is the most practical ancillary test for differentiating melanoma from subretinal blood?

Fluorescein angiography. Most melanomas show hyperfluorescence, and most hemorrhages are hypofluorescent.

7. What is the significance of a mushroom-shaped fundus lesion?

A mushroom-shaped fundus lesion is virtually pathognomonic of choroidal melanoma. Even when the mushroom-shaped lesion is nonpigmented, melanoma is still the most likely diagnosis. It is extremely unusual for any other fundus lesion to assume a mushroom shape.

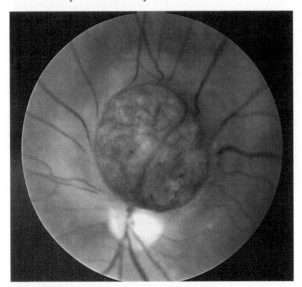

Mushroom-shaped choroidal melanoma.

8. What is the most reliable way to diagnose choroidal melanoma?

The use of binocular indirect ophthalmoscopy by an experienced ophthalmologist who is familiar with the characteristic features of choroidal melanoma and other lesions that simulate choroidal melanoma. Most melanomas can be readily diagnosed by indirect ophthalmoscopy alone.

9. In atypical cases in which the diagnosis is less evident, what are the four most helpful ancillary tests in the diagnosis of uveal melanoma?

- Transillumination
- Ultrasonography
- Fluorescein angiography
- Fine-needle aspiration biopsy

Most melanomas cast a shadow with transillumination, are hyperfluorescent with angiography, and show low internal reflectivity with ultrasonography. Most simulating lesions show different patterns with these modalities. Fine-needle aspiration biopsy is perhaps the most reliable method, but it is an invasive procedure that requires a skilled and experienced physician.

10. What clinical signs suggest that a benign choroidal nevus is likely to grow and eventually evolve into a malignant choroidal melanoma?

- Elevation of the lesion
- Proximity of the lesion to the optic disc
- Orange pigment on the surface of the lesion
- Presence of visual symptoms
- Secondary retinal detachment

11. What clinical signs suggest that a small, suspicious pigmented fundus lesion may eventually metastasize?

- Elevation of the lesion > 2 mm
- Visual symptoms
- Proximity to the optic disc
- Documentation of growth

12. What congenital ocular conditions are clearly associated with a higher incidence of uveal melanoma?

Congenital ocular melanocytosis and oculodermal melanocytosis (nevus of Ota), perhaps because of the excessive melanocytes in their uveal tract, have a greater chance of developing uveal melanoma.

13. Does uveal melanoma have a predilection for sex, age, or race?

Uveal melanoma has no significant predilection for sex. It generally occurs in patients between 40 and 70 years of age and is relatively uncommon in patients under age 20. It has a definite predilection for Caucasians; only 1–2% of cases occur in African-Americans and Asians.

14. What external ocular sign strongly suggests the presence of an underlying ciliary body or peripheral choroidal melanoma?

One or more dilated, tortuous episcleral blood vessels in the ciliary body region (sentinel vessels).

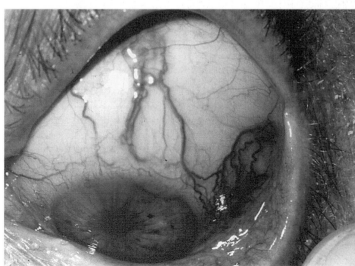

Sentinel vessel over a ciliary body melanoma.

15. What is the main route of distant spread of uveal melanoma?

Melanoma spreads to extraocular locations primarily by hematogenous metastasis to liver. Metastatic uveal melanoma to skin, lung, and other organs is considerably less common. Because there are no lymphatic channels in the eye, lymphogenous metastasis does not occur.

16. What is a melanocytoma?

A melanocytoma is a variant of benign nevus that has distinct clinical and histopathologic features. Clinically, it is usually detected on and next to the optic disc as a deeply pigmented lesion that may have a feathery border because of involvement of the nerve fiber layer of the retina. It also may occur as a deeply pigmented nevus in the choroid, not near the optic disc. Histopathologically, it is composed of round-to-oval cells that have densely packed cytoplasmic melanosomes, small uniform nuclei, and few prominent nucleoli. Like other uveal nevi, it rarely gives rise to uveal melanoma.

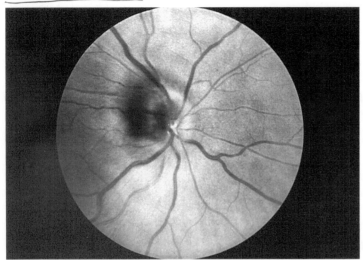

Melanocytoma of the optic nerve.

17. What is the most acceptable method of treating a choroidal melanoma that occupies more than half of the globe and has produced severe visual loss?

Enucleation.

18. What is the most often used alternative to enucleation for a medium-sized melanoma located posterior to the equator?

Brachytherapy with a radioactive plaque.

19. What is the most common treatment for a melanoma that occupies 2 clock hours of the ciliary body?

Resection of the tumor by iridocyclectomy.

20. What is the most acceptable method of management for an asymptomatic pigmented lesions measuring 3 × 3 mm in diameter and 1 mm in thickness and having fine drusen on its surface?

Baseline fundus photographs and examination every 6–12 months. Most such lesions are benign nevi that remain stationary.

BIBLIOGRAPHY

1. Shields CL, Shields JA, Kiratli H, et al: Risk factors for metastasis of small choroidal melanocytic lesions. Ophthalmology 102:1351–1361, 1995.

2. Shields JA, Shields CL: Differential diagnosis of posterior uveal melanoma. In Shields JA, Shields CL: Intraocular Tumors: A Text and Atlas. Philadelphia, W.B. Saunders, 1992, pp 137–153.

3. Shields JA, Shields CL: Diagnostic approaches to posterior uveal melanoma. In Shields JA, Shields CL: Intraocular Tumors: A Text and Atlas. Philadelphia, W.B. Saunders, 1992, pp 155–169.

4. Shields JA, Shields CL: Posterior uveal melanoma. Clinical and pathologic features. In Shields JA, Shields CL: Intraocular Tumors: A Text and Atlas. Philadelphia, W.B. Saunders, 1992, pp 117–136.

5. Shields JA, Shields CL: Introduction to melanocytic tumors of the uvea. In Shields JA, Shields CL: Differential diagnosis of posterior uveal melanoma. In Shields JA, Shields CL: Intraocular Tumors: A Text and Atlas. Philadelphia, W.B. Saunders, 1992, pp 45–49.

6. Shields JA, Shields CL: Melanocytoma. In Shields JA, Shields CL: Intraocular Tumors: A Text and Atlas. Philadelphia, W.B. Saunders, 1992, pp 101–115.

7. Shields JA, Shields CL: Management of posterior uveal melanoma. In Shields JA, Shields CL: Intraocular Tumors: A Text and Atlas. Philadelphia, W.B. Saunders, 1992, pp 171–205.

8. Shields JA, Shields CL, DePotter P, et al: Plaque radiotherapy for uveal melanoma. Ophthalmol Clin 33:129–135, 1993.

9. Shields JA, Shields CL, Ehya H, et al: Fine needle aspiration biopsy of suspected intraocular tumors. The 1992 Urwick Lecture. Ophthalmology 100:1677–1684, 1993.

10. Shields JA, Shields CL, Shah P, Sivalingam V: Partial lamellar sclerouvectomy for ciliary body and choroidal tumors. Ophthalmology 98:971–983, 1991.

11. Territo C, Shields CL, Shields JA, Schroeder RP: Natural course of melanocytic tumors of the iris. Ophthalmology 95:1251–1255, 1988.

X. Neoplasms

55. OCULAR NEOPLASMS

Ralph C. Eagle, Jr., M.D.

1. What is the most common intraocular tumor?

Uveal metastasis, usually from a distant primary carcinoma. An estimated 66,000 patients develop uveal metastases each year. Most of these tumors occur in terminal patients, however, and few are evaluated ophthalmologically or pathologically. In contrast, only 1500 uveal malignant melanomas and 250 retinoblastomas occur in the United States yearly.

Uveal malignant melanoma generally is said to be the most common primary intraocular tumor, but this statement actually applies only to the United States and Europe, because uveal melanoma has a propensity for fair-skinned, blue-eyed persons. Throughout Africa, Asia, and South America, retinoblastoma probably is the most common primary intraocular tumor.

2. What is the characteristic shape of choroidal malignant melanoma?

About 60% of choroidal malignant melanomas have a mushroom or collar-button configuration. Melanomas have a discoid or "almond" shape when they initially arise in the choroid. The mushroom or collar-button configuration develops after the tumor ruptures or erodes through Bruch's membrane and invades the subretinal space, where it forms a round or ovoid nodule.

3. Is a mushroom configuration pathognomonic for choroidal melanoma?

A choroidal tumor that has a mushroom or collar-button configuration is almost always a malignant melanoma. Few things in medicine are pathognomonic, however. Rare mushroom-shaped choroidal metastases have been reported.

4. What features of uveal melanoma are most important from a prognostic standpoint?

Cell type and tumor size. Larger tumors and tumors that contain epithelioid cells have a poorer prognosis. Tumor size generally is expressed in millimeters as the largest tumor diameter (LTD). Other prognostic features include the age of the patient (older patients fare poorer), mitotic activity, the presence of extrascleral extension, certain nucleolar parameters determined cytomorphometrically (called ISDNA and MLN), and the presence of vascular patterns called loops and networks.

5. Describe the cell types found in uveal melanoma.

In 1931 George Callender identified two types of spindle cells, called spindle A and spindle B, and less-differentiated epithelioid cells in uveal melanomas. In 1978 Ian McLean at the Armed Forces Institute of Pathology modified the Callender classification to lump spindle A and B cell tumors together as spindle melanomas. Epithelioid tumors composed largely of epithelioid cells are relatively rare and have the worst prognosis. Many melanomas accessioned in the ophthalmic pathology laboratory are mixed cell tumors composed of a mixture of spindle and epithelioid cells. Callender's original classification also included necrotic and fascicular variants that were deleted from the modified classification.

6. How are melanoma cell types distinguished histopathologically?

Melanoma cells are readily differentiated by the characteristics of their nuclei. Spindle A cells have long, tapering cigar-like nuclei, an absent or indistinct nucleolus, and a characteristic longitudinal stripe caused by a fold in the nuclear membrane. Spindle B nuclei are oval and plumper and have less finely dispersed chromatin and a distinct nucleolus (see figure, next page, left). Epithelioid cell nuclei are typically round and vesicular and have a prominent reddish-purple nucleus (see figure, right). The chromatin is coarse and often clumps along the inside of the nuclear membrane (peripheral margination of chromatin).

Spindle melanoma cells grow as a syncytium. Hence, it is usually difficult to discern the cytoplasmic margins of the bipolar fusiform cells. Epithelioid cells are poorly cohesive and their cytoplasmic margins are readily discernible.

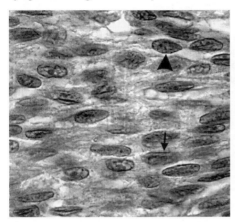 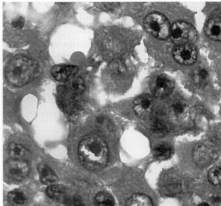

Left, Spindle melanoma cells. This field contains a mixture of spindle A and a few B cells. The spindle A cells are recognized by their slender cigar-shaped nuclei and longitudinal stripe (arrow). The spindle B cell nuclei are more oval with a distinct nucleolus (arrowhead). The margins of individual cells are indistinct. (H&E, original magnification × 250.) *Right,* Epithelioid melanoma cells. The poorly cohesive cells are polygonal in shape and have round nuclei and very prominent nucleoli. (H&E, original magnification × 250.)

7. Which cell type has the worst prognosis?

The presence or absence of epithelioid cells in a uveal melanoma has an important effect on prognosis. If no epithelioid cells are present, the expected survival at 15 years is 72%. If epithelioid cells are present (mixed, epithelioid, or necrotic cell type), the survival at 15 years drops to 37%. A tumor composed entirely of spindle A cells is now considered to be a benign nevus, which is incapable of metastasis. Tumors composed entirely of epithelioid cells have the worst prognosis. Overall, about 50% of patients with uveal melanoma will die from their tumors.

8. What is the most common site of metastatic uveal melanoma?

The liver. Liver metastases occur in 92% of patients who develop metastatic uveal melanoma. The liver is affected initially in 85%.

9. What is the best treatment for uveal malignant melanoma?

Currently there is some controversy about what constitutes the best therapy for uveal melanoma. Today, most small and medium-sized melanomas are treated with the local application of radioactive plaques (plaque brachyradiotherapy). Most plaques are made from radioactive iodine (^{125}I). Irradiation with beams of charged particles (protons or helium ions) is available at several centers. Larger tumors are still enucleated. Other treatment modalities that are used occasionally include local resection, photocoagulation, cryotherapy, and photothermotherapy.

Nonprospective data suggest that the survival after plaque therapy and enucleation are probably similar. Although plaque therapy retains the eye, useful vision is often lost.

10. What is the Zimmerman hypothesis?

In 1978, ocular pathologist Lorenz E. Zimmerman questioned whether melanoma cells were dispersed systemically during enucleation. Zimmerman's hypothesis was based on the observation that the mortality from uveal melanoma rises to about 8% 2 years after enucleation. This contrasts with an estimated 1% per year in patients with untreated tumors. The Zimmerman hypothesis has never been proved or disproved. The publication of the hypothesis stimulated interest in alternate treatment methods such as plaque brachyradiotherapy.

11. Do iris melanomas behave differently?

The prognosis of iris melanoma generally is excellent (4–10% mortality). Most pigmented tumors of the iris are benign spindle cell nevi. Overall, only 6.5% will enlarge during a 5-year period of observation. Although tumors containing epithelioid cells occasionally are encountered, most iris melanomas are low-grade spindle cell tumors.

Clinical features that suggest that a pigmented iris tumor is a melanoma include documented tumor growth, elevated intraocular pressure, hyphema, large tumor size, and tumor vascularity. Although they can occur anywhere, melanomas arise most frequently in the inferior sun-exposed part of the iris.

12. What are the clinical characteristics of uveal metastases?

Uveal metastases usually are creamy yellow amelanotic tumors that have a placoid or nummular configuration. Pigment mottling may occur on the tumor apex. Metastases are often multiple but can be solitary. Metastases usually cause a nonrhegmatogenous serous detachment of the retina with shifting subretinal fluid.

13. What is the most common site of uveal metastasis?

Uveal metastases involve the choroid 81% of the time. They typically are found in the region of the macula where the choroidal blood supply is richest.

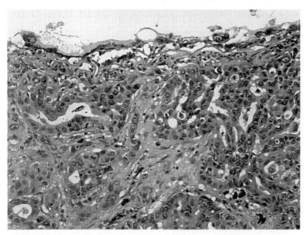

Adenocarcinoma metastatic to the choroid. The metastatic tumor forms gland-like structures in the choroid. The retina is detached. The patient had an occult primary lung carcinoma when he presented with visual loss. (H&E, original magnification × 100.)

14. What are the most common primary neoplasms that metastasize to the eye?

Lung carcinoma in men and breast carcinoma in women. Breast tumors give rise to more than half of all ocular metastases. About one fourth are caused by lung cancer. Most women with uveal breast metastases have a history of mastectomy. In contrast, uveal metastasis often heralds the presence of an occult lung tumor. The incidence of multifocal ocular metastases in patients with metastatic breast and lung carcinoma is 32% and 22%, respectively.

15. What type of hemangiomas occur in the choroid?

Cavernous hemangiomas (see figure, next page). Sporadic lesions tend to be discrete localized elevated reddish orange tumors. The choroidal hemangiomas that occur in patients with Sturge–Weber syndrome are typically diffuse, with indistinct tapering margins. These obscure the underlying choroidal architecture and impart a "tomato ketchup" appearance to the fundus.

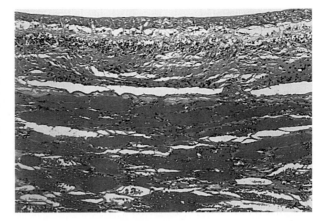

Cavernous hemangioma of the choroid. The choroid is thickened by large oval vascular channels lined by endothelial cells. (H&E, original magnification ×25.)

16. How are uveal melanomas, metastases, and hemangiomas differentiated clinically using B-scan ultrasonography?

Uveal melanomas typically show acoustic hollowness and choroidal excavation on B-scan ultrasonography. In contrast, metastases show moderate to high acoustic solidity and no appreciable choroidal excavation or orbital shadowing. Hemangiomas also show relatively high internal reflectivity and no orbital shadowing.

High internal reflectivity or acoustic solidity reflects the presence of many acoustic interfaces in the tumor. Cords and islands of carcinoma cells in metastases and individual vascular channels in hemangiomas act as acoustic interfaces.

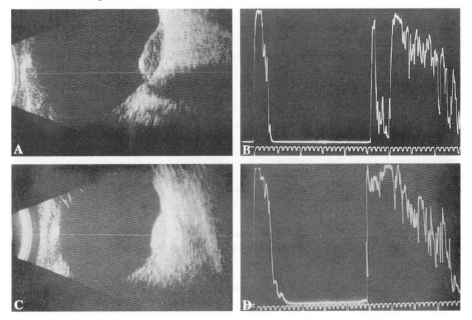

Choroidal malignant melanoma. *A*, The B-scan ultrasound shows the acoustic hollowness of the tumor and choroidal excavation. *B*, the A-scan ultrasound shows characteristic low internal reflectivity. *C*, The B-scan ultrasound reveals the high acoustic solidity of the tumor with no choroidal excavation. *D*, The A-scan ultrasound shows the characteristic high internal reflectivity. (From American Academy of Ophthalmology: Basic and Clinical Science Course, Section 4. San Francisco, American Academy of Ophthalmology, 1992, with permission.)

17. How does retinoblastoma usually present in the United States?

In the United States and Europe, retinoblastoma usually presents with leukocoria (white pupillary reflex). Smaller tumors that involve the macula may initially present with strabismus. All children with strabismus should have a careful fundus examination to exclude retinoblastoma or other significant macular pathology.

In the Third World, children often present in the advanced stages of the disease, which are marked by large orbital tumors secondary to extraocular extension.

18. How old are patients when retinoblastoma is diagnosed?

A mean age of 18 months. Patients who have the familial form of the disease (i.e., who have germ-line mutations) are diagnosed earlier (mean age of 12 months), probably because only a solitary "hit" or gene inactivation is required. Sporadic somatic cases are diagnosed at a mean age of 24 months.

19. What does retinoblastoma look like grossly?

Retinoblastomas arise from and destroy the retina. Grossly, they have a distinctly encephaloid or brain-like appearance, which is not surprising because the retina is a peripheral colony of brain cells. Foci of dystrophic calcification occur in many retinoblastomas. These foci of calcification are evident grossly as lighter flecks.

20. Describe the growth patterns of retinoblastoma.

Exophytic retinoblastomas arise from the outer retina and grow in the subretinal space, causing retinal detachment. Endophytic retinoblastomas arise from the inner layers of the retina, which remains attached. Endophytic tumors invade the vitreous and may seed the anterior chamber, forming a pseudohypopyon of tumor cells. Most large retinoblastomas exhibit a combined endophytic/exophytic growth pattern. The rare diffuse infiltrative growth pattern diffusely infiltrates and thickens the retina without forming a distinct tumefaction.

21. Why do retinoblastomas appear blue, pink, and purple under low-magnification light microscopy?

The blue, pink, and purple areas evident on low-magnification light microscopy of retinoblastoma represent areas of viable, necrotic, and calcified tumor, respectively. Areas of viable tumor appear blue because they are composed of poorly differentiated neuroblastic cells that have intensely basophilic nuclei and scanty cytoplasm. Retinoblastoma cells tend to outgrow their blood supply rapidly and undergo spontaneous necrosis. Loss of basophilic nuclear DNA is responsible for the eosinophilic appearance of the necrotic portions of the tumor. Dystrophic calcification occurs in necrotic parts of the tumor. The calcium has a purple hue in sections stained with hematoxylin and eosin.

22. What is the significance of rosettes in retinoblastoma?

Rosettes are histologic markers for tumor differentiation in retinoblastoma.

Homer Wright rosettes reflect low-grade neuroblastic differentiation. The nuclei of Homer Wright rosettes encircle a central tangle of neural filaments. No lumen is present. Homer Wright rosettes are nonspecific and occur in other tumors such as neuroblastoma.

Flexner-Wintersteiner rosettes represent early retinal differentiation and have a central lumen that corresponds to the subretinal space. The cells enclosing the lumen are joined by a girdle of apical intercellular connections analogous to the retinal external limiting membrane. Cilia, the precursors of photoreceptors, project into the lumen of the rosette. Flexner-Wintersteiner rosettes are highly characteristic for retinoblastoma, but are not pathognomonic. They are also found in some medulloepitheliomas.

Fleurettes are aggregations of neoplastic photoreceptors. Photoreceptor differentiation is the highest degree of differentiation found in retinoblastomas. Fleurettes are composed of groups of bulbous eosinophilic cellular processes that correspond to photoreceptor inner segments. They are often aligned along a segment of neoplastic external limiting membrane in a bouquet-like arrangement.

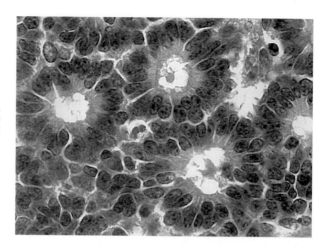

Flexner-Wintersteiner rosettes, retinoblastoma. The tumor cells encircle a lumen. (H&E, original magnification × 250.)

23. What are the most important prognostic features of retinoblastoma?

Important prognostic features of retinoblastoma that can be assessed histopathologically include the presence or absence of optic nerve invasion and uveal invasion and/or extrascleral extension. Unlike uveal melanoma, the size of the tumor does not appear to be important.

Mortality rises as the depth of tumor invasion into the optic nerve increases. In one series, the mortality was 8% if there was no optic nerve invasion and 15% if the tumor had invaded to the lamina cribrosa. Mortality rose to 44% when retrolaminar invasion was present and to 65% when the retinoblastoma extended to the surgical margin or the exit point of the central retinal vessels.

24. How does retinoblastoma kill?

Many children who die from retinoblastoma have some degree of intracranial involvement. This is caused by direct extension of tumor cells along the optic nerve, subarachnoid space, or orbital foramina. Distant hematogenous metastases to bone and viscera can develop after the tumor invades the richly vascularized uvea. Anterior extrascleral extension provides access to conjunctival lymphatics and may be associated with regional lymph node metastases.

25. The retinoblastoma gene is located on what chromosome?

Chromosome 13. It is found in the part of the long, or "q," arm designated the 1–4 band (13q1–4).

26. How is the retinoblastoma gene classified?

The retinoblastoma (Rb) gene is the paradigmatic example of a recessive oncogene. The Rb gene is called a recessive oncogene because both copies of the gene must be lost or inactivated before a tumor can develop. Normal individuals have two functional copies of the retinoblastoma gene, although only one is needed for normal functioning. The gene's protein product, called Rb protein, is found in the nucleus, where it interacts with other transcription factors to control the cell cycle. Absence of Rb protein allows continual cell division and lack of terminal differentiation.

27. If the retinoblastoma gene is recessive, why do cases of familial retinoblastoma appear to be inherited in an autosomal dominant fashion?

Carriers of hereditary retinoblastoma are hemizygous for the retinoblastoma gene (Rbrb). The genotype of carriers includes one functional wild type gene. The second copy of the Rb gene has been lost, inactivated, or produces a defective gene product. A retinoblastoma can arise when a retinal cell loses its remaining functional copy of the Rb gene. A mating between a normal individual (RbRb) and a hemizygous carrier (Rbrb) gives rise to 50% normal offspring and 50% hemizygous carriers—a 50/50 ratio that mimics autosomal dominant transmission perfectly.

28. What does bilateral retinoblastoma signify clinically?

The affected patient carriers a germline mutation in the retinoblastoma gene and is capable of transmitting the tumor to offspring.

29. Can a child with a unilateral retinoblastoma have hereditary disease?

Yes. Unfortunately, the presence of a unilateral tumor does not exclude a germline mutation and transmissible disease. Only about 60% of patients with familial retinoblastoma actually develop bilateral tumors.

30. Are most retinoblastomas familial or sporadic?

Most retinoblastomas occur sporadically in infants who have no family history of the disease. About three-fourths of these sporadic cases are caused by somatic mutations in retinal cells and cannot be passed on to offspring. Such somatic sporadic tumors are invariably unilateral and unifocal. About one-fourth of these sporadic tumors represent new germinal mutations (i.e., new familial cases). The latter can be bilateral and can be passed on to offspring in what appears to be autosomal dominant transmission. Only 5–10% of retinoblastomas occur in patients with a family history of the tumor.

31. Why are sporadic somatic retinoblastomas always unilateral and unifocal?

A sporadic somatic retinoblastoma is caused by the inactivation of both Rb genes in a single retinal cell. The spontaneous mutation rate of the retinoblastoma gene is very low. Hence, the chance of this occurrence in a more than one retinal cell is infinitesimally small. In contrast, it is highly probable that one or more gene inactivations will occur in both retinas of a hemizygous carrier, because the mutation rate is substantially smaller than the number of mitoses involved in the development of the retina. Genes usually are lost during cellular division.

32. Are patients with hereditary retinoblastomas at risk to develop other non-ocular tumors?

Yes. Between 20 and 50% of patients who have a germline mutation in the retinoblastoma gene will develop a second malignant tumor within 20 years. One of the most interesting and characteristic secondary tumors is a retinoblastoma-like tumor of the pineal gland called a pineoblastoma. The association of pineoblastoma and hereditary retinoblastoma has been termed "trilateral retinoblastoma." There is a 500-fold increase in the incidence of osteogenic sarcoma in retinoblastoma gene carriers. Patients also are at risk to develop radiation-induced orbital sarcomas (e.g., osteogenic sarcoma) after radiotherapy for retinoblastoma.

33. What three diseases are confused most often with retinoblastoma clinically?

Persistent hyperplastic primary vitreous, Coats' disease, and ocular toxocariasis.

34. How does Coats' disease differ from retinoblastoma?

Coats' disease is caused by congenital vascular anomalies in the retina that leak, causing an exudative retinal detachment. The subretinal fluid is rich in lipid-laden macrophages and cholesterol crystals, which appear as empty clefts in microscopic sections. Histopathologically, the retina contains abnormal telangiectatic vessels, and its outer layers are massively thickened by hard exudates. A bullous retinal detachment may abut the lens, displacing it anteriorly and causing pupillary block glaucoma. Coats' disease usually occurs unilaterally in boys between age 4 and 10 years. It is usually confused with exophytic retinoblastoma.

35. What are the characteristic features of persistent hyperplastic primary vitreous?

Persistent hyperplastic primary vitreous (PHPV) is a congenital disorder that is present at birth. PHPV is almost always unilateral, and classically is found in a microphthalmic eye. Leukocoria is caused by a fibrovascular plaque of primary vitreous that adheres to the posterior surface of the lens. Attached to the margin of the plaque and drawn centrally, the ciliary processes typically become visible when the pupil is dilated. Although congenital retroblastomas have been reported, on average the tumor is diagnosed at age 18 months.

36. What is the second most common primary intraocular tumor of childhood?

The medulloepithelioma. Medulloepitheliomas probably are derived from anlage of the embryonic medullary epithelium, which lines the forebrain and optic vesicle. Most of these rare tumors become symptomatic around age 4 years and are diagnosed at age 5.

37. Where are most medulloepitheliomas located?

In the ciliary body. Rare medulloepitheliomas of the optic nerve have been reported, however.

38. What is a teratoid medulloepithelioma?

In addition to bands, cords, and rosettes of neoplastic neuroepithelium, teratoid medulloepitheliomas contain foci of heteroplastic tissue including hyaline cartilage, rhabdomyoblasts, striated muscle, and/or brain. More than one third of medulloepitheliomas are teratoid. Nonteratoid medulloepitheliomas lack heteroplastic elements. Both benign and malignant variants of teratoid and nonteratoid tumors occur.

BIBLIOGRAPHY

1. Gamel JW, McLean IW: Modern developments in histopathologic assessment of uveal melanomas. Ophthalmology 91:679–684, 1984.
2. Jakobiec FA, Silbert G: Are most iris "melanomas" really nevi? Arch Ophthalmol 99:2117–2132, 1981.
3. McLean IW, Burnier MN, Zimmerman LE, Jakobiec FA: Tumors of the eye and ocular adnexa. In Atlas of Tumor Pathology, Third Series, Fascicle 12. Washington, DC, Armed Forces Institute of Pathology, Washington, DC, 1994.
4. McLean IW, Foster WD, Zimmerman LE: Modifications of Callender's classification of uveal melanoma at the Armed Forces Institute of Pathology. Am J Ophthalmol 96:502–509, 1983.
5. McLean IW, Foster WD, Zimmerman LE: Prognostic factors in small malignant melanomas of the choroid and ciliary body. Arch Ophthalmol 95:48–58, 1977.
6. McLean IW: Retinoblastomas, retinocytomas and pseudoretinoblastomas. In Spencer WH (ed): Ophthalmic Pathology: An Atlas and Textbook, vol 2, 4th ed. Philadelphia, W.B. Saunders, 1996, pp 1332–1380.
7. McLean IW: Uveal nevi and malignant melanomas. In Spencer WH (ed): Ophthalmic Pathology: An Atlas and Textbook, vol. 3, 4th ed. Philadelphia, W.B. Saunders, 1996, pp 2121–2168.
8. Murphree AL: Molecular genetics of retinoblastoma. In Grossniklaus HE, Margo CE (eds): Advances in Ophthalmic Pathology. Ophthalmol Clin North Am 8:155–166, 1995.
9. Roarty JD, McLean IW, Zimmerman LE: Incidence of second neoplasms in patients with bilateral retinoblastoma. Ophthalmology 95:1583–1587, 1988.
10. Shields JA, Shields CL: Current management of posterior uveal melanoma. Mayo Clin Proc 68:1196–1200, 1993.
11. Shields JA, Shields CL: Intraocular Tumors: A Text and Atlas. Philadelphia, W.B. Saunders, 1992.
12. Shields JA, Shields CL, Parsons HM: Differential diagnosis of retinoblastoma. Retina 11:232–243, 1991.
13. Tso MOM, Fine BS, Zimmerman LE: The Flexner-Wintersteiner rosettes in retinoblastoma. Arch Pathol 88:665–671, 1969.
14. Zimmerman LE, McLean IW: The Montgomery Lecture, 1975. Changing concepts of the prognosis and management of small malignant melanomas of the choroid. Trans Ophthalmol Soc UK 95:487–494, 1975.

56. ORBITAL TUMORS

Jurij R. Bilyk, M.D.

1. Should all orbital capillary hemangiomas be excised?

No. Orbital capillary hemangioma (hemangioma of infancy) should be treated only if there is evidence of amblyopia caused by refractive error (induced myopia or astigmatism) or visually significant ptosis. Treatment usually begins with either corticosteroid injections or systemic therapy; neither modality is completely without risk. Recent studies have shown that capillary hemangioma is highly responsive to interferon alpha-2 therapy. Excision is usually reserved for cases unresponsive to more conservative therapy.

2. What is the differential diagnosis of capillary hemangioma?

The most common cause of proptosis in children is orbital cellulitis. This is usually not confused with capillary hemangioma, which presents in a more indolent fashion. CT or MRI will show a well-circumscribed lesion in cases of capillary hemangioma. Biopsy is reserved for those cases causing a diagnostic dilemma. Orbital dermoid cyst usually presents in the anterior orbit at the superotemporal or superomedial orbital rim. Unlike capillary hemangioma, dermoid cysts exhibit the same radiodensity as fat on CT and as mucus on MRI. **Rhabdomyosarcoma** may be a consideration, especially if the proptosis is rapidly progressive. However, in many cases, cutaneous hemangiomas (e.g., "strawberry patches," "stork bites") are found on examination, and careful review of previous photographs reveals that the proptosis is in fact more longstanding than suspected by the child's parents. Furthermore, because capillary hemangioma is a congenital lesion, it invariably presents within the first 2 years of life, usually within the first 6 months. Although rhabdomyosarcoma may present at any age, the average is about 7 years. Studies have shown that capillary hemangioma is highly proliferative, which explains its rapid growth at an early age. On the other hand, **lymphangioma**, another vascular lesion considered congenital, is static, typically manifesting in the teenage years as proptosis from spontaneous hemorrhage. It usually presents as a poorly defined mass on CT or MRI with "chocolate" cysts if bleeding has occurred. Other considerations include any orbital lesions that present as well-encapsulated masses.

3. When and how does cavernous hemangioma usually present?

Cavernous hemangioma is the most common vascular orbital tumor in adults, typically presenting in the 4th and 5th decades. It is well-circumscribed on imaging, as are fibrous histiocytoma, hemangiopericytoma, and schwannoma, among others. Most orbital tumors, including cavernous hemangioma, are hypointense (dark) on T1-weighted MR images, with a few notable exceptions. Cavernous hemangioma is *not* the adult equivalent of capillary hemangioma. Not only are the lesions distinct histopathologically, but cavernous hemangioma is a slowly proliferating entity. Because of its slow growth, it is usually a well-tolerated lesion, causing few symptoms. Visual loss, if any, is slow and limited to lesions of the orbital apex. Excision is curative.

4. Concerning fibrous histiocytoma and hemangiopericytoma, which of the following statements is false:

(1) Because both are spindle cell tumors, histopathologic diagnosis may be difficult.
(2) Fibrous histiocytoma is the most common mesenchymal tumor of adults.
(3) Histopathologic appearance closely parallels the clinical behavior of hemangiopericytoma.
(4) Hemangiopericytoma is a tumor of pericytes.

Statement (3) is false. One of the more frustrating features of hemangiopericytoma is that histopathologic appearance has little correlation with clinical behavior. In other words, a histologically benign lesion may behave aggressively and recur after excision, whereas a tumor with aggressive features on microscopic examination may never recur. Because fibrous histiocytoma and hemangiopericytoma fall under the rubric of spindle cell tumors of the orbit, diagnostic confusion may occur. Fibrous histiocytoma is easily the most common mesenchymal orbital lesion of adults. Overall, rhabdomyosarcoma is the most common mesenchymal orbital lesion.

5. The most common source of schwannoma of the orbit is the meninges of the optic nerve. True or false?

False. Schwannoma is a tumor of the Schwann cells, which form the lining of peripheral nerves. Within the orbit, most schwannomas arise from sensory nerve sheaths, which may explain their predilection for the superior orbit. The optic nerve is essentially an extension of the central nervous system, surrounded by meninges and bathed in cerebrospinal fluid. The meninges consist of oligodendroglia, not Schwann cells; the equivalent tumor for the optic nerve is therefore an optic nerve meningioma.

6. What are the classic histologic findings in schwannoma?

The Antoni A and B patterns are the classic histologic findings in schwannoma. The A pattern is characterized by abundant, tightly packed spindle cells, whereas the B pattern exhibits fewer cells within a myxoid matrix.

7. Which of the following statements about orbital MRI is true?

(1) Gadolinium and fat suppression are highly effective for T2-weighted images.

(2) Most orbital tumors are iso- or hyperintense to surrounding orbital fat in T1-weighted images.

(3) Computed tomography (CT) is more effective than MRI in determining the presence of hemorrhage within the orbit.

(4) MRI is more effective than CT in imaging orbital bones and is therefore the modality of choice in orbital trauma.

None—all of the above statements are false. Several basic rules must be remembered in interpreting orbital MRI. First, in T1 images, vitreous is dark and fat is bright, whereas in T2 images the reverse is true. Because fat is already dark in T2, there is no reason to suppress it; statement (1) is therefore false. Gadolinium essentially causes any tissues in which it pools to behave more like fat, i.e., to become bright in T1. Thus, if fat were not suppressed in T1, gadolinium might make the orbital tumor disappear into the surrounding fat. It stands to reason that gadolinium injection should always be accompanied by fat suppression in T1 images of the orbit. Second, most orbital tumors are hypointense to fat in T1. Several notable exceptions should be memorized, because they help in the differential diagnosis. The first question to ask the radiologist is whether gadolinium was infused. If the answer is yes, the following exceptions do not apply, because most orbital lesions in fact enhance with gadolinium. If the answer is no and the orbital tumor is bright in T1, suspect:

1. Mucinous lesions, although their appearance depends on viscosity as well as protein and water content. Orbital dermoid cysts and mucoceles extending from the paranasal sinuses may therefore appear bright in T1 without gadolinium enhancement.

2. Lesions containing fat (lipoma, liposarcoma) behave like fat; i.e., they are bright in T1.

3. Tumors containing melanin (melanoma).

4. Subacute hemorrhage (2–5 days). This is extremely helpful in considering lymphangioma, orbital varix, orbital hemorrhage, and hematic cyst. Note, however, that acute hemorrhage (< 2–3 days) is dark on T1.

Based on the above, statement (3) is incorrect: MRI is much more effective than CT in distinguishing blood within the orbit. Statement (4) is not only incorrect, but also potentially dangerous for the patient. One drawback of orbital MRI is that bone is not imaged nearly as well as on CT. Furthermore, because MRI utilizes a powerful magnetic field, metallic foreign bodies may shift during imaging. For example, in one report an unsuspected intraocular metallic foreign body shifted during MRI, resulting in vitreous hemorrhage and retinal detachment. MRI should *never* be used as the initial imaging modality in orbital trauma unless metallic foreign body has been ruled out either by plain films or CT.

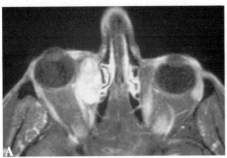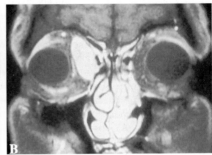

T1-weighted MR images of the orbit with fat suppression.

8. **What is the least likely diagnosis of the lesion shown in the MR image above?**
   (1) Hemangiopericytoma   **(4) Lymphangioma**
   (2) Fibrous histiocytoma   **(5) Cavernous hemangioma**
   (3) Schwannoma

The lesion is well-circumscribed on MRI, which is the usual presentation of all choices except lymphangioma, which typically presents in a more infiltrating pattern with indistinct margins. On surgical exploration, no distinct dissection plane is encountered, because lymphangioma typically grows in what Jakobiec describes as "crab grass" fashion.

9. **Discuss the histologic classification of orbital rhabdomyosarcoma.**

Orbital rhabdomyosarcoma (RMS) is histologically divided into three groups: embryonal, alveolar, and pleomorphic. The embryonal group is further subdivided into classic, botryoid, spindle cell, and anaplastic. The embryonal form is the most common histology in children, whereas the pleomorphic form has a predilection for older adults. The botryoid subtype is defined as an embryonal RMS abutting a mucosal surface (e.g., conjunctiva). The alveolar form appears to affect the inferior orbit most frequently and carries the worst prognosis. Fortunately, recent findings by the Intergroup Rhabdomyosarcoma Study (IRS) indicate that with more aggressive therapy, the prognosis for alveolar RMS approaches the prognosis for the embryonal form.

10. **From what tissue does orbital RMS arise?**

RMS is thought to arise from pleuripotential mesenchymal tissue within the orbit and not from extraocular muscle. Although features of skeletal muscle differentiation are typical in RMS, they do not correspond to a malignant transformation of existing extraocular muscles.

11. **Is RMS the most common cause of proptosis in children?**

No. The most common cause of proptosis in children is orbital cellulitis, and because any treatment delay may be catastrophic, cellulitis must be ruled out first in all children with rapidly progressive proptosis by obtaining orbital imaging.

12. **Is confirmation of RMS by frozen section biopsy an indication for orbital exenteration?**

No. Regardless of the suspected etiology, no patient should undergo special exenteration based on frozen section interpretation; permanent sectioning and special staining must be performed first. With the impressive advances made in chemotherapy and radiation therapy over the past 20 years, exenteration is rarely necessary for effective control of orbital RMS.

13. How is orbital RMS best treated? What is the prognosis?

Much of what is known about the treatment of orbital rhabdomyosarcoma comes from the three Intergroup Rhabdomyosarcoma Studies (IRS). Treatment of orbital RMS consists of a combination of chemotherapy and radiation therapy. Based on recent findings of the IRS-III, cyclophosphamide and doxorubicin may be dropped from the chemotherapeutic regimen in many cases of orbital RMS, leaving vincristine and dactinomycin. Radiation therapy in doses of 4000–6000 cGy definitely carries significant morbidity for the globe, but the IRS-III concluded that it is still necessary for adequate treatment. Anecdotal reports of successful chemotherapy alone for orbital lesions are intriguing but far from conclusive. Lower doses of radiation are currently under study. Orbital and genitourinary RMS carry the best prognosis for unclear reasons. However, local spread from the orbit into the paranasal sinuses or cranial vault decreases survival rates.

14. What is "the rule of 50s"?

The "rule of 50s" summarizes the incidence of lacrimal gland tumors in an orbital referral practice. Fifty percent of lacrimal gland lesions are nonepithelioid, consisting mostly of inflammatory and lymphoproliferative lesions, and 50% are of epithelial origin. Furthermore, 50% of the epithelial tumors are benign pleomorphic adenomas, 50% of the malignant tumors are adenoid cystic carcinoma, and 50% of the adenoid cystic carcinoma is of the basaloid variant. The final rule is important clinically, because a basaloid histopathology for adenoid cystic carcinoma carries the worst prognosis.

In a general opthalmology practice the rule of 50s does not apply. The incidence of infectious and noninfectious inflammatory dacryoadenitis is several times higher than in an orbital referral practice.

15. What factors help to distinguish benign and malignant epithelial lacrimal gland tumors?

1. Lesions present for more than 1 year (possibly more than 6 months) are likely to be benign. Lesions present for less than 3 months are either inflammatory or malignant.

2. The presence of symptoms, especially pain in a lesion causing bony destruction, is ominous, because it points toward the perineural spread along sensory nerves characteristic of adenoid cystic carcinoma. Inflammatory lesions also present with pain, but do not cause bone erosion.

3. The shape of the tumor on CT/MRI may be helpful. Lymphoma tends to mold to the native orbital anatomy, whereas epithelial lesions are more spherical and may distort the shape of the globe. Moreover, lymphoproliferative lesions typically affect both the palpebral and orbital lobes of the lacrimal gland. Epithelial tumors, on the other hand, overwhelmingly begin within the orbital lobe and usually spare the palpebral lobe.

4. Benign epithelial tumors of the lacrimal gland (e.g., pleomorphic adenoma) do not typically cause bony lysis or destruction; their chronicity instead results in a pressure-induced "fossa formation." Conversely, malignant epithelial tumors, typified by adenoid cystic carcinoma, may cause an irregular bony erosion or lysis within the lacrimal gland fossa.

16. Which of the following statements about suspected epithelial tumors of the lacrimal gland is true?

(1) Pleomorphic adenoma is histologically distinct from benign mixed tumor.

(2) Treatment of pleomorphic adenoma consists of incisional biopsy followed by low dose radiation therapy.

(3) Radical cranioorbital exenteration significantly decreases the mortality rates of adenoid cystic carcinoma.

(4) A partially excised pleomorphic adenoma may undergo malignant transformation into a pleomorphic adenocarcinoma.

(5) A partially excised pleomorphic adenoma may undergo transformation into adenoid cystic carcinoma.

Statement (4) is correct. The main point of this question is to differentiate the initial surgical management of benign and malignant epithelial tumors of the lacrimal gland. Because pleomorphic adenoma can recur and undergo malignant degeneration, complete excisional biopsy is indicated in suspected cases. Note that pleomorphic adenoma may transform into its malignant counterpart, pleomorphic adenocarcinoma, and not into adenoid cystic carcinoma. If the lesion is clearly malignant by history and orbital imaging, then incisional biopsy (with or without debulking) is indicated. In unclear cases, excisional biopsy is the better option in case the lesion indeed turns out to be pleomorphic adenoma. Radical cranioorbital resection of adenoid cystic carcinoma has not been conclusively shown to improve long-term prognosis and is avoided by many orbital specialists because of the resultant cosmetic deformity.

Benign mixed tumor is simply another name for pleomorphic adenoma. Both terms hint at the histopathology of the lesion, which consists of two elements present in varying amounts: epithelial (glandular) units and a mesenchymal (stromal) component.

17. What is the most common metastatic tumor to the orbital soft tissue in men and women?

Lung and breast carcinoma, respectively. Note that the question asks specifically about orbital soft tissue. Otherwise, prostate carcinoma would be an acceptable alternative in men, depending on the clinical series. Metastatic prostate carcinoma has a propensity for orbital bone. Breast carcinoma remains the leading metastatic tumor to the orbit in women, although with the increasing frequency of lung cancer among women, this may change in the near future. Of interest, metastatic lesions are about 10 times more common to the uvea than the orbit on autopsy studies. This may be due to the high blood flow through the choroid, which may allow more facile metastatic seeding of uveal tissue.

18. What is the appropriate work-up for orbital lymphoma and lymphoid hyperplasia?

Regardless of the histopathology, any lymphoproliferative lesion of the orbit or ocular adnexa requires a systemic work-up, consisting at least of complete blood count, serum protein electrophoresis, and imaging of the neck, thorax, and abdomen, which should be repeated every 6 months for at least 2 years. Note that Knowles and Jakobiec do not include inflammatory orbital pseudotumor as a lymphoproliferative disorder, because histopathologically the reaction is not limited to lymphocytes. Most orbital lymphomas are of B-cell origin, as confirmed by immunostaining, usually of the so-called MALT type (mucosa-associated lymphoid tissue). Based on their review, Knowles and Jakobiec concluded that tumor location, not histopathology, is the most important factor in determining systemic involvement. Lymphomas of the eyelids had the highest incidence of systemic disease (67%), followed in decreasing order by orbital (35%) and conjunctival lesions (20%). More recent studies by Medeiros and Harris, on the other hand, indicate that histopathologic appearance also may play a role in determining the frequency of systemic disease. The vast majority of lymphoid lesions, whether polyclonal (lymphoid hyperplasia) or monoclonal (lymphoid hyperplasia) are highly radiosensitive.

19. Which of the following statements regarding dermoid cysts of the periocular region is true?

(1) The most common location of these lesions is inferonasal.
(2) They may at times be confused with orbital cellulitis.
(3) Because of their high mucus content, dermoid cysts appear dark in T1-weighted images.
(4) Adult lesions are usually located preseptally, whereas pediatric lesions are postseptal.
(5) Dermoid cysts are considered acquired lesions.

Statement (2) is correct. If a dermoid cyst leaks its contents into the surrounding soft tissue, the resultant inflammatory reaction may be so severe as to mimic orbital cellulitis. Dermoid cysts are congenital lesions formed by a pinching off of ectodermal tissue by two advancing waves of the neural crest. One wave travels over the top of the head toward the orbit from above, whereas the second approaches the orbit from the midface. The two waves meet at the frontozygomatic suture (superolaterally) and frontoethmoidal suture (superomedially). These two areas are, therefore, the most common locations of dermoid cysts, with the lateral area predominating. Most pediatric tumors are preseptal simply because they become apparent sooner and are excised at an earlier age. Postseptal lesions tend to hide within the orbit, causing few, if any, symptoms as they grow slowly over the years and present predominantly in adults. Mucus is one of the few exceptions to the rule that most orbital tumors are dark in T1 images. In fact, the relative hyperintensity of a lesion in the superotemporal orbit is highly suspicious for dermoid cyst.

20. A 37-year-old man presents with a 3-week history of progressive proptosis on the right. His medical history is significant only for perennial allergies and chronic sinusitis. There is no history of tobacco use. He denies fever, nasal discharge or congestion, pain, or visual changes, although he notes recent vertical diplopia. On examination, the patient has a left hypertropia but full extraocular motility, with a nontender, firm, palpable mass noted along the superomedial orbital rim and 4 mm of right proptosis by exophthalmometry. No erythema or tenderness is noted over the eyelids. The remainder of the ophthalmic and systemic exam is unremarkable. A CT obtained by the family physician shows a lesion occupying the right superomedial orbit with extension into the frontal sinus. What is the next step?

An MRI with otolaryngologic consultation may be helpful. Although chronic sinusitis raises the possibility of bacterial orbital abscess, this diagnosis is unlikely given the paucity of ophthalmic and systemic findings. Although a fungal etiology is possible, orbital aspergillosis usually follows an indolent course, not requiring immediate emergency intervention. Mucormycosis is much less likely given the patient's lack of systemic disease (e.g., diabetes) and lack of pain. Dermoid cyst is also a possibility but should never be treated with needle aspiration; leakage may incite a severe inflammatory response. Furthermore, erosion into an adjacent sinus, although not unheard of, is not typical. A paranasal sinus carcinoma is also a distinct consideration, even without a history of tobacco use. However, such lesions are best diagnosed by a transnasal endoscopic approach, which avoids destruction of useful anatomic planes that may slow tumor spread.

The most likely diagnosis in this case is a mucocele of the paranasal sinuses eroding into the orbit. Note that cystic lesions such as mucoceles or dermoid cysts are not necessarily fluctuant on clinical exam. MRI may be particularly useful if mucus can be identified on T1-weighted imaging. Remember that a dermoid cyst also may appear bright on T1 images, as may retained mucus within a sinus blocked by carcinoma. MRI is indicated in this case not to look at bony anatomy but for differential diagnosis. Furthermore, MRI is more sensitive in determining intracranial spread than CT. Otolaryngologic consultation is certainly indicated, because the lesion in all probability may be completely managed by endoscopic sinus surgery.

21. An 8-month-old infant presents with left proptosis. The mother states that the "bulging of the eye" has been present only two weeks and is rapidly progressing. The grandmother does not comment. The child has not been febrile, has been eating and playing normally, and is otherwise healthy. Examination shows quiet eyelids and conjunctiva. Three millimeters of left proptosis is present, without palpable masses. Extraocular motility appears full. There is a question of preferential looking out of the right eye. Retinoscopy reveals an anisometropia of 4 diopters. Vascular lesions are noted on the patient's scalp and right forearm, present since birth. What is the next step?

Attempt to obtain a history from other family members and ask for previous photographs of the child. The absence of systemic (e.g., fever) and local (eyelid erythema, tenderness) findings speaks against orbital cellulitis as the etiology, although very young patients may not mount a significant febrile response. In cases of suspected orbital cellulitis, CT is indicated. Given the fact that the patient is 8 months old and appears to have hemangiomas elsewhere, orbital capillary hemangioma is more likely than rhabdomyosarcoma. Discussion of the duration of the proptosis with other family members as well as close examination of photographs may reveal that the exophthalmos has in fact been present for much longer than 2 weeks. Because the patient appears to be developing anisometropic amblyopia, treatment is indicated. However, imaging should be obtained first to document the location and extent of the lesion. Corticosteroid injection is usually carried out under anesthesia, although some physicians perform it in their office if the child is effectively restrained. Certainly, the parents should be advised of the associated risks of injection, which include globe rupture, eyelid necrosis, and central retinal artery occlusion, among others. Systemic corticosteroids carry other risks, including immunosuppression. If corticosteroids fail, most authorities recommend either surgical debulking or interferon therapy. Debulking may be dangerous at such a young age because of the potential for blood loss. Interferon must be injected intramuscularly on a daily basis for weeks to months and may result in transient fevers, flulike complaints, and retinal hemorrhages. Radon seeds are no longer an acceptable treatment modality.

BIBLIOGRAPHY

1. Alvarez Silván AM, Cantón G, Cuevas P, Gutiérrez A: Successful treatment of orbital rhabdomyosarcoma in two infants using chemotherapy alone. Med Pediatr Oncol 26:186–189, 1996.
2. Ashton N: Epithelial tumors of the lacrimal gland. Mod Probl Ophthalmol 14:306–311, 1975.
3. Avery G, Tang RA, Close LG: Ophthalmic manifestations of mucoceles. Ann Ophthalmol 15:734–737, 1983.
4. Bilyk JR, Adamis AP, Mulliken JB: Treatment options for periorbital hemangioma of infancy. Int Ophthalmol Clin 32(3):95–109, 1992.
5. Bullock JD, Yanes B: Ophthalmic manifestations of metastatic breast cancer. Ophthalmology 87:961–973, 1980.
6. Crist W, Gehan EA, Ragab AH, et al: The Third Intergroup Rhabdomyosarcoma Study. J Clin Oncol 13:610–630, 1995.
7. Croxatto JO, Font RL: Hemangiopericytoma of the orbit: A clinicopathologic study of 30 cases. Hum Pathol 13:210–218, 1982.
8. Ezekowitz RAB, Mulliken JB, Folkman J: Interferon alfa 2a therapy for life-threatening hemangiomas of infancy. N Engl J Med 326:1456–1463, 1992.
9. Font RL, Ferry AP: Carcinoma metastatic to the eye and orbit III. A clinicopathologic study of 28 cases metastatic to the orbit. Cancer 38:1326–1335, 1976.
10. Font RL, Gamel JW: Epithelial tumors of the lacrimal gland: An analysis of 265 cases. In Jakobiec FA (ed): Ocular and Adnexal Tumors. Birmingham, AL, Aesculapius Publishing, 1978, pp 787–805.
11. Font RL, Gamel JW: Adenoid cystic carcinoma of the lacrimal gland: A clinicopathologic study of 79 cases. In Nicholson DH (ed): Ocular Pathology Update. New York, Masson Publishing, 1980, pp 277–283.
12. Font RL, Hidayat AA: Fibrous histiocytoma of the orbit: A clinicopathologic study of 150 cases. Hum Pathol 13:199–209, 1982.
13. Goldberg RA, Rootman J: Clinical characteristics of metastatic orbital tumors. Ophthalmology 97:620–624, 1990.
14. Harris GJ, Jakobiec FA: Cavernous hemangioma of the orbit: An analysis of 66 cases. J Neurosurg 51:219–228, 1979.
15. Harris NL: Extranodal lymphoid infiltrates and mucosa-associated lymphoid tissue (MALT). A unifying concept [editorial]. Am J Surg Pathol 15:879–884, 1991.
16. Henderson JW: Adenoid cystic carcinoma of the lacrimal gland, is there a cure? Trans Am Ophthal Soc 85:312–319, 1987.
17. Iliff CE: Mucoceles in the orbit. Arch Ophthalmol 89:392–395, 1973.
18. Jacomb-Hood J, Moseley IF: Orbital fibrous histiocytoma: Computed tomography in 10 cases and a review of radiological findings. Clin Radiol 43:117–120, 1991.
19. Jakobiec FA: Rhabdomyosarcoma of the orbit. In Fraunfelder F (ed): Current Ocular Therapy. St. Louis, CV Mosby, 1980, pp 267–270.
20. Jakobiec FA, Bilyk JR, Font RL: The orbit. In Spencer WH (ed): Ophthalmic Pathology: An Atlas and Textbook, vol 4. Philadelphia, W.B. Saunders, 1996, pp 2438–2934.
21. Jakobiec FA, Howard G, Jones IS, Tannenbaum M: Fibrous histiocytoma of the orbit. Am J Ophthalmol 77:333–345, 1974.
22. Jakobiec FA, Howard G, Jones IS, Wolff M: Hemangiopericytoma of the orbit. Am J Ophthalmol 78:816–834, 1974.
23. Jakobiec FA, Knowles DM: An overview of ocular adnexal lymphoid tumors. Trans Am Ophthalmol Soc 87:420–444, 1989.
24. Jones IS, Reese AB, Krout J: Orbital rhabdomyosarcoma: An analysis of 62 cases. Am J Ophthalmol 61:721–736, 1966.
25. Knowles DM, Jakobiec FA: Orbital lymphoid neoplasms: Clinical, pathologic and immunohistochemical characteristics. In Jakobiec FA (ed): Ocular and Adnexal immunohistochemical characteristics. In Jakobiec FA (ed): Ocular and Adnexal Tumors. Birmingham, AL, Aesculapius Publishing, 1978, pp 806–838.

26. Knowles DM, Jakobiec FA: Orbital lymphoid neoplasms: A clinicopathologic study of 60 cases. Cancer 46:576–589, 1980.
27. Knowles DM, Jakobiec FA: Ocular adnexal lymphoid neoplasms: Clinical, histiopathologic, electron microscopic, and immunologic characteristics. Hum Pathol 13:148–162, 1982.
28. Kolawole TM, Patel PJ, Boshra Y, Ur-Rahman N: Orbital and intracranial hemangiopericytoma: Case report with a short review. Europ J Radiol 8:106–108, 1988.
29. Loughnan MS, Elder J, Kemp A: Treatment of massive orbital-capillary hemangioma with interferon alfa-2b: Short-term results. Arch Ophthalmol 110:1366–1367, 1992.
30. Maurer HM, Beltangady M, Gehan EA, et al: The Intergroup Rhabdomyosarcoma Study-I: A final report. Cancer 61:209–220, 1988.
31. Maurer HM, Gehan EA, Beltangady M, et al: The Intergroup Rhabdomyosarcoma Study II. Cancer 71:1904–1922, 1993.
32. McNab AA, Wright JE: Cavernous hemangioma of the orbit. Austr N Z J Ophthalmol 17:337–345, 1989.
33. Medeiros LJ, Andrade RE, Harris NL, Cossman J: Lymphoid infiltrates of the orbit and conjunctiva: Comparison of immunologic and gene rearrangement data [abstract]. Lab Invest 60:61A, 1989.
34. Medeiros LJ, Harmon DC, Linggood RM, Harris NL: Immunohistologic features predict clinical behavior of orbital and conjunctival lymphoid infiltrates. Blood 74:2121–2129, 1989.
35. Medeiros JL, Harris NL: Lymphoid infiltrates of the orbit and conjunctiva: A morphologic and immunophenotypic study of 99 cases. Am J Surg Pathol 13:459–471, 1989.
36. Mulliken JB, Glowacki J: Hemangiomas and vascular malformations in infants and children: A classification based on endothelial characteristics. Plast Reconstr Surg 69:412–420, 1982.
37. Mulliken JB, Young AE, Vascular Birthmarks: Hemangiomas and Malformations. Philadelphia, W.B. Saunders, 1988.
38. Mulliken JB: A plea for a biologic approach to hemangiomas of infancy [editorial]. Arch Dermatol 127:243–244, 1991.
39. Newton TH, Bilaniuk LT: Radiology of the Eye and Orbit. New York, Raven Press, 1990.
40. Orchard PJ, Smith CM, Woods WG, et al: Treatment of hemangioendotheliomas with alpha interferon. Lancet 21:565–567, 1989.
41. Quesada JR, Talpaz M, Rios A, et al: Clinical toxicity of interferons in cancer patients: A review. J Clin Oncol 4:234–243, 1986.
42. Regine WF, Fontanese J, Kumar P, et al: Local tumor control in rhabdomyosarcoma following low-dose irradiation: Comparison of group II and select group III patients. Int J Rad Oncol Biol Phys 31:485–491, 1995.
43. Rootman J, Goldberg C, Robertson W: Primary orbital schwannomas. Br J Ophthalmol 66:194–204, 1982.
44. Rose GE, Wright JE: Pleomorphic adenoma of the lacrimal gland. Br J Ophthalmol 76:395–400, 1992.
45. Schmitt E, Spoerri O: Schwannomas of the orbit. Acta Neurochirur 53:79–85, 1980.
46. Shields CL, Shields JA, Peggs M: Tumors metastatic to the orbit. Ophthal Plast Reconstr Surg 4:73–80, 1988.
47. Shorr N, Seiff SR: Central retinal artery occlusion associated with periocular corticosteroid injection for juvenile hemangioma. Ophthalmic Surg 17:229–231, 1986.
48. Sutula FC, Glover AT: Eyelid necrosis following intralesional corticosteroid injection for capillary hemangioma. Ophthalmic Surg 18:103–105, 1987.
49. Van Tassel P, Lee Y, Jing B, De Pena CA: Mucoceles of the paranasal sinuses: MR imaging with CT correlation. Am J Neuro Radiol 10:607–612, 1989.
50. White CW, Wolf SJ, Korones DN, et al: Treatment of childhood angiomatous diseases with recombinant interferon alfa-2a. J Pediatr 118:59–66, 1991.
51. Wirtschafter JD, Berman EL, McDonald CS: Magnetic Resonance Imaging and Computed Tomography. San Francisco, American Academy of Ophthalmology, 1992.
52. Wright JE: Factors affecting the survival of patients with lacrimal gland tumours. Can J Ophthalmol 17:3–9, 1982.

INDEX

Page numbers in **boldface type** indicate complete chapters.

Abducens nerve palsy, 184, 215
Abduction deficits, 191, 215
Abetalipoproteinemia, 195
Abney effect, 27
Abscess
    of nasolacrimal sac, 77
    orbital, 237, 245, 246
    subconjunctival, 200
AC:A ratio. *See* Accommodative
        convergence:accommodation ratio
Acanthamoeba, cultures of, 63
Acanthamoeba infections, corneal, 64, 66, 67
    in contact lens wearers, 62–63
Accommodation
    amplitude of, 12, 23
    range of, 12
Accommodative convergence:accommodation (AC:A)
        ratio, 187, 188, 204
Accommodative insufficiency, 191
Accommodative spasm, 23
Acetazolamide, 136, 138, 141, 155
Achromatopsia, 32, 34, 35, 203
Acid burns, 54
Acne rosacea, 50, 51
Acquired immunodeficiency syndrome (AIDS), ocular
        manifestations of, **267–273**
    aspergillosis infections, 246
    cytomegalovirus retinitis, 267–269, 270–271
    drug toxicity-related, 272
    Kaposi's sarcoma, 271, 272
    malignancies, 271–272
    most common, 267
    optic neuritis, 270
    papillitis, 270–271
    progressive outer retinal necrosis, 269
    relationship to CD4+ T-lymphocyte count, 267
    retinal detachment, 269–270
    retinal microvasculopathy, 267
    retrobulbar optic neuritis, 270
    syphilis-related, 270
Acuity meters, false-positive readings with, 21
Acute retinal necrosis syndrome, 307
Acyclovir, 70, 71
Adduction, Duane syndrome-related deficits of, 191, 192
Adenocarcinoma, 252, 334
Adenoid cystic carcinoma, 343, 343
Adenoma, pleomorphic, 343–344
Adenovirus, as uveitis cause, 60
Adherence syndrome, 200
Adolescents
    convergence insufficiency in, 190, 191
    idiopathic infantile nystagmus in, 205
    myopia in, 102
Adrenergic agonists, 123, 136, 137, 138
"After-cataract" membrane, 173
Afterimages, 27
Albinism, 202, 204, 205
Alcohol use, as hyphema cause, 151, 154
Allergic reactions, to drugs, 48, 79, 141
Altitudinal defects, 218
Amaurosis
    fugax, 306
    Leber's congenital, 32, 34, 96, 202

Amblyopia, **176–182**
    anisometropic, 176, 177, 190
    astigmatism-associated, in children, 21
    classification of, 176
    congenital esotropia-associated, 185
    congenital fibrosis syndrome-associated, 194
    crowding phenomenon of, 181
    definition of, 176
    treatment of, 179–181
        prior to congenital esotropia surgery, 185
American Academy of Ophthalmology, 177, 181
Aminocaproic acid, adverse effects of, 155
Aminoglycosides, 78, 286
    as red eye cause, 48
    as retinopathy cause, 277
    synergistic action of, 79
    effect on tear production, 85
Amplitude, accommodative, 12, 23
Anderson procedure, 204
Anemia, as hyphema cause, 151
Anesthesia, for cataract surgery, 165–166
    retrobulbar injection of, 1, 165, 166
Aneurysm
    as chiasmal visual field defect cause, 221
    as cranial neuropathy cause, 213
    intracavernous, 196
    Leber's miliary, 279
    third-nerve palsy-associated, 209, 212
Angiography
    carotid, 233
    fluorescein, 290, 328
        for age-related macular degeneration evaluation, 290,
            291
        for choroid visualization, 5
        for cilioretinal arteries visualization, 5
        for Coats' disease evaluation, 279
        for diabetic retinopathy evaluation, 304
    magnetic resonance, 233
Angiomatosis retinae, 280
Angular magnification, 18
Anhidrosis, 209
Aniridia, 134
Aniscoria, 208
Aniseikonia, 18–19, 212
Anisometropia
    as amblyopia cause, 176, 177, 178, 190
    without amblyopia, 181
    Duane syndrome-related, 192
    Prentice's rule of, 15
Ankylosing spondylitis, 57, 59
Anophthalmos, 249
Anterior chamber
    angle of, 3
        central, in plateau iris, 126
        closure classification of, 120–121
        dilation of, 120
        gonioscopic visualization of, 3, 114, 118–120
        landmarks of, 117
        recession of, 159–160, 161
    blood in. *See* Hyphema
    cells of, 61
    depth of, relationship to refraction, 102
    flares of, 61

Anterior chamber *(cont.)*
  flat, 146, 148–149, 171
  in herpes simplex infections, 49
  inflammation of, corneal ulcer-related, 61
  effect of pilocarpine on, 140
  in primary angle closure glaucoma, 125
Anterior chamber tap, 64–65
Anterior inferior cerebellar artery syndrome, 216
Anterior segment
  ischemia of, 319
  necrosis of, 319
  neovascularization of, 313–314
Antibiotics
  intraocular injection of, as retinopathy cause, 277
  topical, **76–83**
Anticholinergic medications, contraindication in narrow
    angle glaucoma, 126
Antidepressants, effect on tear production, 85
Antifibrinolytic agents, as hyphema treatment, 154
Antifungal agents, as corneal ulcer treatment, 65
Antiglaucoma medications, as corneal ulcer treatment, 65
Antihistamines, as dry eye syndrome cause, 49
Antihypertensive drugs, effect on tear production, 85
Antimetabolites, use in trabeculectomy patients, 143,
    147–148
Anulus of Zinn, 1, 8
Aphakia, 169
Apoplexy, pituitary, 196, 221
Apraclonidine, 48, 136, 141
Apraxia, congenital motor, 196
Aqueous humor, obstruction of, 112
Aqueous misdirection syndrome. *See* Glaucoma,
    malignant/ciliary block
Aqueous suppressants, 127
Arachnodactyly, 163
Arcuate defects, 218
Arden ratio, 35
Argon lasers, 3, 127, 130, 133, 142, 151, 313, 314
Argyle-Robertson pupil, 211
Argyrosis, 277
Arrhythmias, 309
Arterioles, retinal, talc-related closure of, 276, 277
Arteritis, giant cell, 213, 222–223, 246, 308, 309
Arthritis, neonatal conjunctivitis-related, 74
Artificial tears, 56, 85, 87–88
Aspergillosis, orbital, 246
Aspirin, 143, 151, 154, 303
Asteroid hyalosis, 42, 43
Astrocytoma, juvenile pilocytic, 237
Asthenopia, 21, 190–191
Asthma, keratoconus-associated, 96
Astigmatic axis, 23
Astigmatism
  acquired, 22
  as amblyopia cause, 179
  circle of least confusion in, 16
  corneal, 102
  definition of, 102
  as diplopia cause, 212
  keratoconus-related, 99–100
  lenticular, 102
  of oblique angle, 17
  of oblique incidence, 17
  post-cataract surgery, 16, 22
  post-corneal transplant, 108
  with-the-rule versus against-the-rule, 16
Atopy, 45, 96, 100
Atropine, 21, 23, 48, 85
Auscultation, use in orbital inflammation evaluation, 244

Autoimmune disorders, as corneal ulcer cause, 61
Axenfeld's anomaly, 134

Bacillus cereus, as posttraumatic endophthalmitis cause,
    286
Bacitracin, 77, 80
Basal cell carcinoma, of the eyelid, 253–254, 255
Basal cell nevus syndrome, 255
Bassen-Kornzweig syndrome, 195
Batten-Mayou-Vogt-Spielmeyer disease, 308
Behçet's disease, 59
Bell's palsy, 49
Bell's phenomenon, 251
Benedicki's syndrome, 216
Best's disease, 36
Beta blockers, 85
  action mechanism of, 137
  contraindication in trabeculectomy patients, 149
  contralateral effects of, 139
  as corneal ulcer treatment, 65
  as dry eye syndrome cause, 49
  as glaucoma treatment, 123, 136, 137–138, 139
  as hyphema treatment, 154
Betaxolol, as glaucoma treatment, 136, 137, 138
Bezold-Brucke phenomenon, 26–27
β-galactosidase deficiency, 308
Bifocals, 15, 19, 205
Binocular vision, in congenital esotropia, 183–184
Biometry, 38
Biomicroscopy, ultrasound, 44
Biopsy
  corneal, 66
  for eyelid lesion evaluation, 254
  frozen section, for orbital rhabdomyosarcoma evluation,
    342
  incisional, for adenoid cystic carcinoma evaluation,
    343–344
  for sebaceous cell carcinoma evaluation, 255–256
  of the temporal artery, 9
Blebs, 145, 146, 147, 149, 150
Blepharitis, 50, 67, 77, 85, 86
Blepharoconjunctivitis, chronic, 255
Blepharophimosis syndrome, 250
Blepharotomy, transverse, 9
Blindness. *See also* Vision loss
  glaucoma-related, 111, 115–116
  inflammatory orbital pseudotumor-related, 246
  as light/near dissociation cause, 211
  neonatal conjunctivitis-related, 72
  orbital inflammation-related, 246
  retinopathy of prematurity-related, 295
Bloch-Sulzberger syndrome, 298
Blood-retinal barrier, 4
Blurred vision
  age-related macular degeneration-related, 289
  corneal dystrophy-related, 89
  desferrioxamine-related, 278
  digitalis-related, 277
  granulomatous uveitis-related, 257
Bone marrow transplantation, 86
Bowman's layer, corneal dystrophies of, 89, 90, 93
"Box-carring" phenomenon, 307
Brachytherapy, 330
Brainstem tumors, 197
Breast cancer, metastatic, 334, 344
Brimonidine, 123, 136
Brown's syndrome, 192–194, 199, 215
Brucellosis, 258
Bruch's membrane, 4, 284, 290

Bruits, 244
Buerger's disease, 246
Burns
    acid-related, 54
    conjunctival, 86
    as keratocanthoma cause, 253
    ultraviolet, 50
Busacca nodules, 257

Calcification
    orbital, 231, 232
    retinal detachment-related, 42
    of retinoblastoma tumors, 264, 335, 336
    ultrasound appearance of, 39, 43
Canaliculo-dacryocystorhinostomy, 229
Cancer, as aminocaproic acid contraindication, 155
Canthoxanthine, as retinopathy cause, 276
Capillary nonperfusion, interferon-related, 277
Capsulotomy, 168, 173, 174
Carbachol, 136, 143
Carbonic anhydrase inhibitors
    action mechanisms of, 137
    contraindication in sickle cell disease, 155
    as corneal ulcer treatment, 65
    discontinuation prior to trabeculectomy surgery, 143
    as glaucoma treatment, 123, 136, 141
    as hyphema treatment, 154
Carotid artery occlusive disease, 121, 306, 308, 309
Carteolol hydrochloride, 136, 137
Cataracts, **162–164**
    congenital, 162, 176, 179
    as diplopia cause, 212
    glassblowers', 163
    Morganian, 163
    nonsurgical management of, 165
    nuclear sclerotic, 162
    pigmentation of, 162
    posterior subscapular, 162
    preoperative evaluation of, 40
    radiation therapy-related, 255
    "sunflower", 286
    topical steroids-related, 80–81
    trabeculectomy-related exacerbation of, 142
    traumatic, 153, 163
    vitrectomy-related, 305
Cataract surgery
    astigmatism following, 16, 22
    complications of, 16, 22, 133, **171–175**, 316
    indications for, 163–164
    with preexisting filters, 148
    as rhegmatogenous retinal detachment cause, 316
    techniques of, **165–170**
Cautery, as puncta closure technique, 88
Cavernous sinus syndrome, 216
Cecocentral lesions, 45
Cefazolin, 64, 66
Cefotaxime, 74
Ceftriaxone, 74
Cellulitis
    orbital, 235, 236, 245, 344
        in infants, 345
    preseptal, 245
    strabismus surgery-related, 200
Central nervous system disease, disseminated, 74
Cephalosporin, 78
Cerebellopontine angle tumor, 216
Chalazion, 22, 50, 212, 255
Chalcosis, 134, 286
Chandler's syndrome, 92, 112, 121, 134

Chelating agents, as maculopathy cause, 278
Chemicals
    as neonatal conjunctivitis cause, 72, 73
    as open-angle glaucoma cause, 134
    as ophthalmia neonatorum cause, 73
    as superficial punctate keratopathy cause, 50
Chemoreduction, as retinoblastoma treatment, 323
Chemosis, 77, 235, 284
Chemotherapy, 324, 342–343
Cherry-red spots, 308
Chiasm. *See* Optic chiasm
Children
    adverse effects of eye drops in, 115
    amblyopia screening of, 177
    astigmatism in, spectacle prescriptions for, 21
    conjunctivitis in, 54
    craniopharyngioma in, 221
    cycloplegic agents for, 21
    developmentally-delayed, rectus muscle recession in, 1
    medulloepithelioma in, 338
    optic nerve glioma in, 237
    orbital cellulitis in, 245
    proptosis in, 342
    radiation therapy-related orbital deformity in, 255
    retinoblastoma in. *See* Retinoblastoma
    rhabdomyosarcoma in, 237
    spontaneous hyphema in, 265
    third-nerve palsy in, 209
Chin-up head posture, 180, 193, 194, 203
Chlamydial infections, 54, 55, 72, 73
Chlorolabe, 25
Chloroquine, 35, 274–275, 276
Chlorpromazine, as retinopathy cause, 275
Chorioretinitis, syphilitic, 260
Chorioretinitis sclopetaria, 284
Choroid
    detachment of, 148, 149
    effusions from, 3, 121
    fluorescein angiographic visualization of, 5
    hemangioma of, 334, 335
    infiltrates of, primary intraocular sarcoma-related, 264
    metastatic tumors of, 334
    neovascularization of, 260, 288, 289–290, 291
    nevus of, 41, 327, 328
    osteoma of, 38
    rupture of, 153, 284
    tumors of, 38, 316
    as uveal metastases site, 334
Choroidal excavation, 41
Choroideremia, 32
Choroiditis, 46, 259, 261
Choroidretinopathy, central serous, 316
Chromatic aberration, of thick lens, 17
Chronic progressive external ophthalmoplegia, 194–195,
    196, 197
Cidofovir, toxicity of, 269
Ciliary bodies
    anterior, angle recession of, 152
    melanoma of, 329
    sentinel vessels' relationship to, 329
    swelling or anterior rotation of, 112, 120–121
    as trabeculectomy site blockage cause, 148
Ciliary body band, 117
Cilioretinal arteries, 5, 278, 307
Ciliospinal center of Budge, 206
Ciprofloxacin, 65, 68, 78, 80
Circle of least confusion, 16
Clear lens extraction, 109
Clindamycin, 286

Clotting disorders, 151, 155
Coats' disease, **279–282**
    differentiated from retinoblastoma, 231, 322, 338
Cocaine test, 211
Cogan's lid, 250
Cogan-Reese syndrome, 112, 121
Cold sores, 49, 69
Collagen vascular diseases, 49, 56, 85, 218, 287
Coloboma, 176, 192, 221
Color, attributes and properties of, 25–26, 27
Color vision, **24–29**
    defects of
        amblyopia-related, 180
        digitalis-related, 277
        inheritance of, 29
        optic neuritis-related, 218
        orbital inflammation-related, 244
    evaluation of, 244
Coma, 17
Commotio retinae, 283
Cones, 24–25, 26
    contact lens-induced, 95
Congenital abnormalities. *See also* specific congenital
        abnormalities
    as exudative retinal detachment cause, 316
Congenital fibrosis syndrome, 194
Conjunctiva
    foreign bodies in, 52–53, 73
    intraepithelial neoplasia of, 53
    Kaposi's sarcoma of, 271, 272
    lymphoma of, 344
    in primary acute angle glaucoma, 121
    scarring of, dry eye-related, 49, 86
    slit lamp examination of, 244
    squamous cell carcinoma of, in AIDs patients, 272
    tarsal follicles of, 48
    in trabeculectomy surgery, 143, 145
Conjunctival injection, proptosis associated with, 235, 236
Conjunctivitis
    chlamydial, 54, 55
    chronic, 54–55, 77
    dry eye-related, 86
    follicular, 54, 69, 73, 253
    giant papillary, 51
    gonococcal, 48–49, 68–69, 77
    herpes simplex, 70, 74
    hyperacute bacterial, 77
    Lyme disease-related, 261
    neonatal. *See* Ophthalmia neonatorum
    Parinaud's oculoglandular, 54, 55
    as red eye cause, 48
    syphilitic, 260
    tuberculosis-related, 259
    vernal, 96
    viral, 77
Conjunctivo-dacryocystorhinostomy, 229
Connective tissue disorders, 57, 96
Contact lens
    aniseikonia associated with, 18–19
    as corneal infection cause, 52, 62–63
    corneal infiltrates associated with, 67–68
    decentered, as monocular diplopia cause, 21
    as keratoconus cause, 95
    as keratoconus treatment, 99–100, 101
    Koeppe, 118
    effect on nystagmus, 205
    power of, 12
    prismatic effect alleviation with, 15
    as red eye cause, 51–52

Contact lens *(cont.)*
    steepening the fit of, 22–23
Contact lens solutions, 67–68
Contact lens warpage syndrome, 95
Contrast sensitivity test, 165, 218
Contrecoup mechanism, 283
Convergence
    accommodative. *See also* Accommodative
            convergence:accommodation (AC:C) ratio
        effect on nystagmus, 205
        fusional, effect on nystagmus, 205
Convergence insufficiency, 23, 190–191, 217
Corectopia, 92
Cornea
    abrasions of, 52, 73, 153
    dystrophies of, 52, **89–94**, 96, 109
    edema of, 124
    endothelial cells/dendrites of, 70, 81
        effect of refractive surgery on, 109
    epithelial cells of
        non-healing defects of, in diabetic patients, 305
        pre-cataract surgery assessment of, 165
    erosion of, 235
    filaments of, in superior limbic keratoconjunctivitis, 56
    foreign bodies in, 52–53
    infections of, **61–71**
        differentiation among types of, 62–63
        gonococcal, 68–69
        herpes simplex, 70–71
        herpetic, 69–71
        predisposing conditions for, 62
    innervation of, 5
    irregular surface of, effect on potential acuity meter
            readings, 21
    irritation of, as tearing cause, 227
    keratometric measurements of, 20
    neonatal cloudy, 5
    opacity of, as amblyopia cause, 176
    pannus of, sebaceous gland carcinoma as mimic of, 255
    in primary angle closure glaucoma, 121, 125
    refractive function of, 102
    scarring of
        corneal ulcer-related, 66
        herpetic keratitis-related, 70
        thyroid-related ophthalmopathy-related, 241, 242
        topical steroid treatment for, 79, 80–81
    topography of, in refractive surgery patients, 103
    traumatic injury to, as red eye cause, 48
    ulcers of, 51, **61–71**, 78, 79
Cornea guttata, 92, 93
Corneal haze, 109
Corneal nerves, in keratoconus, 97
Corneal scrapings, 63
Corneal transplantation, 98–99, 100, 101, 108, 173
Corticosteroids
    injection of, as neonatal proptosis treatment, 345–346
    as optic neuritis treatment, 218–219
    topical
        as corneal ulcer treatment, 67
        as glaucoma risk factor, 113
        as herpes simplex keratitis treatment, 70
Cotton-wool spots, 267, 277, 287, 301
Couching, 166
Coumadin, 143, 151, 154
Cranial nerve palsies
    fifth, 196
    fourth, 192, 196, 213
    Lyme disease-related, 261
    multiple, 196–197

Cranial nerve palsies *(cont.)*
  sixth, 184, 213, 215
    congenital, 185
  third, 196, 209, 212–216, 227, 249
Cranial nerve III, aberrant regeneration of, 213
Cranial nerve V, divisions of, 7
Cranial neuropathies, isolated, 213
Craniopharyngioma, 221
Crede prophylaxis, for neonatal conjunctivitis, 73
Critical angle, 13
Crocodile tears, 192
Crowding phenomenon, 181
Crutches, eyelid, 251
Cryocyclodestruction, 128
Cryopexy, 283
Cryotherapy
  as Coats' disease treatment, 280, 281, 282
  as retinoblastoma treatment, 323, 324
  as retinopathy of prematurity treatment, 296, 297
  as uveal malignant melanoma treatment, 333
Cryptococcal infections, in AIDS patients, 267, 270, 271
Cyanoacolaid adhesives, 88
Cyanoacrylate, 65, 146
Cyanolabe, 25
Cyclodestruction, 128
Cyclodialysis, 152, 153, 159–160
Cyclodialysis cleft, 160
Cyclogyl, 21
Cycloplegic agents
  as corneal ulcer treatment, 65
  length of effectiveness of, 21
  as malignant glaucoma treatment, 127
  as systemic intoxication cause, 21
Cyst
  dermoid, 232, 344–345
  hemorrhagic, 341
  intraretinal, 42, 284
Cysticercosis, 246, 264
Cystinosis, 91
Cytomegalovirus infections, in AIDS patients, 267–269, 270–271

Dacryoadenitis, 246, 259, 343
Dacryocystitis, 54, 55, 73, 77, 229
Dacryocystorhinostomy, 229, 230
Dark adaptation, 31, 36
Deafness, Duane syndrome-related, 192
Decompression, orbital, 242
Dendrites, corneal, 70, 81
Dental floss syndrome, 140
Dermatitis, radiation therapy-related, 255
Descemet's folds, 125
Descemet's membrane, 3, 97, 98, 286
Desferrioxamine, as maculopathy cause, 278
Deuteranopia, 28–29
Diabetes mellitus, 22, 121, 253, 313. *See also* Retinopathy, diabetic
Dialysis
  cyclo-, 152, 153, 159–160
  renal, 287
  retinal, 152, 283
Dichlorphenamide, 136
Dichromatism, congenital, 28
Digitalis, 138, 277
Dilation, for anterior chamber angle visualization, 120
Diopters, 12, 14, 15, 20
Dipivefrin hydrochloride, 136, 138
Diplopia, **212–217**
  acute acquired comitant esotropia-related, 189

Diplopia *(cont.)*
  evaluation of, 244
  inflammatory orbital pseudotumor-related, 246
  intermittent, 212
  intermittent exotropia-related, 190
  monocular, 21, 212
  proptosis-related, 234
  thyroid ophthalmopathy-related, 242
Disc. *See* Optic disc
Disciform degeneration, peripheral, 328
Disciform lesion, ultrasound evaluation of, 41
Dissociated vertical deviation (DVD), 186
Divergence insufficiency, 191
Divergence paresis, 217
Doll's eyes, 215
Doppler studies, 245, 308
Dorsal midbrain syndrome. *See* Parinaud's syndrome
Dorzolamide, as glaucoma treatment, 136, 137–138, 140–141
Down's syndrome, 96, 99, 100
Doxycycline, 50, 67
Double elevator palsy, 193
Drugs. *See also* specific drugs
  allergic reactions to, 48, 79, 141
Drusen, 43, 222, 288, 289, 292
Dry eyes. *See* Keratoconjunctivitis sicca
Dry mouth, 85, 246
Duane's retraction syndrome, 185, 191–192
Dyschromatopsia, 275
Dysproteinemias, 91
Dystrophy
  cone, 32, 33–34, 35
  corneal, 52, **89–94**, 96, 109
  endothelial, 5, 96
  muscular, 249
  myotonic, 35
  ocular pharyngeal, 195, 249
  vitelliform macular, 36

Eaton-Lambert syndrome, 196
Echothiophate iodide, 136, 143
Eclampsia, 287
Ectopia, macular, 294
Ectropion
  as corneal infection cause, 62
  definition of, 228
  ptosis surgery-related, 251
  repair of, 228
  as superficial punctate keratopathy cause, 50
Eczema, 96
Edema
  Berlin's, 283
  corneal, 61
    acute hydrops-related, 98
    cataract surgery-related, 172–173
    corneal membrane dystrophy-related, 92
    as corneal ulcer risk factor, 62, 63
    malignant glaucoma-related, 148
  of eyelids, 236
  of inner canthus, 73
  macular
    acute retinal necrosis-related, 261
    clinically significant, 302
    cystoid, 173, 276, 277
    diabetic, 300, 301, 302–304
    interferon-related, 277
    effect on potential acuity meter readings, 21
    refractory, as vitrectomy indication, 305
    retinal vein occlusion-related, 312–313, 314
    syphilitic, 260

Edema *(cont.)*
  of the optic disc, 287
  posterior polymorphous, 134
  retinal, traumatic hyphema-related, 153
Edinger-Westphal nucleus, 206
Ehlers-Danlos syndrome, 96
Electromagnetic spectrum, 24
Electro-oculogram (EOG), 35–36, 274, 276
Electrophysiologic evaluation, of toxic retinopathies, 274, 276
Electroretinogram (ERG), 30–35
  relationship to electro-oculogram, 36
  for iron toxicity evaluation, 285–286
  for toxic retinopathy evaluation, 274, 276
  relationship to
Embolism
  amniotic fluid, 309
  of carotid artery, 306
  retinal, 278, 306–307
Emmetropia, 11, 12
Endophthalmitis
  cataract surgery-related, 132, 173
  differential diagnosis of, 323
  keratitis-related, 65
  paracentesis-related, 309
  postoperative, 172, 200, 258
  posttraumatic, 286
  sterile, rifabutin-related, 272
  trabeculectomy-related, 142
  as uveitis mimic, 60
  vitrectomy-related, 319
Enophthalmos, 228, 235, 249
Entropion, 9, 50, 62, 228, 255
Enucleation
  as choroid melanoma treatment, 330
  as Coats' disease treatment, 281
  as retinoblastoma treatment, 323
  as uveal melanoma treatment, 333–334
EOG. *See* Electro-oculogram
Epikeratophakia, 100
Epinephrine, 48, 136, 138, 155
Epiphora. *See* Tearing
Episclera, in primary acute angle glaucoma, 121
Episcleral venous pressure, 133
Episcleritis, 48, 56–57, 261
Epitheloid cells, in melanoma, 332, 333, 334
Epitheloid tumors, 332, 343–344
ERG. *See* Electroretinogram
Erythema, acne rosacea-related, 50
Erythrolabe, 25
Erythromycin, 73, 74, 77, 80
Eschars, orbital, 246
Escherichia coli, as neonatal conjunctivitis cause, 72
Esodeviations, **183–189**
Esophoria, 183
Esotropia, 178, 180
  accommodative, 184, 186–187
    as amblyopia cause, 180
    early-onset, 185
    nonrefractive, 188
    partial or decompensated, 188
    refractive, 187
    relationship with congenital esotropia, 188
  acute acquired comitant, 189
  congenital, 180, 183–186, 190
  cyclic, 188
  definition of, 183
  differential diagnosis of, 184–185
  as divergence insufficiency, 191

Esotropia *(cont.)*
  Duane syndrome-related, 192
  infantile, 183
  in neurologically-impaired patients, 185
  sensory, 185
Estrogens, effect on tear production, 85
Ethambutol, 250–260, 270, 272
Ethmoid bone, 1
Ethylene glycol, 276
Examination room, red eye transmission in, 48
Exenteration
  cranioorbital, of adenoid cystic carcinoma, 343, 344
  orbital, frozen section as indication for, 342
  of recurrent eyelid tumors, 255
Exfoliation syndrome, 114, 115, 163
Exophoria, 190, 191
Exophthalmometer, Hertel, 244
Exophthalmos, 44, 246
Exotropia
  binocular lens-related, 19
  congenital, 190
  constant, as amblyopia cause, 180
  differential diagnosis of, 190
  Duane syndrome-related, 192
  intermittent, 180, 190
  neonatal, 183
  post-rectus recession, 1
External beam radiotherapy, 324
Extracapsular cataract surgery, 166, 167
Eye
  clinical anatomy of, **1–6**
  color perception ability of, 26
  schematic, 14
Eye drops, 76. *See also* Topical medications
  general rules for prescription of, 139
  safety of, 115
Eyelid crutches, 251
Eyelids
  anatomy of, 8–10
  crease of, 249, 251
  crusty, blepharitis-related, 50
  deformities of, 49
  edema of, 236
  fissure of, in ptosis patients, 250
  "floppy", 50, 96
  full-thickness lower-lid laceration of, 9
  inflammation of, 85
  lag of, 239
  lower, laxity of, 226–227
  papillae of, 56
  retraction of, thyroid ophthalmopathy-related, 236, 239, 240, 243
  schematic cross-section of, 2
  sensory nerve supply of, 9
  telangiectasia of, 50
  tumors of, 212, **252–256**
Eye rubbing, 50, 96, 100

Familial amyloid polyneuropathy type IV, 91
Farber syndrome, 308
Farsightedness. *See* Hyperopia
Fat pads, 2, 9
Fetal hyaloid vasculature, 4
Fever, 69
Fiber layer of Henle, 4
Fibrohistiocytoma, 232, 238, 340, 342
Fibroplasia, retrolental, 277
Fibrosis syndrome, congenital, 194

Field vision, iron overload-related loss of, 278
Filters
    neutral density, 180–181
    preexisting, in cataract surgery, 148
    translucent, 179
Fistula
    arteriovenous, 196
    carotid-cavernous, 235, 244
Fixation preference testing, 177, 178, 185
Flashes, retinal break-related, 316
Fleischer ring, 97, 98, 100
Fleurettes, retinoblastoma-related, 323, 336
Flexner-Wintersteiner rosettes, 323, 336
Floaters, 60, 257, 267, 316
Floppy eyelid syndrome, 50, 96
Fluorescent light, appearance of color under, 28
Fluoroquinolones, 64, 78
5-Fluorouracil, 147, 148
Focal points, 11, 12, 14
Forced ductions, 198
Foreign bodies, intraocular
    copper, 285
    imaging detection of, 285
    iron, 278, 285–286
    as neonatal conjunctivitis cause, 73
    as open-angle glaucoma cause, 134
    orbital, 53, 232, 341–342
    as red eye cause, 52–53
    removal of, 285
    retinal, 40
    as scleritis cause, 57
    as superficial punctate keratopathy cause, 50
    traumatic hyphema-associated, 153
    ultrasound detection of, 38, 40, 43
    as uveitis masquerade syndrome, 60, 258, 263, 266
Foreign body sensation
    acne rosacea-related, 50
    dry eye condition-related, 49, 85
Foscarnet, 268, 269
Fovea
    anatomy of, 5
    as center of visual field, 45
Foveal avascular zone, 304
Foville's syndrome, 216
Fractures, blowout, 1, 7, 194, 249
Freckle, Hutchinson's melanotic, 256
Frontal nerve, location of, 8
Frontomaxillary suture, 7
Frontozygomatic suture, 7
Full-threshold testing, 45
Fundus
    in diabetic retinopathy, 300
    examination of, in pediatric strabismus, 335
    pigmentation/pigmented lesions of, 4, 327–331
    traumatic injury to, 283–287
Fungal infections
    corneal, 63, 64, 65
    as granulomatous uveitis cause, 258
    orbital, 246

Galactosidase deficiency, 308
Ganciclovir, 261, 267, 268
Gangliodisease GM1-type 2, 308
Ganglion cell disease, retinal, 32
Gas, intraocular, 319
Gaucher's disease, 308
Geneva lens clock, 20, 22
Gentamycin, 79, 286
Glands of Kraus, 5, 6

Glands of Wolfring, 5, 6
Glare/contrast sensitivity testing, 165
Glaucoma, 111–116
    acute primary closed-angle, 111
    angle closure, 117–129
        acute, 48, 121–122
        aqueous misdirection syndrome associated with,
            127–128
        chronic, 121, 122
        inflammation-related, 128
        intermittent, 122
        nanophthalmos-related, 129
        pilocarpine treatment of, 140
        plateau iris presenting as, 126–127
        primary, 121–126
        retinopathy of prematurity-related, 297
        scleral buckling-related, 319
        secondary, 159
        synechiae as risk factor for, 58
    angle recession, 130, 160–161
    "best" treatment for, 115
    in cataract patients, 174
    ciliary block. See Glaucoma, malignant/ciliary block
    congenital, 73, 111
    corneal membrane dystrophy-related, 92
    definition of, 111
    evaluation of, 115
    focal, 111
    ghost-cell, 134, 159
    hemolytic, 134, 159
    hemosiderotic, 159
    herpes zoster ophthalmicus-related, 69
    hyphema-associated, 156, 158–159, 160
    lens-particle, 132
    low-tension, 111
    malignant/cilliary block, 120, 124–125, 127–128, 133, 148
    medical treatment of, 136–141
    narrow angle, 126
    neovascular, 121, 128, 281, 310, 313–314
    open-angle, 111
        secondary, 130–135
    pathogenesis of, 113–114
    peripheral vision loss associated with, 112–113
    phacoanaphylactic, 132
    phacolytic, 163–164
    phacomorphic, 163–164
    postoperative, 133
    predisposing factors for, 111–112
    primary open-angle, 160
    as red eye cause, 48
    referrals for evaluation of, 116
    retinoblastoma-related, 323
    as ring scotoma cause, 46
    secondary, hyphema-related, 265
    steroids-related, 80–81, 159
    trabeculectomy surgery for, 124, 142–150
    treatment goals in, 114
    treatment-related stabilization of, 115–116
    vasospastic, 113–114
    visual field findings in, 46
Glaucomatocyclitic crisis, 60
Glaukomflecken, 121, 122, 125
Glioma, 221, 232, 237
Globe
    Duane syndrome-related retraction of, 191, 192
    lacerated, 286
    rupture of, 3, 52–53, 153, 286
        as hyphema cause, 151
        scleral suture-related, 200

Globe *(cont.)*
  ultrasound evaluation of, 38, 39
  vertical displacement of, 194
Glycerin, as glaucoma treatment, 123, 136
Goldberg syndrome, 308
Goldenhar's syndrome, 192
Goldman-Favre syndrome, 32
Goldmann gonioscope, 119
Goldmann three-mirror lens, 118
Goldmann visual field, 45–46
Goldmann-Weekers adaptometer, 36
Goniolens, 118–119
Gonioscopy, 59, 114, 140
  for anterior chamber angle visualization, 3, 118–120
  for hyphema evaluation, 159
  indentation, 123
  for primary angle closure glaucoma evaluation, 125
  for secondary open-angle glaucoma evaluation, 130, 131, 132
  technique of, 119
  for traumatic hyphema evaluation, 153
Goniosynechiolysis, 124
Gonococcal infections, 48–49, 68–69, 72, 73, 74
Gout, 56, 57
Gradenigo's syndrome, 216
Granulocyte colony-stimulating factor, 268
Granuloma
  choroidal, 259
  eosinophilic, 232
Graves' disease, 88, 234, 236, 244–245
Green light rays, refraction of, 17
Guarded filtering procedure. *See* Trabeculectomy
Guillain-Barré syndrome, 197
Gumma, 260
Guttate conditions, corneal membrane dystrophy-related, 92
Gyrate atrophy, of the retina and choroid, 32

HAART (highly active antiretoviral therapy), 269
Haemophilus, cultures of, 63
Haemophilus influenzae infections, 54, 72, 236
Hallevorden-Spatz disease, 308
Harada's disease, 316
Harada-Ito procedure, 215
Hay fever, 96
Hemangioma
  as acquired astigmatism cause, 22
  capillary, 232
  cavernous, 232, 237, 238, 340, 342
  choroidal, 41, 316, 334, 335
  orbital capillary, 340, 345
  ultrasound evaluation of, 335
Hemangiopericytoma, 238, 340, 342
Hemianopia, 45, 46
Hemoglobin A_1C, correlation with diabetic retinopathy, 301
Hemorrhage
  cataract surgery-related, 171, 172
  choroidal, 41, 172
  of optic disc, 271
  of optic nerve sheath, 171
  orbital, 341
  postoperative, 151, 171, 172
  preretinal, 287, 300
  recurrent, hyphema-related, 156, 157
  retinal
    cytomegalovirus retinitis-related, 267, 268
    fundus trauma-related, 287
    interferon-related, 277
    in leukemia, 265

Hemorrhage *(cont.)*
  retinal *(cont.)*
    retinal arterial obstruction-related, 307, 313
    retinal venous obstruction-related, 310
  retrobulbar, 171, 235, 251
  subchoroidal, 121
  subconjunctival, 53, 55
  subretinal, differentiated from choroidal melanoma, 328
  suprachoroidal, 121
  vitreous, 287
    as amblyopia cause, 176, 179
    contrast-enhanced magnetic resonance studies of, 231–232
    diabetic retinopathy-related, 134, 300, 303, 304–305, 304–305
    retinal vein occlusion-related, 312, 313, 314
    scleral rupture-related, 284
    talc retinopathy-associated, 276
    traumatic hyphema-related, 153
    ultrasound evaluation of, 42
Heneralopia, 277
Hepatic disease, as aminocaproic acid contraindication, 155
Herpes simplex infections, 49
  as acute retinal necrosis cause, 261
  as conjunctivitis cause, 74
  as corneal infection cause, 65, 80
  as keratitis cause, 62
  as neonatal conjunctivitis cause, 72
  recurrence of, 69
  as uveitis cause, 60
Herpesvirus infections
  as granulomatous uveitis cause, 258
  as ophthalmia neonatorum cause, 72, 74
Herpes zoster virus infections, 3
  in AIDS patients, 267
  as corneal infection cause, 65, 80
  as episcleritis cause, 56
  as multiple ocular nerve palsy cause, 197
  as scleritis cause, 57
Herring's law, 251
Histiocytoma, fibrous, 232, 238, 340, 342
HLA-B 27 test, 59
Homatropine, 21
Homer Wright rosettes, 336
Homocystinuria, 120, 146
Homonymous visual field defects, 45
Horner's syndrome, 209, 210, 211, 215, 249
Horseshoe tears, 153, 283
Hruby lens, 20
Hurler syndrome, 308
Hutchinson's melanotic freckle, 256
Hutchinson's sign, 3, 69
Hydatid disease, orbital, 246
Hydrops, acute, 98–99
Hydroxychloroquine, as retinopathy cause, 274, 275
Hypercholesterolemia, 253
Hyperemia, conjunctival, 77
Hypermetropia, 179
Hyperopia
  absolute, 23
  accommodative esotropia-associated, 184
  accommodative requirements in, 18
  acquired, 22
  as cycloplegic refraction indication, 21
  definition of, 102
  direct ophthalmoscopic image size in, 19
  facultative, 23
  4-D, amplitude of accommodation in, 12
  latent, 23

Hyperopia *(cont.)*
  manifest, 23
  nanophthalmos-associated, 129
  round-top versus flat-top reading lens for, 15
  secondary focal point in, 11
  undercorrection of, 23
Hyperosmotic agents
  action mechanism of, 136, 137
  as acute hydrops treatment, 99
  as aqueous misdirection syndrome treatment, 127
  contraindication in sickle cell disease, 155
  as glaucoma treatment, 123, 127, 136
Hyperplasia, lymphoid, work-up of, 344
Hypersensitivity, staphylococcal, 50, 61, 67
Hypertension, 301, 312, 313
Hyperthyroidism, 239
Hypertropia
  Brown's syndrome-related, 199
  differential diagnosis of, 192
  far point in, 12
  superior oblique palsy-related, 213–214
Hyperviscosity syndromes, 313
Hyphema, **151–161**
  cataract surgery-related, 172
  definition of, 151
  eight-ball, 157, 159
  recurrent hemorrhage associated with, 156–157
  spontaneous, in children, 265
  traumatic, 152–154, 156, 160
Hypopyon, 64
Hypothyroidism, 239
Hypotony, 171
Hypotropia, 249
Hypoxia, 61, 67–68
Hysteria, 46, 222

ICE (iridocorneal endothelial) syndrome, 92, 121, 134
Image displacement, 15
Image jump, 15
Image point, 25 cm to the left of a +5.00 lens, 14
Imaging, orbital, **231–233**. *See also* Magnetic resonance imaging; Ultrasonography
  for thyroid-related ophthalmopathy evaluation, 240
Immunocompromised conditions. *See also* Acquired immunodeficiency syndrome (AIDS), ocular manifestations of
  as corneal ulcer risk factor, 62
Immunosuppression, as recurrent herpes simplex infection cause, 69
Incadescent light, 28
Incontinentia pigmenti, 298
Indocyanine green videoangiography, 231, 290
Infants. *See also* Neonates
  amblyopia screening of, 177
  cataracts in, 162
  Coats' disease in, 279, 281
  glaucoma in, 116
  herpes simplex infections in, 69
  myopia in, 102
  nystagmus in, 202
  premature
    oxygen therapy toxicity in, 277
    retinopathy in, 190, 194
  proptosis evaluation in, 345–346
  retinoblastoma in, 322, 335, 337
  visual acuity, 5
Infarction, ischemic, 212
Infection
  as chiasmal visual field defect cause, 221

Infection *(cont.)*
  orbital, 245–246
  strabismus surgery-related, 200
Inferior oblique overaction (IOOA), 186
Inferior oblique palsy, 193
Infiltrates
  choroidal, 264
  corneal, 67–68
  retinal, 264
Inflammation
  as angle closure cause, 128
  corticosteroid-refractory, 264
  definition of, 244
  as exudative retinal detachment cause, 316
  granulomatous, 286
  intraocular lens-related, 174
  melanoma-related, 265
  of the optic nerve. *See* Neuritis, optic
  orbital, **244–247**
    idiopathic, 232
  postoperative, 172
  as retinal arterial obstruction cause, 307, 308
Inflammatory bowel disease, 60
Influenza, as uveitis cause, 60
Infratrochlear nerve, in Hutchinson's sign, 3
Interference principle, 21
Interferon, 277–278, 292
Intracapsular cataract surgery, 166
Intracorneal ring, 107
Intraocular lens implants, 169–170
  complications of, 174
  insertion of, 165
  power calculations for, 17–18, 169–170
Intraocular pressure
  elevated, 112
    acute retinal necrosis-related, 261
    angle closure glaucoma-related, 121, 122, 123, 124, 125
    control of, with trabeculectomy, **142–150**
    as glaucoma risk factor, 111, 113
    laser peripheral iridotomy-related, 124
    steroids-related, 82
    trabeculotomy-related, 149, 313
  measurement of, 114
  medically "uncontrolled", 155, 156
  normal, 113
  post-trabeculectomy, 149, 150, 313
Iopidine, 140–141
Iridectomy
  laser, 151
  during trabeculectomy surgery, 143
Iridocorneal endothelial (ICE) syndrome, 92, 121, 134
Iridocyclectomy, 330
Iridocyclitis, Fuchs' heterochromatic, 133
Iridodialysis, 152, 153, 163
Iridotomy
  laser, 125, 126, 127
  peripheral, 123–124, 126
Iris
  adhesion to trabecular network, as glaucoma risk factor, 112
  as anterior chamber angle landmark, 117
  atrophy of, as diplopia cause, 212
  darkening of, 278
  injury to, as unilateral dilated, poorly reactive pupil cause, 209
  melanoma of, 334
  microhemangioma of, 151
  neovascularization of, 59, 151, 310

Iris *(cont.)*
  nodules of, 257
  peripheral configuration of, 120
  in primary angle closure glaucoma, 121, 125
  progressive atrophy of, 121
  prolapse of, cataract surgery-related, 171
  root insertion of, 120
  sphincter tears of, 152, 153
  trabeculectomy site blockage by, 148
Iris bombe, 128
Iris dilator muscle, 206
Iris sphincter muscle, 206
Iritis, 59, 272
Iron, toxicity of, 285–286
Irritation
  chronic, 53
  topical medication-related, 141
Ischemia
  anterior segment, 200, 201
  microvascular, as third-nerve palsy cause, 209
  of the optic nerve, 113, 114
  retinal arterial obstruction-related, 307, 308, 310
Ischemic tissue, retinal, "rescue" of, 310
Ischemic vascular disease, 197
Ishihara color plates, 244
Isoniazid, toxicity of, 259–260
Isosorbide, as glaucoma treatment, 136

Jackson cross, 23
Joint hypermobility, keratoconus-associated, 96
Jones, Lester, 9
Jones dye test, 228–229

Kaiser Fleischer ring, 286
Kaposi's sarcoma, 271, 272
Kawasaki's disease, 246
Kearns-Sayre syndrome, 194, 195
Kellman, Charles, 167
Keratectomy
  lamellar, 90
  photorefractive, 103, 105–106, 107, 108, 109–110
Keratitic precipitates, 61
Keratitis
  acanthamoeba, 63, 65
  disciform stromal, 70
  filamentary, 86
  fungal, 62
  herpetic, 49, 62, 69
    corneal membrane dystrophy-related, 92
    differentiated from herpes zoster ophthalmicus, 70
    recurrence of, 81–82
    steroid-related exacerbation of, 81
  interstitial, 259, 260
  Lyme disease-related, 261
  punctate superficial, 88
  superior limbic, 255
Keratoacanthoma, 253
Keratoconjunctivitis
  atopic, keratoconus-associated, 96
  superior limbic, 56, 244
  vernal, 99
Keratoconjunctivitis sicca, 49, 50, **84–88**, 85, 246
  as corneal ulcer cause, 61
  radiation therapy-related, 255
  tearing associated with, 227
  topical medication-related, 141
Keratoconus, 93, **95–101**
  as acquired myopia cause, 22
  as diplopia cause, 212

Keratometer, 20
Keratometry, 17, 18
Keratopathy
  corneal membrane dystrophy-related, 92
  exposure, proptosis-related, 234
  neutrophilic, 61
  superficial punctate, 49, 50, 54
Keratoplasty, penetrating, 91, 100, 101
Keratosis, 252
Keratotomy
  astigmatic, 108
  excimer laser photo-astigmatic, 108
  radial, 103, 104, 105, 106, 107, 109
Keratouveitis, 70, 81–82
Kestenbaum procedure, 204
Knapp procedure, 193
Knapp's rules, 215
Koeppe nodules, 257
Kollner's rule, 29
Krukenberg spindles, 130, 131

Lacrimal bone, 1
Lacrimal glands
  accessory, 5, 6
  inflammation of. *See* Dacryoadenitis
  removal of, lack of tear deficiency following, 5
  sarcoid infiltration of, 49
  stenosis of, radiation therapy-related, 255
  tumors of, 49, 235, 343–344
Lacrimal nerve, location of, 8
Lacrimal pump mechanism, orbicularis oculi muscle
  involvement in, 10
Lacrimal system, **226–230**
  anatomy of, 226
  obstructions of, 228–229
Lacrisert, 87
Lagophthalmos, 4–5, 62
Lamina cribosa, retinoblastoma invasion of, 336
Large cell sarcoma, as uveitis masquerade syndrome, 258
Lasers (light amplification by stimulated emission of
  radiation), 22
  as anterior stromal puncture treatment, 90
  use in cataract surgery, 168
  use in capsulotomy, 173, 174
  as corneal dystrophy treatment, 90
  as corneal erosion treatment, 52
  use in cyclodestruction, 128
  use in hyaloidotomy, 127
  use in iridectomy, 151
  use in iridoplasty, 127
  use in iridotomy, 123–124, 125, 127
  use in photocoagulation
    as age-related macular degeneration treatment,
      291–292
    in darkly pigmented fundi, 4
    panretinal, 310
    as retinal detachment treatment, 318
    as retinal dialysis prophylaxis, 283
    as retinoblastoma treatment, 323, 324
    as retinopathy of prematurity treatment, 296–297
  use in photoreactive keratectomy, 105
  as puncta closure technique, 88
  use in trabeculectomy surgery, 142, 143–144
Latanaprost, 136, 138–139
Lateral inhibition, in color perception, 27
Lattice degeneration, 316, 317
Leber's congenital amaurosis, 32, 34, 96, 202
Leber's miliary aneurysm, 279
Leber's optic atrophy, 45, 225

Lens. *See also* Spectacles, lens of
anterior subscapular region of, orange deposits in, 278
capsule of
leakage through, 132
opacity of, 212
dislocated, 22, 163
extraction of, as aqueous misdirection syndrome
treatment, 128
Hruby, 20
innervation of, 5
intraocular decentration of, as diplopia cause, 212
in primary angle closure glaucoma, 121, 125
refractive function of, 102
subluxation of, 120, 153, 212
Lens-iris diaphragm, anterior displacement of, 112
Lensmeters, 20
Lentigo maligna, 256
Leprosy, 258
Leukemia
as hyphema cause, 151
retinal involvement in, 265
as uveitis masquerade syndrome, 258, 263
Leukemic infiltrates, orbital, 232
Leukocoria, 338
retinoblastoma-related, 231, 263, 322, 335
Levator muscle
congenital maldevelopment of, 249
dehiscence of, 196, 248
function measurement of, in ptosis patients, 250–251
Levobunolol, as glaucoma treatment, 136, 137, 138
Light
spectrum of, 24
transmission to the brain, 25
visual perception of, 24
Light/near dissociation, 211
Light rays, vergence of, 14
Light reflex test, 190, 194
Limbus, surgical, 3
Lincoff balloon, 318
Liposarcoma, 341
Liver, as uveal melanoma metastasis site, 333
Loupes, as low vision aids, 19
Lower lid retractors, 9
Low vision aids, 19, 293
Lung cancer, metastatic, 334, 344
Lye burns, 54
Lyme disease, 56, 59, 60, 258, 260–261
Lymphadenopathy, preauricular, 69
Lymphangioma, 232, 340, 341, 342
Lymphatics, absence of, from the orbit, 344
Lymphoma
orbital, 235, 237–238, 344
primary intraocular, 264
as uveitis masquerade syndrome, 258, 263
Lymphoproliferative disorders, 232

Macula
anatomy of, 5
cherry-red spots of, 308
clinical, 288
ectopia of, 294
edema of, effect on potential acuity, 21
holes in, 283
representation in the visual cortex, 6
retinoblastoma of, 335
scars of, as amblyopia cause, 176
vertical dsiplacement of, 194
Macular degeneration, age-related, **288–293**, 328
electroretinographic evaluation of, 32

Macular degeneration, age-related *(cont.)*
effect on potential acuity meter readings, 21
Maculopathy
bull's eye, 274
chelating agent-related, 278
ischemic, 276, 312, 313
Magnetic resonance imaging (MRI)
of cavernous hemangioma, 340
of dermoid cysts, 344, 345
fat suppression, 341, 342
for idiopathic infantile nystagmus evaluation, 203
for intraocular foreign body detection, 285
for multiple sclerosis prediction, 219
orbital, 231–233, 245, 341–342
of orbital inflammation, 245
of proptosis, 236
of retinoblastoma, 326
of sinusitis, 345
Magnification, 18
Magnification formula, for telescopes, 18–19
Magnifiers, hand-held, 19
Malingering, 46
Malnutrition, as glaucoma risk factor, 111
MALT (musoca-associated lymphoid tissue) lymphoma,
344
Mannitol, as glaucoma treatment, 136
Marcus Gunn jaw winking syndrome, 249, 251
Marfan's syndrome, 120, 146, 163
Marginal reflex distance, measurement of, in ptosis
patients, 250
Marijuana, effect on tear production, 85
Masquerade syndromes, 258, **263–266**
Maxillary nerve, 9
McLean, Ian, 332
Measles, as uveitis cause, 60
Medulloepithelioma, 338
Meibomian glands, 6, 84, 227
infections of, 67, 85
Meibomianitis, 50
Melanocytoma, 330
Melanoma
choroidal, 316, 317, 328
differentiated from hemorrhagic retinal detachment,
231–232
malignant, 329, 332
mushroom-shaped, 328, 332
peripheral, 329
ultrasound evaluation of, 40–41
of ciliary bodies, 329
cutaneous, 323
of the eyelid, 252, 256
as hyphema cause, 151
imaging of, 341
inflammatory response associated with, 265
of the iris, 334
spindle cells in, 332, 333
uveal, 329, 330, 332, 333, 335
as uveitis masquerade syndrome, 60, 258, 263
Melanoma cells, histopathologic differentiation of,
332–333
Mellaril (thioridazine), as retinopathy cause, 275
Meningioma, 197, 221
Meningitis, 54, 74, 271
Meniscus
normal, 49
tears of, as red eye cause, 49, 56
Meretoja's syndrome, 91
Metallosis, electroretinographic findings in, 35
Metals, ocular toxicity of, 285

Metamorphopsia, 212, 289
Metapranolol, as glaucoma treatment, 137
Metastases
    as hyphema cause, 151
    orbital, 232
    of orbital soft tissue, 344
    ultrasound evaluation of, 41, 335
    uveal, 332, 334
Meters, relationship to diopters, 14
Methazolamide, as glaucoma treatment, 136, 141
    in surgical patients, 138
Methoxyfluorane anesthesia, as retinopathy cause, 276
Methylphenidate hydrochloride, talc component of, 276
Microaneurysms, diabetic retinopathy-related, 300, 302
Microhemangioma, of the iris, 151
Micropannus, corneal, superior, 56
Microphthalmos, 249
Migraine, 209, 249
Millard-Gruber syndrome, 216
Miosis, Horner's syndrome-associated, 209, 210
Miotics, 136
    action mechanism of, 136, 137
    as glaucoma treatment, 123, 138–139
    implication for cataract surgery, 174
    as plateau iris treatment, 127
    as refractive accommodative esotropia treatment, 187
    topical, contraindication in narrow-angle glaucuoma, 126
Mirrors
    convex, vergence of, 19
    reflecting power of, 20
Mitomycin C, 147, 148
Mitral valve prolapse, 96
Mobius syndrome, 185, 194, 194
Mohs' lamellar resection, 254
Molluscum contagiosum, 54, 55, 253
Monochromatism, rod. See Achromatopsia
Morning glory disc syndrome, 316
Morphine, effect on tear production, 85
Mucin, as tear film component, 5, 227
Mucocele, 194, 197, 345
Mucormycosis, 235, 246, 345
Multiple myeloma, 91
Multiple sclerosis
    as diplopia cause, 212
    as internuclear ophthalmoplegia cause, 197
    optic neuritis as risk factor for, 218–220
    as ptosis cause, 249
    uveitis associated with, 266
    as uveitis masquerade syndrome, 258, 263
Mumps, as uveitis cause, 60
Munson's sign, 97
Muscle, slipped, 200
Muscle surgery, as thyroid-related ophthalmopathy
    treatment, 242, 243
Muscular dystrophies, 249
Mutton-fat keratic precipitates, 257
Myasthenia gravis, 216
    as diplopia cause, 212, 213, 215, 216
    as hypertropia cause, 192
    mimics of, 196
    as multiple cranial nerve palsy mimic, 197
    as ptosis cause, 196, 216, 249, 250
    signs and symptoms of, 250
Mycobacteria, cultures of, 63
Myopathy, as diplopia cause, 212
Myopia
    acquired, 22
    axial, 12
    Bruch's membrane defects-related, 4

Myopia (cont.)
    cataracts-related, 165
    corrective lens for, refraction of, 17
    definition of, 102
    direct ophthalmoscopic image size in, 19
    far point in, 12
    4-D, amplitude of accommodation in, 12
    nuclear sclerotic cataract-related, 162
    prevention of overcorrection of, 17
    refractive, 12
        surgical treatment for, 102, 103–107, 108–109
    residual, post-refractive surgery, 108–109
    retinopathy of prematurity-related, 297
    as rhegmatogenous retinal detachment risk factor, 316
    round-top versus flat-top reading lens for, 16
    secondary focal point in, 11
    as surgery-related vitreous loss risk factor, 146
Myositis, 246
Myotonic dystrophy, 35

Nanopthalmos, 129, 316
Nasolacrimal duct, obstruction of, 228
    congenital, 73, 229, 230
Nasolacrimal sac, abscess of, 77
Nasopharyngeal carcinoma, 197
Natamycin, 65
Near point, 12
Near point exercises, 191
Near reflex, spasm of, 212
Nearsightedness. See Myopia
    nuclear sclerotic cataracts-related, 162
Necrosis, retinal, 261, 269
Neisseria, cultures of, 63
Neisseria gonorrhoeae infections, 48–49, 72
Neomycin, 80
Neonates
    amblyopia screening of, 177
    esotropia in, 183
    glaucoma in, 111
    orthotropia in, 183
    strabismus in, 183
Neoplasms, ocular, 332–339
Neosynephrine test, 251
Neuralgia, postherpetic, 69
Neurilemoma, orbital, 232
Neuritis, optic, 218–220, 246. See also Neuropathy, optic
    in AIDS patients, 270
    as central retinal artery obstruction cause, 306
    definition of, 218
    as multiple sclerosis risk factor, 218–220
    retrobulbar, in AIDS patients, 270
    visual outcome in, 218–219
Neurofibroma, 134, 232, 238
Neurologic disturbances, miscellaneous, 221–225
Neuromuscular junction disorders, as diplopia cause, 212
Neuromyotonia, ocular, as diplopia cause, 212
Neuropathy, optic, 221–225
    as diplopia cause, 212
    ischemic, 222
    Leber's hereditary, 225
    radiation therapy-related, 255
    retinal necrosis-related, 261
    toxic/nutritional, 45, 259–260, 270
    traumatic cataract-related, 163
Neuroretinitis, 25, 261
Nevus
    choroidal, 41, 327, 328
    of Ota, 329
    uveal, 330

Nicotinic acid, as cystoid macula edema cause, 276
Niemann-Pick disease, 308
Night blindness, 32, 34, 35, 36
Night vision, 24
Nocardia, cultures of, 63
Nodal point, 14
Nodules
    Busacca, 257
    Koeppe, 257
    preauricular, 48, 54
Nonsteroidal antiinflammatory drugs, 58, 109, 151, 154
Null point, of periodic alternating nystagmus, 204
Null zone, in idiopathic infantile nystagmus, 202, 203
Nutrition, as age-related macular degeneration treatment, 292
Nyctalopia, 275, 278
Nystagmus, **202–205**
    congenital esotropia-related, 186
    convergence retraction, 212
Nystagmus blockage syndrome, 185, 188, 202

Obesity, as glaucoma risk factor, 111
Occlusion, vascular retinal. *See also* Retinal arterial
        occlusion; Retinal venous occlusion
    drug-induced, 277
Ocular deviations
    congenital esotropia-associated, 184
    miscellaneous, **190–197**
Oculocerebrorenal syndrome, 134
Oculomotor nerve palsies. *See* Cranial nerve palsies, third
Ofloxacin, 64, 68
Oguchi's disease, 35
Ophthalmia, sympathetic, 60, 258, 260, 286–287
Ophthalmia neonatorum, **72–75**
Ophthalmic artery
    in acute angle closure glaucoma, 121
    obstruction of, 34, 306, 308
Ophthalmic nerve, 9
Ophthalmicus, herpetic, 69
Ophthalmoplegia
    chronic progressive external, 249
    internuclaer, 197, 316
Ophthalmoscope/ophthalmoscopy, 114
    direct, 18, 19, 20
    indirect, 20, 285, 319
    use in orbital inflammation evaluation, 244
Opsins, 25
Optic chiasm
    crossed and uncrossed fibers of, 4
    lesions of, 208, 221
Optic disc
    choroidal nevus of, 327
    edema of, 287
    hypoplasia of, 202
    neovascularization of, 300, 301–302, 303, 304, 312, 314
    papillitis of, 270–271
    tilted, as bitemporal field defect mimic, 221
Optic nerve
    bilateral swollen, 223
    compression of, 234, 241, 242
    in cytomegalovirus retinitis, 268
    in glaucoma, 113, 115, 122, 126
    glioma of, 221, 237
    HIV infection of, 270
    injury to
        as central retinal artery obstruction cause, 306
        traumatic hyphema-related, 153
    lesions of
        as afferent pupillary defect cause, 208
        differentiated from optic nerve sheath lesions, 233

Optic nerve *(cont.)*
    in Lyme disease, 261
    melanocytoma of, 330
    meninges of, 341
    in papillitis, 270–271
    retinoblastoma invasion of, 323, 336, 337
    in syphilis, 260
Optic pits, as exudative retinal detachment cause, 136
Optics, **11–23**. *See also* Refraction
Optic tract, lesions of, as afferent pupillary defect cause,
        208
Optociliary shunt vessels, 223
Oral contraceptives, 49, 278
Orbicularis oculi muscle, three portions of, 9, 10
Orbit
    absence of lymphatic vessels and nodes from, 2
    adnexal trauma to, 284
    anatomy of, 7–8
    bones of, 1, 7, 341
    cellulitis of, 344
    complete examination of, 244
    degenerative diseases of, 244
    fat/fat pads of, 2
    foreign bodies in, 53
    imaging of, **231–233**
        for thyroid-related ophthalmopathy evaluation, 240
    infections of, 245–246
    inflammatory conditions of, **244–247**
    lesions of, as multiple cranial nerve palsy mimic, 197
    lymphoma of, 237–238, 344
    retinoblastoma invasion of, 323
    schematic cross-section of, 2
    septum of, 2
    structural disorders of, 244
    in thyroid-related ophthalmopathy, 241
    trauma to, 192
    tumors/cancer of, 244, **340–347**
        contrast-enhanced magnetic resonance evaluation of,
                232–233
        thyroid disease-related, 241
    vascular disorders of, 244
Orbital disease, as central retinal artery obstruciton cause, 306
Orbital foramina, retinoblastoma invasion of, 337
Orbital inflammatory pseudotumor, 192, 196
Orbital rim, weak areas of, 7
Orthophoria, 190, 192
Orthotropia, 183, 185
Osteogenesis imperfecta, 96
Osteoma, choroidal, 38
Osteosarcoma, retinoblastoma associated with, 323
Otitis media, 54, 73
Oxalosis, 276

Pachymeter, 20
Pain, orbital, evaluation of, 244
Paint pigments, 28
Palatine bone, 1
Palpebral fissure, measurement of, in ptosis patients, 250
Pancreatitis, 287, 309
Panophthalmitis, 260, 261
Papillae, superior palpebral, 56
Papilledema, 223, 227, 271
Papillitis, in AIDS patients, 270–271
Papules, acne rosacea-related, 50
Paracentesis, 143, 148, 157, 309
Paralysis
    divergence, 217
    pharmacologic, as unilateral dilated, poorly reactive
            pupil cause, 209

Parinaud's syndrome, 197, 211, 217
Parkinsonism, 217
Parotid duct transfer, 88
Pars plana, vitrectomy of, 318, 319
  failure of, 320
Pars planitis, 60, 264
Patching
  as amblyopia treatment, 179
  as corneal dystrophy treatment, 90
  as hyphema treatment, 154
  pressure, contraindication in corneal abrasions, 52
  risks of, 179
Penalization, as amblyopia treatment, 179
"Pencil push-ups", 191
Penicillin, allergic responses to, 79
Perfluoropropane, 319
Perimetry, 47
Peripheral vision, glaucoma-related loss of, 112–113
Peter's anomaly, 5
Phacodenesis, 163
Phacoemulsification, 109, 167–168
Phenothiazines, 35, 49, 275, 276
Photocoagulation. See also Lasers (light amplification by
    stimulated emission of radiation), use in
    photocoagulation
  as Coats' disease treatment, 280
  panretinal, 303–304
  as uveal malignant melanoma treatment, 333
Photodynamic therapy, for age-related macular
    degeneration, 292
Photons, 24
Photophobia
  corneal dystrophy-related, 89
  corneal ulcer-related, 61
  dry eyes-related, 85
  herpes simplex virus-related, 49
  idiopathic infantile nystagmus-related, 205
  in infants, 116, 205
  superior limbic keratoconjunctivitis-related, 56
  uveitis-related, 58
Photoreceptor response, 31
Photoreceptors, 24, 316
Photothermotherapy, as uveal malignant melanoma
    treatment, 333
Phthisis bulbi, 44, 249
Phylectenulosis, 50, 259
Physiologic blind spot, 45
"Pie-in-the-sky" lesions, 45, 227–228
Pigment dispersion syndrome, 114, 115, 131–132
Pigmented lesions, of the ocular fundus, **327–331**
Pigment, 25, 28
Pilocarpine, 87
  adverse effects of, 22, 48, 137–138, 139
  discontinuation prior to trabeculectomy surgery, 143
  as glaucoma treatment, 136, 137–138, 139–141
  Ocuserts of, 139
Pilocarpine HS ophthalmic gel, 140
Pinealoblastoma, 322, 338
Pingueculum, 53
Pinhole diameter, most effective, 21
"Pink eye", 48
Pituitary tumors, 221
Plaque brachyradiotherapy, 323, 324, 333
Plateau iris syndrome, 112, 120, 126–127
"Plus disease", 295
Pneumonia, 54
Pneumonitis, 73
Polyarteritis nodosa, 57, 246
Polyarthropathy, 278

Polycoria, 212
Polymyxin B, 77, 80
Polysporin, 77
Posner four-mirror lens gonioscope, 118
Posner-Schloss syndrome, 132–133
Potential acuity testing, 21, 165
Power (P), of schematic eye, 14
Preauricular nodes, 48, 54
Prednisolone, 81, 82, 146
Prednisone
  contraindication in optic neuritis, 219
  as optic neuritis treatment, 218–219, 220
Pregnancy
  as acyclovir contraindication, 71
  as aminocaproic acid contraindication, 155
  as diabetic retinopathy risk factor, 301
  as doxycycline contraindication, 50
  as retinal arterial obstruction risk factor, 309
  as tetracycline contraindication, 50
Prentice's law, 15
Preoperative examination, of ptosis patients, 250
Presbyopia, 102, 103
Pressure patches, containdication in corneal abrasions, 52
Primary focal point, 11
Prince rule, 23
Principal plane, 14
Prisms, 14–15, 24, 242
Progressive outer retinal necrosis, 269
Progressive supranuclear palsy, 197, 217
Prolactinoma, 221
Propionibacterium acnes, as granulomatous uveitis cause,
    258
Proptosis, **234–238**
  bilateral, 235, 236
  cavernous hemangioma-related, 237
  classification of, 244
  contrast-enhanced magnetic resonance studies of, 232–233
  evaluation of, 244
  Graves' ophthalmopathy-related, 236
  magnetic resonance imaging of, 232
  paranasal sinus mucocele-related, 345
  pediatric, 342, 345–346
  thyroid-related ophthalmopathy-related, 239, 240, 241
  unilateral, 236
Prostaglandins, 136, 137
Pseudoesotropia, 183, 185
Pseudoexfoliation, 120, 130, 146, 163
Pseudo-Foster-Kennedy syndrome, 225
Pseudoguttae, 92
Pseudohypertropia, 192, 194
Pseudohypopyon, 263–264
Pseudomonas infections
  as conjunctivitis cause, 72, 74
  in contact lens wearers, 62–63
  as corneal infection cause, 66
  as ophthalmia neonatorum cause, 74
  as red eye cause, 52
Pseudopapilledema, 227
Pseudoproptosis, 235
Pseudoptosis, 193, 249
Pseudoretinoblastoma, 322
Pseudostrabismus, 190, 190
Pseudotumor, 235, 246
Pseudotumor cerebri, 223–224, 261
Pseudoxanthoma elasticum, 4
Pterygium, 53
Ptosis, **248–251**
  acquired, 248
  as acquired astigmatism cause, 22

Ptosis *(cont.)*
  as amblyopia cause, 176, 178–179, 180
  aponeurotic, 248
  chronic progressive external ophthalmoplegia-
    associated, 194, 195
  classification of, 248
  congenital, 248–249
  congenital fibrosis syndrome-associated, 194
  double elevator palsy-associated, 193
  Horner's syndrome-associated, 209, 210, 211
  myasthenia gravis-associated, 196
  nonsurgical correction of, 251
  orbital inflammation-associated, 246
  surgical correction of, 251
    eye closure difficulty after, 49
  third nerve palsy-associated, 213
Puncta, closure of, in dry eye conditions, 87–88
Pupil, **206–211**
  abnormalities of, in syphilis, 260
  Adie's tonic, 209, 210
  afferent defects of, 180, 207–208, 284
  aneurysm of, 212
  Argyle-Robertson, 211
  innervation of, 206
  muscular control of, 206
  nonreactive, as diplopia cause, 212
  unilateral dilated, poorly reactive, 209
Pupillary block, 120
  as angle closure glaucoma cause, 159
  as flat anterior chamber cause, 148
  relative. *See* Glaucoma, angle closure, primary
Pupillary dilation, of cataracts, 165
Pupillary light reflex, 207
Pustules, acne rosacea-related, 50

Quadrantanopia, 46
Quinine intoxication, 35
Quinine sulfate, as retinopathy cause, 275, 276

Radiation therapy
  as basal cell carcinoma treatment, 255
  complications of, 255
  as orbital rhabdomyosarcoma treatment, 342–343
  as orbital sarcoma cause, 338
  as retinoblastoma treatment, 323, 338
  as thyroid-related ophthalmopathy treatment, 241
Radio waves, 24
Recess-resect procedure, 198
Rectus muscles
  inferior, entrapment of, 194
  medial, slipped or lost, 194
  recession of, 1, 204, 243
  resection of, 193, 194
  in strabismus surgery, 198, 198, 199
  in thyroid-related ophthalmopathy, 234, 240
Recurrent erosion syndrome, 62
Red eye, **48–60**
  central retinal vein occlusion-related, 313
  conjunctivitis-related, 53–55, 56
  in contact lens wearers, 51–52
  corneal ulcer-related, 61
  dry, 49
  foreign body-related, 52–53
Red-green duochrome test, 17
Red light rays, refraction by plus lens, 17
Reese Ellsworth classification system, for retinoblastoma,
    324–325
Referrals, 55, 116
Reflection, total internal, 13

Refraction, **11–23**
  critical angle of, 13
  cycloplegic
    in accommodative insufficiency, 191
    in acquired myopia, 22
    indications for, 21
    in neonates, 190
    in uncorrection of hyperopia, 23
  of green light rays, 17
  plus cylinder conversion to minus cylinder form of, 16
  spherical equivalents in, 16
  in with-the-rule astigmatism, 16
Refractive elements, of the eye, 102
Refractive errors
  congenital esotropia-associated, 184
  corrective lens for, 12
Refractive index, 12–13, 14
Refractive surgery, **102–110**
  as astigmatism treatment, 102, 108
  as hyperopia treatment, 109
  indications and contraindications for, 96, 102–103
  as myopia treatment, 102, 103–107, 108–109
Refsum's disease, 195
Reiter's syndrome, 59
Relative luminosity curves, 27
Renal disease, 71, 155, 301
Reticulum cell sarcoma, 263, 264
Retina
  in acute angle closure glaucoma, 122
  attachment mechanisms of, 316
  breaks of, 316–317
  degenerative conditions of, 32
  disorders of, electroretinographic evaluation of, 31
  dragging of, retinopathy of prematurity-related, 297, 298
  holes in, 283, 297
    horseshoe tears, 153, 283
  infiltrates of, primary intraocular sarcoma-related, 264
  lesions of
    as afferent pupillary defect cause, 208
    as monocular diplopia cause, 21
  leukemic involvement of, 265
  necrosis of, 258, 283
  neovascularization of
    diabetic retinopathy-related, 300, 301–302, 303, 304
    oxygen therapy-related, 277
    retinal vein occlusion-related, 312, 314
    talc retinopathy-related, 276
  photoreceptors of, 24, 316
  in primary angle closure glaucoma, 126
11-cis Retinal, 25
Retinal arterial obstruction, **306–311**
  acute retinal necrosis-related, 261
  bilateral, 309
  branch type, 278, 306
    Lyme disease-related, 261
    symptoms of, 307
  central type, 278, 306
    as angle closure cause, 121
    appearance of, 308
    cianretinal artery in, 4
    electroretinographic findings in, 35
    emergency treatment for, 310
    symptoms of, 307
  combined type, 310
  differentiated from retinal venous obstruction, 310
  drug-induced, 278
  late complications of, 310
  prophylactic treatment for, 309
  treatment for, 309–310

Retinal arterioles, structure of, 6
Retinal artery, central
  in acute angle closure glaucoma, 121
  structure of, 6
Retinal capillary occlusion, 287
Retinal detachment, **315–321**
  in AIDS patients, 269, 270
  as angle closure cause, 121
  cataract surgery-related, 173
  chronic, 42
  Coats' disease-related, 280, 281
  cytomegalovirus retinitis-related, 269, 270
  definition of, 315
  dialysis-related, 283, 284
  exudative, 128, 315, 316, 317
  hemorrhagic, differentiated from choroidal melanoma,
    231–232
  iatrogenic, 319
  laser capsulotomy-related, 173
  peripheral, as uveitis masquerade syndrome, 258, 263,
    266
  repair of, 317–318
    failure of, 320
  retinoblastoma-related, 325
  retinopathy of prematurity-related, 294, 295–296, 297
  rhegmatogenous, 315
    predisposing factors for, 316
    repair of, 317, 319
    retinal vein occlusion-related, 312, 313, 314
  total, electroretinographic findings in, 35
  traction, 312, 315
    combined with rhegmatogenous retinal detachment,
      305
    diabetic retinopathy-related, 305
    proliferative vitreoretinopathy-related, 320
    repair of, 317–318, 320
    retinal vein occlusion-related, 313, 314
  traumatic cataract-related, 163
  ultrasound evaluation of, 41–42
  vitrectomy-related, in diabetic patients, 305
  vitreous loss-related, 173
Retinal pigment epithelium, 316
  age-related macular degeneration-related changes in,
    288, 289
  in choroidal ruptures, 284
  congenital, 327, 328
  desferrioxamine-related changes in, 278
  in scleral blunt trauma, 283
  tamoxifen-related, 277
  thioridazine-related changes in, 275
Retinal vein occlusive disease, **312–314**
  acute retinal necrosis-erlated, 261
  branch type, 4, 312–313
  central type, 313–314
    electroretinographic findings in, 34, 35
    ischemic, 314
  differentiated from retinal arterial obstruction, 310
  drug-induced, 278
Retinitis
  cytomegalovirus-related, in AIDS patients, 267–269, 270
  herpetic, as retinal arterial obstruction cause, 307
  progressive peripheral, acute retinal necrosis-related, 261
  syphilitic, 260
Retinitis pigmentosa, 32, 96, 266
  clinical features of, 32–33
  conditions which mimic, 32
  electro-oculographic findings in, 36, 36
  electroretinographic findings in, 33, 34
  as ring scotoma cause, 46

Retinitis pigmentosa *(cont.)*
  sector, as bitemporal field defect mimic, 221
  as uveitis masquerade syndrome, 263
  X-linked, female carriers of, 33
Retinitis pigmentosa sine pigmento, 32
Retinitis punctate albescens, 32
Retinoblastoma, 231, **322–326**, 337
  bilateral, 337
  classification of, 324–325
  definition of, 322
  differentiated from Coats' disease, 231, 279–280
  familial, 324, 335, 337, 338
  as hyphema cause, 151
  imaging studies of, 231
  low-magnification light microscopic appearance of, 336
  as mortality cause, 337
  as most common primary intraocular tumor, 332
  prognostic features of, 336
  second cancers associated with, 323
  signs and symptoms of, 335
  sporadic, 335, 337–338
  trilateral, 322
  ultrasound evaluation of, 38
  unilateral, 337
  as uveitis masquerade syndrome, 60, 258, 263–264
Retinoblastoma gene, 322, 338
Retinopathy
  cancer-associated, 35
  crystalline, 276
  decompression, 126
  diabetic, **300–305**
    cataract surgery-related exacerbation of, 174
    proliferative, 320
    ultrasound evaluation of, 42
  hypertensive, 304
  pigmentary, iron overload-related, 278
  of prematurity, 190, 194, 277, **294–299**
  Purtscher's, 287
  radiation-related, 255, 304
  toxic, **274–278**
Retinoplexy, pneumatic, 318, 320
Retinoschisis, X-linked, 32, 33, 35, 36, 298
Retinoscopy, "with" movement during, 20
Retrobulbar injection, of anesthesia, 1, 165, 166
Rhabdomyosarcoma, 232, 237, 340, 342–343, 345
Rheumatoid arthritis, 49, 57, 61, 62, 85
Rhinophyma, 50
Rhodopsin, 25
Rieger's anomaly, 134
Rifabutin, 272
Rimexolone, 82
Ritalin, talc component of, 276
Rods, 24–25, 27
Rosettes, in retinoblastoma, 336
Roth spots, 265
Rubella syndrome, congenital, 33, 134
"Rule of 50s", 343

Salicylates, as retinopathy cause, 276
"Sand in the eyes" sensation, 50
Sandoff disease, 308
Sarcoid, as uveitis cause, 60
Sarcoidosis, 131
  definition of, 259
  differentiated from diabetic retinopathy, 304
  as granulomatous uveitis cause, 258
  optic neuritis associated with, 218
  orbital, 246
  as scleritis cause, 57

Sarcoma, 323, 338
Schirmer test, 86–87, 227
Schlemm's canal, 117
Schwalbe's line, 3, 117
Schwannoma, 238, 341, 342
Sclera
    blunt trauma to, 283
    in globe ruptures, 3
    rupture of, 153, 284
    thinnest area of, 3
Scleral buckling, 318, 319
    as acquired myopia cause, 22
    failure of, 320
        in AIDS patients, 270
    as retinal detachment cause, 284
Scleral flaps, 143–144
Scleral spur, 117
Scleritis
    acute retinal necrosis-related, 261
    differentiated from episcleritis, 56
    necrotizing, 57, 58
    nodular anterior, 57
    posterior, 57, 316
    as red eye cause, 48, 56, 57–58
    syphilitic, 260
    tuberculosis-related, 259
Sclerocornea, 5
Scleroderma, 85
Scleromalacia perforans, 58
Sclerosis
    nuclear, 22
    systemic, 85
Scopolamine, 21, 85
Scotoma
    central, 218, 221, 289
    definition of, 45
    granulomatous uveitis-related, 257
    junctional, 221
    mascular, effect on potential acuity meter readings, 21
    paracentral, 277
    parafoveal, 274
    ring, 46, 278
Sebaceous cell carcinoma, of the eyelid, 255–256
Sebaceous gland carcinoma, 255
Secondary focal point, 11
Secondary membrane, 173
"Second sight", 162, 165
Sentinel vessels, 329
Sepsis, neonatal conjunctivitis-related, 74
Short wavelength automated perimetry (SWAP), 47
Shunts, aqueous tube, 128
Sickle cell disease, 153, 154, 155, 158, 304
Siderosis, 134, 285
Siderosis bulbi, 285–286
Silver, as retinopathy cause, 277
Silver nitrate drops, 56, 72, 73
Sinuses, paranasal, mucocele and carcinoma of, 345
Sinusitis, 236, 345
Sjögren's syndrome, 49, 85, 246
Skew deviation, 192, 217
Skin cancer, metastatic, 196
Skin lesions, herpes zoster, 69
Skin pigmentation, relationship to age-related macular
    degeneration, 288
Sky, color of, 28
Slit lamp examination, 97, 244
Smears, for corneal ulcer evaluation, 65–66
Smoking, as thyroid-related ophthalmopathy cause, 239
Snellen visual acuity test, 23, 165

Snell's law, 13
Snow blindness, 50
Solumedrol, as optic neuritis treatment, 218–220
Spectacles
    aniseikonia with, 18–19
    base curve determination of, 20
    for cataract patients, 165, 169
    as keratoconus treatment, 99
    lens of
        antireflective coatings on, 21
        binocular high-power single-vision, 19
        minus, effect on strabismic deviation measurements,
            15
        plus, 15–16, 17, 19
        round-top versus flat-top, 15–16
        spherical deviations of, 17
        strabismic deviation measurement of, 15
        thick, aberrations of, 17
        vertex distance measurement of, 21
    new, patients' dissatisfaction with, 21–22
    postoperative, patients' dissatisfaction with, 22
    power of
        comparison with contact lens, 12
        lensmeter measurement of, 20
    for ptosis correction, 251
Spherical aberration, of thick lens, 17
Spherical equivalents, 16
Sphingolidiposes, 308
Spindle cells, 332, 333
Spiraling, 46
Squamous cell carcinoma, 272
SRK formula, for intraocular lens implant calculation,
    17–18
Staphylococcal infections
    as conjunctivitis cause, 54, 72
    as orbital cellulitis cause, 236
    as posttraumatic endophthalmitis cause, 286
Steroids. See also Corticosteroids
    long-term, adverse effects of, 50
    post-trabeculectomy use of, 146
    subconjunctival injections of, contraindication in
        scleritis, 58
    as thyroid-related ophthalmopathy treatment, 241
    topical, 76–83
        as angle closure glaucoma treatment, 123
Steven-Johnson syndrome, 86
"Stork bites", 340
Strabismus
    as amblyopia cause, 176, 181
    astigmatism-associated, in children, 21
    cyclic, 188
    as cycloplegic refraction indication, 21
    measurement of, Prentice's rule of, 15
    myasthenia gravis-associated, 196
    neonatal, 183
    paralytic, 199
    retinal detachment repair surgery-related, 319
    retinoblastoma-related, 263, 335
    small-angle, 198
    surgical treatment of, 198–201
        in amblyopia patients, 181
        as monocular diplopia cause, 21
"Strawberry patches", 340
Streptococcal infections, 54, 63, 236
Streptomycin, toxicity of, 259–260
Stroma, keratoconus-related thinning and scarring of, 97, 98
Stromal haze, post-surgical, 105, 106
STUMPED mnemonic, for neonatal cloudy corneas, 5
Sturge-Weber syndrome, 133, 134, 334

Subarachnoid space, retinoblastoma invasion of, 337
Submacular surgery, 292, 293
Sulfacetamide, 77, 80
Sulfa medications, as red eye cause, 48
Sulfonamides, as acquired myopia cause, 22
Sulfur hexafluoride, 319
Superficial temporal artery, surgical landmarks of, 9
Superior oblique palsy, 213–215
Superior orbital fissure, 1, 8
Superior orbital fissure syndrome, 216
Superior temporal field loss, 221
Suprathreshold testing, 45
Surgery, intraocular. *See also* specific types of surgery
    as ptosis cause, 249
Surgical patients, glaucoma medical treatment for, 138
Sussman four-mirror lens gonioscope, 118
Swinging flashlight test, 207, 208
Sympathetic ophthalmia, 60, 258, 260
Sympathomimetics, contraindication in narrow angle
    glaucoma, 126
Synechiae
    as angle closure glaucoma risk factor, 58, 59
    corneal ulcer-related, 65
    granulomatous uveitis-related, 257
    peripheral
        anterior, 121, 122, 123, 125
        corneal membrane dystrophy-related, 92
        posterior, 65
Syphilis
    diagnostic tests for, 260
    ocular manifestations of, 260
        in AIDS patients, 270
        episcleritis, 56
        granulomatous uveitis, 258
        optic neuritis, 218
        orbital, 246
        scleritis, 57
    as surgery-related vitreous loss risk factor, 146
    uveitis, 60, 260
Systemic lupus erythematosus, 57, 218, 309

Talc, as retinopathy cause, 276, 277
Tamoxifen, as retinopathy cause, 276, 277
Tarsorrhaphy, 70, 88
Tay-Sachs disease, 308
Tear break-up time, 86, 227–228
Tear drainage system, anatomy of, 226
Tear film
    abnormalities of, as corneal ulcer risk factor, 62
    debris-filled, 49
    in dry eyes, 86
    layers of, 5–6, 227
    precorneal, 84–85
Tearing
    causes of, 226
    lagophthalmos-related, 4–5
Tear pump, 226–227
Tear replacement therapy, 87
Tears
    adequate volume of, 227
    artificial, 56, 85, 87–88
    inadequate composition of, 227–228
Telangiectasia, 279, 281, 301, 304
Telescopes, 18–19
Temporal artery, superficial, surgical landmarks of, 9
Tenon's capsule
    in strabismus surgery, 198, 200
    in trabeculectomy, 143, 145
Tenon's cyst, 149, 150

Tensilon test, 196, 216
Tetracycline, 50, 73, 80
Thalassemia major, 278
Thalidomide, 292
Thermiography, 324
Thermokeratoplasty, 100–101, 109
Thermotherapy, as retinoblastoma treatment, 323
Thioridazine (Mellaril), as retinopathy cause, 275
Third-nerve palsy. *See* Cranial nerve palsies, third
13q deletion syndrome, 322
Three-step test, 213–214
Thrombosis, cavernous sinus, 196, 245
Thymoma, 196
Thyroid-related ophthalmopathy, 192, **239–243**. *See also*
    Exophthalmos; Graves' disease
    as bilateral proptosis cause, 235
    differentiated from Brown's syndrome, 194
    as diplopia cause, 212, 215
    myasthenia gravis-associated, 196
    as orbital inflammation cause, 244
    as orbital tumor cause, 241
    strabismus surgery in, 199
    ultrasound evaluation of, 44
Thyroiditis, autoimmune, 278
Thyroid-stimulating hormone, 240
Tight lens syndrome, 52
Timolol, as glaucoma treatment, 115, 136, 137, 141
Tissue glue, for corneal ulcers, 65
Tobramycin, 64, 65, 66, 79, 277
Tolosa-Hunt syndrome, 197
Tonometry, 114
Topical medications, **76–83**
    antibiotics, **76–83**
    as corneal ulcer risk factor, 62
    as dry eye cause, 85, 141
    as eye irritation cause, 141
    steroids, **76–83**
        use in refractive surgery, 109–110
    as superficial punctate keratopathy cause, 50
Total internal reflection, 13
Toxicity, ocular, differentiated from conjunctivitis, 54
Toxins, as retinopathy cause, **274–278**
Toxocariasis, ocular, 264
    differential diagnosis of, 323
    as pseudoexotropia cause, 190
    as retinoblastoma mimic, 322, 338
    as vertically displaced macula cause, 194
Toxoplasmosis, ocular, 258, 264
    in AIDS patients, 267, 271
    diagnosis of, 258–259
    as granulomatous uveitis cause, 258–259
    as retinal arterial obstruction cause, 307
    treatment for, 259
Trabecular meshwork
    as anterior chamber angle landmark, 117
    inflammatory cell blockage of, 131
    injury/tears to, 152, 160–161
    obstruction of, 159
Trabeculectomy, 124, **142–150**
    antimetabolite use in, 147–148
    failure of, 142
    flaps in, 143–145
    fornix versus conjunctival approach in, 142–143
    indications for, 142
    intraocular pressure effects of, 149–150
    as neovascular glaucoma treatment, 128
    postoperative care in, 146
    preexisting, 148
    wound leaks associated with, 146, 150

Trabeculoplasty, argon laser, 3, 142
Trace elements, as age-related macular degeneration
    treatment, 292
Trachoma, 54, 55
Transposition procedure, in strabismus surgery, 199
Transverse magnification, 18
Transsynaptic degeneration, 35
Trauma
    as angle-recession glaucoma cause, 130
    as cataract cause, 163
    as chiasmal visual field defect cause, 221
    as corneal ulcer cause, 62
    to the fundus, **283–287**
    as hyphema cause, 152–154, 156, 160
    as internuclear ophthalmoplegia cause, 197
    as recurrent herpes simplex infection cause, 69
    as third-nerve palsy cause, 209
    ultrasound evaluation of, 43
Trichiasis, 50, 62
Trichinosis, orbital, 246
Trichromatism, 28, 29
Trifluorothymidine, as red eye cause, 48
Trigeminal nerve, herpes zoster lesions of, 3
Trochlear nerve, location of, 8
Trochlear nerve palsy, 213, 215
Tropicamide (Mydriacyl), 21
Tuberculosis
    ocular manifestations of, 259
        granulomatous uveitis, 258
        orbital, 246
        scleritis, 57
        uveitis, 60
    treatment for, 259–260
Tumors, ocular, **332–339**
    as exudative retinal detachment cause, 316
    of the eyelid, **252–256**
    as hyphema cause, 151
    morpheaform, 253, 254
    most common, 332
    nodular, 253–254
    orbital, 235, **340–347**
    as third-nerve palsy cause, 209
    ultrasound evaluation of, 40

UGH (uveitis, glaucoma, hyphema) syndrome, 60, 133
Ulcers
    corneal, **61–71**, 78
        biopsy of, 66
        contact lens-related, 51
        definition of, 61
        diagnostic smears and cultures of, 63–64, 65–66
        infectious versus sterile, 61, 62
        topical corticosteroid treatment for, 67
    dendritic, 49
    genital, uveitis-related, 59
    oral, uveitis-related, 59
    "rodent", 253
Ultrasonography, **38–44**
    for calcification evaluation, 43
    for choroidal melanoma evaluation, 40–41
    for foreign body detection, 285
    for lesion feature evaluation, 39–40
    orbital, 44
    for retinal detachment evaluation, 41–42
    for retinoblastoma evaluation, 231, 325
    for tumor/neoplasm evaluation, 231, 335
Ultrasound biomicroscopy, 44
Ultraviolet radiation, 50, 53, 69
Urethral pain, uveitis-related, 59

Uvea
    effusions of, 128
    retinoblastoma invasion of, 336, 337
    scleral attachments of, effect of choroidal effusions on,
        3
Uveitis, 58–59
    as angle closure cause, 121
    anterior, 48, 58–59
    chronic, intraocular lens-related, 174
    classification of, 257
    as convergence insufficiency exacerbating cause, 190
    differential diagnosis of, 323
    granulomatous, **257–262**, 286
    herpes zoster ophthalmicus-related, 69
    Lyme disease-related, 261
    masquerade syndromes as mimics of, 60, **263–266**
    posterior, severe, 136
    spectacle lens-induced, 60
    syphilitic, 260

Valsalva maneuver, 55, 244
Vancomycin, 79, 286
Van Herrick technique, 119
Varicella zoster virus infections, 69, 261
Varix, orbital, 235, 341
Vasculitides, orbital inflammation-associated, 246
Vasculitis
    orbital, 235
    retinal, 259, 261, 306
Vasoconstrictors, as red eye cause, 57
Vergence, 14, 19
Vertex distance, 21
Videokeratography, computer-based, 103
Vision loss
    age-related macular degeneration-related, 288, 290
    angle closure glaucoma-related, 121
    congenital, 34
    corneal ulcer-related, 66, 71
    diabetic retinopathy-related, 300
    optic neuritis-related, 218
    orbital inflammation-related, 244, 246
    retinal arterial occlusion-related, 307, 308
    retinal venous occlusion-related, 312–313
    retinopathy of prematurity-related, 294
    thyroid-related ophthalmopathy-related, 241
    trabeculectomy-related, 142
Visual acuity
    in amblyopia, 176, 177, 180–181
    in diabetic retinopathy, 302–303
    in infants, 5
    in nystagmus, 205
    in optic neuritis, 218, 219
    in retinal arterial obstruction, 308
Visual development, delayed, 202
Visual fields, **45–47**
    defects of, 45, 218, 221
    restricted, 222
Visual field testing, 47
Visual pigments, 25
Vitamin A deficiency, 46, 49
Vitamins, as age-related macular degeneration treatment,
    292
Vitrectomy
    as diabetic retinopathy treatment, 304–305
    as endophthalmitis treatment, 64–65
    for foreign body removal, 285
    pars plana, 128, 318, 319, 320
    with silicone oil, as AIDS-related retinal detachment
        treatment, 270

Vitreoretinal degeneration, lattice-like, retinopathy of
    prematurity-related, 297
Vitreoretinopathy
    familial exudative, 298
    proliferative, 320, 321
Vitreous
    cataract surgery-related loss of, 173
    hemorrhage of. *See* Hemorrhage, vitreous
    persistent hyperplastic, 322, 338
    trabeculectomy surgery-related loss of, 146
Vitreous cavity, antibiotic injection into, as endophthalmitis
    treatment, 64–65
Vitreous tap, for endophtalmitis evaluation, 64–65
Vitritis
    iron overload-related, 278
    Lyme disease-related, 261
    primary intraocular sarcoma-related, 264
    syphilic, 260
von Hippel-Lindau syndrome, 280
Vogt-Koyanagi-Harada syndrome, 258, 260, 265
Vogt's striae, 97

Waldenstrom's macroglobulinemia, 91
"Wall eyes", 190
Weber's syndrome, 216
Wegener's granulomatosis, 57, 85, 218, 235
Wegener's syndrome, 246
Welder's flash, 50

Whitnall's superior suspensory ligament, bony attachments
    of, 9
Willebrand's knee, 4, 221
Women
    Coats' disease incidence in, 279
    dry eyes in, 85

Xanthelasma, 253
Xanthogranuloma
    as hyphema cause, 151
    juvenile, 258, 263, 265
Xanthopsia, 277
Xerostomia, 85, 246
X-rays, 24

Yellow vision, 277

Zeiss goniolens, 118–119
Zimmerman hypothesis, 333–334
Zonules
    in primary angle closure glaucoma, 125
    tears of, 152
Zovirax ointment, 70
Zygoma bone, 1
Zygomaticomaxillary suture, 7
    in primary angle closure glaucoma, 125
    tears of, 152
Zovirax ointme